DISABILITY'S CHALLENGE TO THEOLOGY

DISABILITY'S CHALLENGE TO THEOLOGY

Genes, Eugenics, and the Metaphysics of Modern Medicine

DEVAN STAHL

University of Notre Dame Press
Notre Dame, Indiana

CONTENTS

PREFACE

After years of failing to conceive, my first pregnancy was an occasion for celebration, but it brought with it many difficult choices. Before conceiving naturally, my husband and I considered whether we should try in vitro fertilization (IVF). Many couples who struggle with infertility are presented with an array of assisted reproductive technologies, but we felt a particular urgency to our choice, because I had gone off my multiple sclerosis medication for several years during our attempts to conceive. With relapsing-remitting MS, relapses compound, and I worried that forgoing my medication for so long would have lasting implications. Having taught bioethics for many years, I was well aware of the controversies surrounding IVF, including various religious objections to the practice. Thankfully, my denomination, the Presbyterian Church (USA), carefully considered the ethical nature of IVF in its 1983 resolution "The Covenant of Life and the Caring Community."[1] In this long and rich document, the denomination explores the nature of infertility (including the social injustices that may lead to infertility), the indignities that can accompany fertility evaluations, the stress of infertility on a marriage, the cost of fertility treatments, the difficulties of adoption, the goods of medical treatment, and the possible commodification of children.[2] The document asserts parenting as a covenant invitation that ought to be considered carefully. In its 2012 resolution "On Providing Just Access to Reproductive Health Care," the PCUSA urges couples considering assisted reproductive treatments to be guided by "individual conscience" in consultation with "families, pastors, health-care professionals, and scientifically accurate medical information."[3] Understanding IVF as permissible, I began to consider whether it was right for me and my husband.

We were spared the difficult choice of whether to use IVF when I unexpectedly conceived, but then a new set of questions came our way. Early on in my pregnancy, I was offered genetic testing. Because of my age and chronic illness, I had an "at-risk" pregnancy and required oversight by a specialist, who encouraged me to consider genetic screenings. A simple cell-free fetal DNA test (done through a blood draw) in my first trimester could show me signs of Down syndrome, trisomy 18, or trisomy 13, as well as increased chances for other genetic and chromosomal conditions. As a disability advocate, I could not imagine terminating a viable pregnancy because my child had (or might have) a genetic or chromosomal disability. Just as I value my own life, I would value the life of my child. Still, I considered whether it was prudent to get genetic testing when it was offered. Those same Presbyterian resolutions that guided my thinking on IVF struck me as problematic for discussing genetic technologies. In the 1983 resolution, genetic "problems" (i.e., disabilities) are described as "tragic" and "catastrophic," children born with them as a "burden" and "damaged," and the detection of such problems in utero as an occasion to decide whether to continue with a pregnancy.[4] Genetic counseling, screenings, and future therapies are described as implicit goods and even "a wondrous gift."[5] The PCUSA advocates pastoral counseling for future parents and congregational support and prayer for families contemplating these difficult choices,[6] but I feared the document fell into the trap of understanding genetic disability as inherently bad.

Nearly all parents will face the choice of whether to use genetic technologies, but in my experience such choices are rarely discussed in our churches. In the medical world, genetic screenings and various genetic technologies are understood as obvious goods. Yet the animating metaphysical and ethical assumptions that guide medico-scientific research and application do not always align well with the

classic Christian tradition. Christians ought to be careful not to conflate the goods of medicine with the goods of Christian life. It is all
too easy to understand "health" as an ultimate good in modern society, but Christians have a different ultimate good: friendship with
God. In our quest to achieve the goods of health, we may overlook
other goods that God presents to us: goods that enable to us to love
and accept others as gifts. By current medical standards, my chronic
illness disqualifies me from the ideal healthy life, but a multitude of
goods have come from my illness journey—goods I would have never
achieved if I had sought health above all else. Learning to accept myself prepared me to accept others as they are, without first trying to
change them. I knew this was how I was called to welcome my child
as well. Within this frame, the use of genetic screenings became more
complicated. Could I simultaneously accept and screen my child?
Would screening help prepare me for the child I would receive, or
would it give me a false sense of control? And if my child did have a
disability, would accepting that child prohibit me from considering
genetic interventions? My lingering questions were not addressed by
my denomination's resolutions or by most of my theological texts.

As this book shows, liberal Protestants within various denominations, including the PCUSA, have almost always been enthusiastic
adopters of new biomedical technologies, even ones that have devastating consequences for persons with disabilities. As I explore in
chapter 1, the liberal Protestant embrace of the American eugenics
movement should give many of us pause when we consider genetic
technologies today. I question many Protestants' acceptance of biomedical progress and its general neglect of people with disabilities.
The voices of persons with disabilities have been (and continue to be)
marginalized in theology and bioethics, but we cannot seriously consider the appropriate use of technologies that would surveil, ameliorate, prevent, or eradicate disability without the input of persons who
live with the very bodies and minds such technologies target. I do not
think it is too strong a statement to say that we have entered a new
era of "soft" eugenics. Our government is no longer forcing "unfit"
members of society to be sterilized, but there is tremendous social
pressure for parents to *choose* genetic screening, selective abortion,

and preimplantation genetic diagnosis. In the near future, we will likely also need to consider the appropriate uses of gene editing, such as CRISPR, on human embryos.

As the PCUSA's 1983 resolution rightly points out, genetic technologies pose deep questions about how much we can know of God through the current ordering of the natural world, the limitations of our human dominion over nature, the inability of science to qualify the goods of human life, and eschatological concerns over the future of our species.[7] This book seeks to explore these questions in detail, paying particular attention to how such questions are answered by the classic Christian tradition as well as contemporary disability theologians and scholars. By seeking out marginalized perspectives, Christians can better consider the ethical implications technologies pose.

Theological Genethics Assessed

Liberal Protestants typically consider themselves adept at evaluating and incorporating the insights of modern science into their theologies, particularly when compared to evangelical and fundamentalist Christians. Philip Clayton goes so far as to call the Christian engagement with the sciences the "birthright" of liberal Christianity.[8] Given liberal theology's openness toward science and scientific progress, one would assume that mainline Protestant denominations would be skilled at critically evaluating the use of genetic science and the use of genetic technologies in medical care. A historical review of the twentieth century, however, reveals that liberal Protestants' openness toward science has been much more accommodating than critical. In fact, liberal Protestants have championed some of the most dangerous scientific programs of the past century. Scholars such as Christine Rosen and Amy Laura Hall have skillfully traced how liberal Protestants came to embrace the American eugenics movement and how America's most well-educated and elite Christians were so easily beguiled by eugenics propaganda. For various reasons, however, Roman Catholics and conservative Protestants rejected eugenics. How did liberal Protestants go so wrong?

This book argues that engagement with metaphysics and a theology of nature is crucial for Christians to evaluate genetic science as well as the moral use of genetic technologies, such as human genetic engineering, gene therapy, genetic screenings, preimplantation genetic diagnosis, and gene editing. Theologically liberal Protestants who sided with modernism during the Fundamentalist-Modernist Controversy in the late nineteenth century were easily led into the eugenics movement of the early twentieth century because they maintained a positive attitude toward developments in the medical and natural sciences, while at the same time lacking the theological tools necessary to critically assess them. Modern science has an implicit metaphysics that liberal Protestants have generally failed to recognize and, therefore, have not attempted to critically assess. At the turn of the twentieth century, most liberal Protestants had excised metaphysics from their theologies, focusing instead on subjective experience and social ethics. Opposed to natural law theories and generally unconcerned with natural theology, they lacked the critical skills necessary to oppose eugenics. Roman Catholics, on the other hand, never insulated themselves from science. They have maintained a robust engagement with metaphysics and a rich natural law theology, which has enabled them to evaluate the moral use of medical technologies with far more precision than Protestants.

Little has changed in either the theological or political concerns of most Protestants. Many mainline denominations continue to use overly simplistic criteria when evaluating medical technologies. Simplistic evaluations will fail to serve Christians well as medical technologies advance and we continue to live longer and with more disabilities. The church—the place where supportive, compassionate people come together to share their faith and values—should be the ideal place for people to grapple with difficult medical-moral decisions. Unfortunately, most Christians will make medical decisions apart from their religious communities. At best, congregations pray for parishioners when they become ill, but important medical decisions are placed on individuals, rather than on the body of Christ.

As a theological bioethicist, I desire to ground my ethical claims in Christian theology. For the most part, the book will mine the classic

Christian tradition for answers to the questions posed by genetic technologies. I do not believe Christians need to invent a new theology to respond to advanced medical technologies; rather, they will need to relate older theological tenets to new discussions. At the same time, I use the lens of disability theory to question how classic Christian formulations have smuggled in cultural conceptions of normalcy. Importantly, the book prioritizes the experience of disability to help the church be more authentic to its own mission in the world.

The relationship between theology, metaphysics, and ethics is consistently addressed within this work. Although many Protestant theologians have questioned the appropriateness of developing a Christian metaphysics, a metaphysical account of the world will enable Christians to see where their understandings of the world align with or are contradicted by the basic assumptions of the modern medical and natural sciences. Without a critical metaphysics, liberal Protestants all too easily accept the implicit metaphysics of the sciences, which led them to support the eugenics movement of the early twentieth century. Several chapters in the book address the metaphysical discrepancies between our modern scientific accounts of the natural world, including human nature, and those of the classic Christian tradition. Ultimately, I hope to show that metaphysics is an important task for theological bioethicists because it reveals some essential differences between the Christian message and the aims of medical science. Roman Catholic bioethics exemplifies the usefulness of metaphysics in theological bioethics, but there are alternative metaphysical constructions of the world that may be more appealing to liberal Protestants whose understanding of nature is informed by their account of divine creation.

CHAPTER OUTLINES

The book begins with a historical account of American churches' involvement in the eugenics movement. To understand why liberal Protestants were attracted to eugenic science in the past, we must understand why the topics of nature and metaphysics fell out of favor within Protestantism in the twentieth century. Without the theological resources to adequately assess the goals and means of eugenics, Protestants were easily seduced by a science that promised to improve society through good reproductive practices. In the twenty-first century, the eugenics movement of the early twentieth century has been almost universally condemned as both bad science and discriminatory, but few Protestant churches have formally apologized for their involvement in the eugenics movement. Moreover, eugenics is rarely mentioned in documents that discuss the moral implications of contemporary genetic technologies. Protestants must dissect how they could have entered into such harmful alliances in the past before they can begin to examine how they should approach genetic technologies in the present.

Chapter 2 takes a step back to examine the historical relationship between what we now call "science" and "religion." Today, the "conflict myth," which asserts that science and religion have always been discrete disciplines in conflict, is prevalent. The conflict myth is entirely mistaken, however. Reforms in theology were influential to reforms in natural philosophy, which led to the Scientific Revolution. Moreover, after the Reformation, western Europe experienced an unprecedented convergence between theology and natural philosophy, which had the unintended consequence of collapsing the natural and supernatural as well as placing natural philosophy and theology onto the same explanatory territory. A God who could be collapsed into nature was easy to discard within the scientific method. Once Protestants began to drop the investigation of nature out of their theologies, modern science became the only legitimate way to understand the natural world. The result tends to be an enthusiastic endorsement of technologies that promise to end suffering and maximize choice, without critically engaging the harms such technologies might pose to vulnerable persons.

Chapter 3 uncovers the implicit metaphysics undergirding contemporary genetic science. Developments in biology and genetics in the nineteenth and twentieth centuries changed the relationship between science and religion in such a way that the importance of theology in understanding the creation and meaning of human life began to be sidelined within the biological sciences. Not only does genetic science retain a metaphysics, it frequently functions as a secular theology, taking up questions that were once reserved for theological speculation. The source and meaning of human life have now been reduced to scientific explanation. The result is that the human being is understood as nominal, the sum of her parts, and no part of the human being lies beyond science's reach. Critically examining the metaphysical and theological elements of contemporary genetic science is important for Christian theologians because many Christians falsely assume they share medicine's purposes and goals for human life.

Chapter 4 further examines the metaphysical divergence between theology and medical science by putting forth a Christian metaphysical understanding of nature, or "creation." Modern genetic science generally assumes that genetic "defects" are harmful to the human species and, therefore, must be corrected. I contend, on the other hand, that this cannot be taken as obviously true for Christians who believe in God's providence. Theologians must first explain how God interacts with the natural world before they can begin to evaluate whether a natural occurrence is against God's purposes. Chapter 4 examines the Christian understanding of God the Creator and the presence of "natural evil" in the world. Whereas many theologians believe genetic disabilities are connected to the Fall and represent a form of natural evil to be overcome or prevented, there is reason to believe this is an ill-fitting category for disability. Such thinking led to the eugenics movement and continues to support the idea that genetic technologies are obviously good and even salvific for persons with disabilities.

Chapter 5 narrows the discussion of God's relationship to creation to God's relationship to human nature, to analyze how God interacts with humans in particular and how humans are related to the rest of nature. Defining ontological personhood in relation to God is essential for determining how Christians should understand human nature and its relation to genetic disability. Using a Christian conception of the *imago Dei*, I show how a theological account of personhood differs from secular accounts that place many persons with disabilities outside of the human community. Understanding the inherent dignity of all persons then helps one understand how human nature is fallen and prone to sin as well as the promise of resurrection. Chapter 5 explicitly rejects the understanding of genetic defect and disability as directly related to human sin and, instead, positions them as part of the natural course of finite human life.

Taking for granted the naturalness of human limitation, chapter 6 reexamines the place of natural law within a Protestant theology and argues that there is a relationship between human beings' essential nature and their moral obligations. Building upon the Christian metaphysics and ontology of the previous two chapters, chapter 6 explores the nuances of a Christian genethic (genetic ethic) that takes seriously God's relationship to creation and to human nature. I explore the usefulness of natural law in both the Roman Catholic and liberal Protestant traditions to show how liberal Protestants have much to learn from their Catholic counterparts, even if their natural law arguments may ultimately rely more upon a biblical foundation than some Roman Catholic constructions. Of course, to address moral obligations with any particularity, theologians must move beyond natural law when determining the ethical use of particular genetic technologies.

Chapter 7 addresses the value of the virtues and embodied experience within the process of moral discernment. The cultivation of practical wisdom, or prudence, is crucial for moral decision-making in any context. In moral evaluations of genetic technologies, the wisdom of disability experience ought to be prioritized, not only because genetic technologies tend to target the bodies of persons with genetic disabilities, but also because the rationale for their use often makes false assumptions concerning what it is like to live with a disability. Nondisabled persons are notoriously bad at determining what it is like to live with impairment and therefore have limited moral imaginations when it comes to envisioning the good life for those with genetic disabilities. This chapter supplies various accounts of nondisabled bioethicists and geneticists misunderstanding and misrepresenting the experience of disability. The chapter counters these accounts with alternative understandings of disability and the human person offered by disability theorists and theologians. Ultimately, understanding the experience of genetic disability and the wisdom garnered from it will be crucial for Christians who wish to provide normative guidance on the use of genetic technologies.

Finally, chapter 8 examines how the prioritization of disability experience can transform, rather than merely inform, policies concerning genetic technologies as well as the communal life of the church. The choice to use genetic technologies is often constrained by societies that refuse to properly accommodate and welcome people with disabilities. Parents who belong to welcoming communities will be better able to imagine how their children will be positively received. Creating welcoming communities will require a liturgical transformation, which can reorient congregations to the value of all persons within the body of Christ. Only once people with disabilities are welcomed, are cared for, and feel as though they belong in church can pastors and congregations aid in the work of moral discernment concerning the ethical use of genetic technologies. As the body of Christ, congregations must learn to care for another's physical, mental, and spiritual needs so that medical decisions are never merely individual.

This book does not attempt to provide a single Christian response—a yes or no answer—to the use of particular genetic technologies. Instead, I provide a theological account of Christian metaphysics and ontology that can serve as the foundation for genethical teaching within the church and encourage theological reflection. Far too often, genethics debates occur between those who believe that altering nature is "playing God" and those who believe that, as "cocreators," Christians are obligated to pursue nearly every medical endeavor. I hope to avoid these kinds of debates by thoughtfully examining how Christians understand nature as well as their obligations to one another. I also hope the book will serve as a starting point for deeper discussions about disability within the human life span. Few theologians writing on genetics consider how these discussions will affect persons with genetic disabilities. The neglect of the experience of disability betrays a larger neglect in much of Christian theology. By prioritizing the experience of disability, I hope to refocus the debate on genetic technologies.

ACKNOWLEDGMENTS

This book is a labor of love that has taken many years to complete. Undoubtedly, doing work at the intersections of theology, bioethics, and disability is a difficult task. In one way or another, each discipline has been in dispute with the others over the years. If this book at all succeeds in bringing these discourses together, it is because of the incredible mentorship I have received over the course of my scholarly life. Many thanks to Jeffrey Bishop for convincing me to do an interdisciplinary PhD in health care ethics and for mentoring my dissertation as well as many other scholarly works over the years. Thanks also to Tom Tomlinson, who never let me believe that religion was irrelevant to the field of bioethics. When I felt out of my depth, particularly when engaging Roman Catholic thought and Thomas Aquinas, I could also count on my colleagues Jason Eberl and Christopher Ostertag for guidance. I apologize in advance for any misunderstandings and unfair critiques that may have found their way into this book despite your valiant efforts.

I also owe a debt of gratitude to the Institute of Theology and Disability, where I have been welcomed over the past decade. It was at the Institute where I first presented portions of this work and received feedback from colleagues as well as the great disability theologian Hans Reinders. It was at the Institute where I met my fellow disability theologians Sarah Barton and Bethany McKinney Fox. Thank you for your continual support and friendship over the years. My work is much improved by engaging with your work.

This book would have not have been completed without the support of the Religion Department at Baylor University. Making the transition from a medical school to a religion department was made easy through the support and confidence of the faculty at Baylor University. Thank you for finding room in religion for a bioethicist.

And finally, thank you to my loving and supportive family. To my wonderful husband Chris, who endured many cross-country moves and late-night writing sessions so that I could pursue my dreams, I owe you so much. I hope this book makes you and Theo proud.

CHAPTER ONE

Science, Religion, and the Ideal Eugenic Man

If you were lucky enough to walk through the newly opened Bronx Zoo in New York City in September 1906, you may have stumbled upon the exhibition of Ota Benga, a Congolese pygmy living in the zoo's monkey house. At four feet eleven inches, 103 pounds, and showing finely sharpened teeth, Benga was a remarkable sight, and over forty thousand New Yorkers flocked to see him. His easy interaction with the zoo's primates, particularly Dohong the orangutan, enhanced what many New Yorkers already saw as Benga's "exotic" and "primitive" appearance. Upon seeing such a strange man, you may have laughed at him or even poked him in the ribs and chased him around the zoo grounds along with other New Yorkers at the time.[1] Or perhaps you would have protested his exhibit, but to do so, you would have found yourself embroiled in a debate that had less to do with the demeaning exhibition of a person (after all, freak shows were a common attraction at the time) and more to do with the rising tensions between science and religion. A number of clergymen protested Benga's display as inhuman, but what was equally disconcerting to the clergymen was what Benga's display suggested about Darwin's theory of evolution. "The exhibition evidently aims to be

1

a demonstration of the Darwinian theory of evolution," protested Reverend James H. Gordon. "The Darwinian theory is absolutely opposed to Christianity, and a public demonstration in its favor should not be permitted."[2] For Reverend Gordon and other members of the Colored Baptists Ministers' Conference, the problem was not simply that the zoo was claiming Benga, and by extension other "Negroes," to be akin to apes but that all humans were akin to apes.[3] The zoo's director, William T. Hornaday, confirmed the ministers' fears, noting, "I am a believer in the Darwinian theory. . . . [I am] giving the exhibitions purely as an ethnological exhibit."[4] Like Hornaday, journalists at the *New York Times* were baffled by the protests against Benga's display:

> We do not quite understand all the emotion which others are expressing in the matter. . . . It is absurd to make moan over the imagined humiliation and degradation Benga is suffering. The pygmies . . . are very low in the human scale, and the suggestion that Benga should be in a school instead of a cage ignores the high probability that school would be a place . . . from which he could draw no advantage whatever. The idea that men are all much alike except as they have had or lacked opportunities for getting an education out of books is now far out of date.[5]

For many white liberal elites in the early twentieth century, adherence to Darwin's theories fit comfortably with theories of racial superiority. A decade later, many of those who supported Benga's display, including many liberal Protestants, became prominent racial anthropologists and eugenicists. Ota Benga's exhibit was short-lived, but it revealed how entrenched the religious debates concerning Darwin's theories had become. "The Pygmy at the Zoo" incident would not be the last time Christians allowed their acceptance of "Darwinist science" to obscure society's exploitation of marginalized people. Within two decades, many Protestants were preaching eugenics sermons from their pulpits and advocating for the sterilization of society's "unfit" members.

The history of churches' interaction with Darwinism and the early eugenics movement reveals the underlying theological and

ethical commitments of many prominent American Christian traditions. In this chapter, I examine how and why liberal Protestants, conservative evangelical and fundamentalist Protestants, and Roman
Catholics responded differently to the eugenics movement. In particular, I focus on how each tradition's understanding of "nature" and
interaction with the natural sciences influenced their acceptance or
rejection of eugenics. If contemporary mainline Protestants wish to
be open to dialogue with the natural and medical sciences while avoiding the eugenic logic they accommodated in the past, they must recover and rearticulate the theological resources that will enable them
to do so. Ultimately, as later chapters reveal, for Protestants to engage
with medical technologies aimed at altering nature, they must first
supply an account of nature and humans' place in it.

To show why a theological account of nature is necessary for
Protestantism, I begin by exploring how this theological lacuna first
developed. Against the notion that "science" and "religion" have always been discrete and conflicting disciplines, Protestant thinkers
were influential in the rise of the Scientific Revolution because of a
unique convergence between theology and natural philosophy that
occurred in the sixteenth and seventeenth centuries. Theologians in
the eighteenth and nineteenth centuries, however, progressively diminished the study of nature in their theological investigations,
making it difficult for theology to seriously engage scientific developments in the twentieth century. Next, I compare the theological resources Protestants and Roman Catholics drew upon when assessing
the American eugenics movement. Whereas Roman Catholics were
able to use their natural law tradition and continued engagement with
the sciences to reject many aspects of eugenics, liberal Protestants
who lacked a theology of nature were more easily swayed to believe
that they could usher in the Kingdom of God through eugenic
projects. Conservative evangelical and fundamentalist Protestants, on
the other hand, rejected eugenics because they saw it as a companion
to Darwinism, which challenged their scientific reading of scripture.
Finally, I explore Roman Catholic and Protestant responses to advances in genetic engineering in the late twentieth and early twenty-
first centuries to reveal how little has changed in each tradition's
fundamental orientation toward medico-scientific progress. Before

mainline Protestants weigh in on moral debates concerning genetic engineering, they must first come to terms with their enthusiastic adoption of eugenics programs in their not-so-distant past. Only by understanding how they could have formed such a destructive alliance in the first place can mainline Protestants hope to avoid the same mistakes in the future. To engage in scientific dialogue productively, Protestants must once again shore up a theology of nature that is capable of practical application.

Theological Engagements with Nature

A historical review of Protestantism's interaction with the sciences in the twentieth century reveals a consistent tendency of modern liberals to embrace science at the expense of a consistent and coherent theology. As the religion scholars Christine Rosen and Amy Laura Hall show, modern liberal Protestants eagerly embraced the eugenics movement to stay relevant in an increasingly secularized and scientific culture. Subsequently, Protestants who were the most willing to embrace scientific programs and scientific logic became the least able to combat the encroachment of science into the religious realm. Conservative evangelical and fundamentalist Protestants, on the other hand, accepted the importance of science but rejected any science that contradicted their own biblical interpretation, instead opting for a "biblical science" that was generally incapable of seriously engaging scientific advancement. Little has changed in either the theology or the overall concerns of Protestants. Liberal Protestants continue to champion accommodationism, which can lead them to embrace scientific findings and biotechnologies uncritically, whereas conservative evangelicals and fundamentalists continue to reject much of contemporary science in the name of biblical literalism and biblical science. Clearly, these are generalizations that overlook many of the nuances in contemporary theology and theological bioethics; however, such characterizations serve as cautionary warnings for Protestants. Neither wholesale approval nor wholesale rejection of biotechnologies will serve Christians well in the twenty-first century.

To help Christians navigate an increasingly complicated medical system, which offers an array of biotechnologies, including genetic and reproductive technologies, theologians must revive a theology of nature that is capable of responding to advancements in medicine.

The Protestant Reformation and the Scientific Revolution

Protestantism's near neglect of the topics of nature and technology over the past two hundred years has made the task of supplying a clear and robust critique of genetic technologies exceptionally difficult. According to religious historians, however, this disengagement from nature is unique in the history of Protestantism. In chapter 2, I delve more deeply into the changes in theology and natural philosophy that led to the Scientific Revolution, but for now it is worth briefly exploring how closely connected these reforms were in the sixteenth and seventeenth centuries. Historian Peter Harrison argues that theological changes precipitated by the Reformation created the groundwork for the Scientific Revolution to occur. In particular, Harrison notes that the reformers' focus on literal readings of texts and a renewed focus on humans' fallenness laid the foundation for a different approach to the natural world.[6] Reforms in theology eventually gave way to new methods in natural philosophy, including the empirical method and induction, as well as new motivations for studying the natural world—namely, redeeming or improving nature. Protestants helped transform the task of natural philosophy from discovering the meaning of creation to discovering its purpose. In particular, Protestants sought to discover God's original intentions for the universe so they could help fulfill those intentions and thus redeem nature. Protestant reformers could not have predicted that their attention to the earth would eventually allow for an expulsion of religion from natural science.

Deeply suspicious of the teachings of the Catholic Church, first- and second-generation reformers turned to the early, uncorrupted church (through the canonical texts) as their authority for both theology and natural philosophy. Interpreting scripture without the aid of the Roman Catholic Church required a standardized reading to ensure that infinite interpretations would not abound. For this reason, the reformers chose to elevate the literal or plain interpretation of scripture above all others. According to Harrison, the result was the demise of allegorical readings of scripture and eventually allegorical readings of nature as well. Whereas in the medieval tradition all physical objects pointed beyond themselves toward a shared series of resemblances, the reformers focused on the literal interpretation of both scripture and the natural world, stripping physical objects of their allegorical meanings and symbolic, spiritual truths. Natural philosophers and natural historians found meaning within objects rather than beyond them, and one had to break objects open to reveal how God made them. Only arduous empirical investigation could show how objects were designed and what use they might be to humans.[7] Even creatures themselves were objects to be used or investigated for human purposes.

The sixteenth century also witnessed a revival of Augustinian anthropology, which emphasized the limitations of human cognition.[8] Through the work of theologians such as John Calvin, epistemological debates were reignited. For Calvin, God is amply manifest in nature, but humans are too stupid and superstitious to realize it.[9] The Fall damaged the human will, making it difficult to choose the good, as well as our intellectual faculties, making it difficult to know the good. Calvin writes, "But although we lack the natural ability to mount up unto the pure and clear knowledge of God, all excuse is cut off because the fault of dullness is within us."[10] After the sixteenth century, no serious project that sought to advance human knowledge could do so without addressing the ability of the human mind to discern truth. Rather than diminishing interest in the natural world or other scientific pursuits, however, the focus on how to attain knowledge took on a new urgency and birthed new methods of inquiry, such as experimentalism. The human mind was fallen, but working together, humans could acquire knowledge gradually by meticulously gathering evidence about the earth. Emphasis on the fallenness of the world also gave rise to a sustained motivation for transforming and ultimately redeeming the world. Whereas the goal of philosophy had always been to transform the philosopher, the new, true end of philosophy was to transform the world.[11]

What many now view as the exploitation of the natural world began as a theological endeavor to redeem the natural world through human dominion. For later thinkers such as Francis Bacon, the sciences could even help restore Adam's prelapsarian abilities: "The glory of God is to conceal a thing, but the glory of the king is to find it out; as if, according to the innocent play of children, the Divine Majesty took delight to hide his works, to the end to have them found out; and as if kings could not obtain a greater honour than to be God's playfellows in that game, considering the great commandment of wits and means, whereby nothing needeth to be hidden from them."[12] Bacon was more optimistic than many of his reformed predecessors, such as Calvin, that the effects of the Fall could be remedied through the sciences. Even anatomy and physiology became means of studying the body and understanding humanity's fallenness. At the University of Wittenberg, Philipp Melanchthon opened up education in anatomy and medicine to all students (not simply medical students) through his work *Liber de Anima* (1540). Melanchthon believed knowledge of the body was a way to "know thyself" and thereby to know God.[13] Physical limitations were also thought to be a result of the Fall, so that overcoming the body's limitations was seen as a reversal of the Fall. Life extension, therefore, became another scientific pursuit influenced by a reformed anthropology.[14]

Beginnings of the Science/Religion Split

The sixteenth and seventeenth centuries experienced an unprecedented mutuality between theologians and natural philosophers. Whereas many philosophers contend that the scientific revolution separated the fields of science and theology, the historian Amos Funkenstein has shown this period to be a unique point of convergence between them. Encouraged by the Reformation's elevation of the laity, the natural philosophers of the sixteenth and seventeenth centuries came to be seen as secular theologians, helping to reveal the mind of God in the realm of the natural world.[15] The mutuality between scientific and religious pursuits, however, began to break down in the seventeenth century. Once the scientific method became entrenched within experimentalism and inductive reasoning, its link to the Fall began to dissolve. By the end of the seventeenth century, explicit theological justifications for this new experimentalism were already being ignored in accounts of the scientific method.[16] In the eighteenth century, thinkers such as David Hume continued to defend experimentalism as an appropriate method to account for the imperfections of human nature.[17] Yet eventually the link between experimentalism and human limitation also faded from scientific reflection, and experimentalism was taken for granted as the appropriate method for scientific pursuits.

Meanwhile, in the late eighteenth century, Immanuel Kant dealt a serious blow to God's place within natural philosophy. Before Kant, most theologians who spoke of God's revelation in nature did so already assuming God's reign over nature. Any knowledge about God that could be gleaned from nature already presumed God's presence in nature. For Kant, however, there was no way to reason to God from the natural world because we cannot experience anything in nature that would lead us to find God. If we want to find God, we must look not to "the starry heavens above" but to the "moral law within."[18] Influenced by both Kant and Pietism, Friedrich Schleiermacher devoted the majority of his work to relating the thought of God to the experience of self, characterized by "the feeling of absolute dependence." In *The Christian Faith*, Schleiermacher allows for a doctrine of God as creator and preserver of nature but believes propositions about God and the world must be "authenticated as expressions of religious emotions."[19] By focusing primarily on subjective experiences, or what many have termed "the subjective turn" in philosophy, Protestant theology gave a theology of nature scant attention apart from safeguarding science's autonomous realm. Subsequently, some of Schleiermacher's later followers, including Albrecht Ritschl and his disciples, went even further in giving priority to the ethical over the natural and subsequently rallied to expel metaphysics from theology altogether. Not all theologians followed Ritschl's expulsion of metaphysics, but most Protestant theologies in the nineteenth and twentieth centuries tended to prioritize ethics over metaphysics and thus failed to see how one was necessarily related to the other.

At the same time that Protestant theologians were moving away from a theology of nature, the Industrial Revolution was relocating American churchgoers away from the countryside and into cities. The theme of nature was largely irrelevant to a population that worked twelve hours or more in a factory and lived in crowded slums. In an agrarian society, the seasonal rhythms of nature set the conditions of labor, and it was not difficult to see labor as mirroring God's continual action in creation. In an industrial society, however, nature came to be seen as a reservoir of materials and resources to be exploited by scientific technology for human advantage. Francis Bacon's understanding of nature as a human resource and science as necessary for the relief of the human condition became the predominant orientation toward nature in the late nineteenth and twentieth centuries.

Scientists Pull Away from Religion

In the second half of the nineteenth century, the moral and religious frameworks that had once guided scientific pursuits were no longer referenced explicitly. "Science" came to be seen as its own field, a conceptual object to be practiced and unified around a common method and identity for practitioners. To establish science as a field unto itself, scientists needed to distinguish their realm from that of nonscientific activities. The establishment of the professional scientist, with a unique scientific method and a new designation ("scientist" as opposed to natural philosopher or historian), helped to distance science from its social origins. Around this same time, "religion" also came to be understood as a conceptual object that could be critiqued using the logic of other disciplines.[20]

By the twentieth century, thinkers had all but forgotten the role the Protestant Reformation had played in early modern science. Whereas once the natural sciences relied upon religion for social legitimacy, when religion itself became less central in the Western landscape, science pulled away from religion. Soon, myths that science and religion had always been in conflict emerged. "Religion" was associated with inflexibility, dogmatism, and institutional authority, which was antithetical to scientific progress. Whereas "progress" for thinkers such as Bacon was embedded within an understanding of God's providential plan, without underlying theological values, "progress" became an end in itself.[21]

Even after the natural sciences were considered disciplines distinct from religion, few theologians criticized scientific methods. Until the twentieth century, theology itself was considered a science—perhaps even the queen of the sciences—and clergy exerted widespread intellectual and cultural influence. Even though most Protestant denominations in the nineteenth century contained both liberal and conservative wings, the question of accepting or rejecting the natural sciences was not a widespread concern among Protestants until the twentieth century.

THE RISE AND FALL OF THE EUGENICS MOVEMENT

The Great Protestant Divide and Eugenics

A deep and lasting divide between liberal and conservative (many of whom would become fundamentalist) Protestants began with their antithetical responses to revolutionary developments in science, technology, and psychology at the turn of the twentieth century. Throughout most of the nineteenth century, the majority of Protestants held out a reasonable hope that America could establish itself as a cohesive Christian nation.[22] At the dawn of the twentieth century, however, American Protestants experienced a profound spiritual and cultural crisis. In response to their quickly changing world and declining church attendance, many Protestants reacted by embracing modernism, hoping to remain relevant in a society that seemed to be losing its religious essence.[23] Since they had been supportive of the claims of modern science, the popularity of John William Draper's *History of the Conflict between Science and Religion* (1874) and Andrew Dickson White's *A History of the Warfare of Science with Theology in Christendom* (1896) came as a blow. Both Draper and Dickson maintained that religion had always struggled against science, a claim that gave new urgency to many theologians' need to ally themselves with modern science, including Darwinian evolution. Having virtually ignored any explicitly theological account of nature for generations, many Protestants who embraced modernism ceded the exploration of the natural world almost entirely to the natural sciences, believing natural philosophy could produce theological truths. This rendered the relationship between natural science and religion distant but amiable at the turn of the twentieth century. As a result, liberal Protestants became all too eager to affirm the findings and endeavors of modern science. Without a theology of nature to draw upon and with a scientific naturalism that guided their thinking, Protestants' ability to evaluate new medical and scientific technologies theologically was attenuated. Neglecting nature had devastating practical consequences for Protestants in the early twentieth century. Concerned not to appear as though they were "antiscience," and optimistic that their Social Gospel movement would help usher in the Kingdom of God, many liberal Protestants in the 1920s found themselves natural allies with the American Eugenics Society.

More concerned with finding the "historical Jesus" than outlining Christian dogma or metaphysics, liberal Protestants such as Walter Rauschenbusch developed a "Ritschlian liberalism," which promoted progressive social, economic, and political programs.[24] Rauschenbusch's concerns made him the defining figure of the Social Gospel movement in the early twentieth century. As postmillennialists, many liberal Protestants saw it as their duty to help save society to ensure Christ's return. The Social Gospel movement encouraged social action—often through cooperation with secular organizations—to help eliminate what many in the middle class saw as society's essential problems: poverty, crime, disease, drunkenness, and prostitution. Eugenicists too, sought to build a healthier society by eliminating the root causes of society's suffering: bad genes. Eugenics offered liberal Protestants a scientific route to improving humankind. The renowned minister Rev. Harry Emerson Fosdick praised the eugenics movement for its "humanitarian desire to take advantage of the scientific control of life so as to change social conditions that mankind may be relieved from the crushing handicaps which now press it."[25] For Fosdick, joining the eugenics crusade made him "both an intelligent modern and a serious Christian."[26] With the support of popular ministers, eugenicists staged sermon competitions to spread their salvific message, and ministers from a wide range of Protestant denominations eagerly participated. In 1928, for example, Rev. Edwin Bishop won third place in a sermon contest sponsored by the American Eugenics Society, declaring:

> Jesus . . . plainly taught that individuals differed widely in their innate capacities, that there were one-talent men and two-talent men and five-talent men, and that capacity self-fulfillment would come in realizing the inherent endowment. . . . Enter therefore eugenics. This advancing science proposes capacity self-fulfillment for the individual by giving him a better physical chance, better mental faculties, and better moral endowments. . . . [Isn't it true] that if we used as much intelligence in human mating as we use in breeding horses and cows, we could surely breed out some of the ills as well as breed in some of the excellencies now inhering in our flesh? Shall we humans not realize what God is trying to do for us and how He suggests that we participate with Him in conscious evolution? Should not the church following the lead of Jesus, who preached capacity self-fulfillment for the individual, be mightily interested in any program that would aid children to be physically well-born? And it is but a step from anatomical structure and physiology to mental faculties and moral endowments.[27]

By the 1920s, many religious leaders were willing to reinterpret charity to include eugenics. Churches sponsored Fitter Family contests, held Race Betterment conferences, issued eugenic marriage licenses, and supported government sterilization programs. When given a part to play in eugenics propaganda, liberal Protestants became eager promoters of the eugenics agenda.[28] Amy Laura Hall contends, "Protestants who were most accustomed to their role as well-educated citizens had the fewest theological resources to resist the messages of eugenics. The oldest and most unquestionably American of the Protestant churches were the first to jump on the eugenics bandwagon."[29] Because of their easy accommodation of the eugenics movement, liberal Protestants wound up promoting the values of white, elite, productive, native-born families at the expense of America's most vulnerable citizens.

In opposition to Protestants who embraced modern liberalism, conservative evangelicals and members of the bourgeoning fundamentalist movement were predominantly premillennialists and resisted scientific teachings when these appeared to challenge biblical doctrines, such as the Virgin Birth, the bodily resurrection of Christ, and God's creation of the earth as described in Genesis.[30] Eventually, many began to rebel against Darwinism as well as the eugenics movement, seeing the two as intimately related. Unlike their more liberal counterparts, conservatives decided it was of the utmost importance to hold fast to the biblical foundations of American civilization, which they believed were under assault by modernism.[31] As they attempted to hold on to their tradition against the encroachment of science, their emphasis on biblical infallibility grew, and they ended up supporting a reading of the biblical text that was essentially scientific: the Genesis story, they insisted, could be read as a scientific account of the origins of the earth.

Although many assume that these conservative Protestants were simply anti-intellectual and antiscience, historian George Marsden believes the debate over evolution was really the result of the clash of scientific worldviews. Fundamentalists remained loyal to the first scientific revolution; they stood in the intellectual tradition of Francis Bacon, who was committed to careful observation and the classification of facts.[32] Yet it was not only conservative fundamentalists who rejected Darwinism. Christians with more liberal leanings were also concerned that the acceptance of Social Darwinism would justify the denigration of the weak in favor of the strong. In his crusade against evolution, for example, the progressive politician William Jennings Bryan proclaimed both that Darwinism was simply not scientific enough and that Darwin's theory would undermine Christian morality by prioritizing the strong over the weak.[33] Even public theologians who did not proclaim themselves fundamentalists worried that Social Darwinism would negatively affect the poor and disenfranchised.[34]

Bryan's contention that Darwinism was not scientific enough was preceded by early modern Christians looking to natural philosophy to prove biblical events. "Creationism," which places scientific and theological accounts of nature's origins on the same explanatory terrain, follows from an earlier era that witnessed the convergence of theology and natural philosophy, as I will explore in more detail in chapter 2. In the seventeenth and early eighteenth centuries, theologians and natural philosophers alike looked to prove the authenticity of biblical events through empirical evidence. Darwin's theory of natural selection did away with the centrality of the biblical account of creation and the necessity of the God of creation, but it was not empirically verifiable—it did not depend on fact and demonstration and so could not be considered scientific using the standards of the empirical method.[35] Whereas a Newtonian worldview could still account for the supernatural, Darwinism could not. Darwin's theory was far from impregnable, but it eliminated the need for a "god of the gaps" science. The Darwinist revolution created the expectation that science could now explain the entirety of natural history without reference to God. One could still believe that evolution manifested God's providence, but to do so was now an act of faith. Initially, there were liberal and conservative Christians on both sides of the creation-evolution debates. As I will show, it was only later that conservative Protestants came together in their insistence that a true battle between science and religion was happening in classrooms that were teaching Darwinian evolution.

The Great Depression, the rise of fascism in Europe, and the signs of another world war on the horizon helped curb debates surrounding the Christian embrace of modernity. In his essay "Ten Years That Shook My World," Reinhold Niebuhr wrote of his "rejection of almost all of the liberal theological ideals and ideas with which I ventured forth in 1915."[36] The rise of neo-orthodoxy was a response to the failure of liberal Protestantism in the nineteenth and early twentieth centuries. The neo-orthodox did not embrace modern science as earlier liberals had done, but they also did not challenge it; instead, they focused their critique on the optimism and triumphalism liberalism had embraced. Neo-orthodox theologians stressed the dialectical nature of theology by emphasizing the tensions, paradoxes, and ambiguities of Christian existence, as well as the infinite distance between God and humans. Against rationalism, they claimed God is unknowable except through divine grace and revelation. The neo-orthodox turn toward revelation, however, distanced theologians even further from nature. Karl Barth, one of the most influential theologians of the twentieth century, rejected natural theology, including any notion that God could be understood from nature (apart from divine revelation), that humans have a natural knowledge of God, or that there is a natural morality. Barth's theology, including his neglect of natural theology, remains influential in mainline and evangelical Protestantism today.

The Roman Catholic Response to Eugenics

In opposition to their liberal Protestant counterparts, many Roman Catholics were wary of eugenics from its inception and were some of the movement's most intellectually rigorous opponents. Unlike conservative Protestants, however, Roman Catholics did not reject Darwinist science along with eugenics. Guided by their natural law tradition and sexual ethic, Roman Catholics leaders opposed eugenics, particularly as it involved sterilization.[37] Attacks ranged from the scientific merits of eugenics, to its consequences for the poor and marginalized, to the evils of sterilization.

In the early twentieth century, prominent Catholic figures believed they could make their case against eugenics most powerfully if they did not appeal directly to their religious tradition (which might be divisive in countries where they were not the dominant religion) but instead relied upon rational argument. Catholic writers attacked the scientific merit of eugenics and its political consequences. G. K. Chesterton, for example, claimed eugenicists could not prove heredity was primarily responsible for human behavior. He was also concerned that eugenics allowed governments to override the individual rights of its citizens.[38] He wisely predicted that the poor would suffer the most from eugenics.[39] Chesterton's harsh critiques of eugenic science helped to curtail government support of the eugenics movement in

Britain. Roman Catholics in the United States were also able to defeat some legislative proposals to allow forced sterilization at the turn of the twentieth century, particularly in states heavily populated by Roman Catholics, but they were ultimately unsuccessful in preventing eugenic sterilization from becoming legalized after the Supreme Court ruling in *Buck v. Bell* (1927). Like Chesterton, the heads of Catholic organizations tried to persuade non-Catholics that eugenics was wrong using scientific and legal arguments rather than directly appealing to Catholic social doctrine.

Not all Roman Catholics were convinced that eugenics was altogether wrong. Some Catholic clergy even served as members of the American Eugenics Society.[40] What they could not tolerate, however, was the use of sterilization or artificial contraception, which became integral means to achieving the ends of eugenics. In *Casti connubii* (1930), Pope Pius XI officially condemned eugenic sterilization, declaring, "Christian doctrine establishes, and the light of human reason makes it most clear, that private individuals have no other power over the members of their bodies than that which pertains to their natural ends; and they are not free to destroy or mutilate their members, or in any way render themselves unfit of their natural functions, except when no other provision can be made for the good of the whole body."[41] Rather than using social justice arguments or appeals to eugenics as a discriminatory practice, Pius XI limited his condemnation of eugenics to natural law arguments aimed at upholding the dignity and natural ends of human beings (procreation), which he believed were undermined through sterilization and artificial contraception. Even as genetic technologies have become more prolific, the magisterium has maintained its teachings on sexual ethics and its understanding of the moral order of nature, which I will detail more carefully in chapter 6.

After the Eugenics Movement

By the 1940s, critics of the eugenics program were rising up from within the scientific community. Particularly after the world learned of Hitler's atrocities, the idea of "eugenic sterilization" and racial purity became increasingly suspect. To distance themselves from Hitler's eugenic program, eugenicists began calling themselves "population scientists" and "human geneticists," and eugenics organizations changed their names. A growing number of scientists began to criticize the eugenics movement for being essentially racist, classist, and anti-immigrant. Hermann Muller, one of the most popular population geneticists in the late 1940s and 1950s, proclaimed, "Eugenics has become 'hopelessly perverted' into a pseudoscientific façade for 'advocates of race and class prejudice, defenders of vested interests of church and state, Fascists, Hitlerites, and reactionaries generally.'"[42] Although the majority of geneticists in this period no longer believed behaviors could be patterned in "races," they were still concerned with protecting the "genetic quality" of society. Muller believed advancements in agriculture and medicine prevented genetically unfit people from being expelled naturally from the gene pool. Those who might have otherwise died in their youth were living to reproductive age and increasing society's "genetic load."[43] Instead of advocating that certain people should forgo having children, Muller urged men who recognized their "inferior status" to allow their wives to receive artificial insemination from men with "more outstanding genetic qualities."[44] Many population biologists and geneticists assumed people would flock to sperm banks if they were educated about heredity.[45] They were mistaken.

Meanwhile, tremendous strides were being made in the basic science of genetics. Scientists discovered that genes are codes found on the double-helical strands of DNA, and later they recognized the four base chemicals that form the "alphabet" of the genetic code. By sequencing genes, scientists were able to identify risk factors for genetic and chromosomal disorders. In 1959, for example, researchers in France and England discovered that Down syndrome resulted from the possession of three copies of chromosome 21 instead of two. Advances in biochemistry and cytogenetics (the branch of genetics concerned with the study of the structure and function of cells, particularly chromosomes) bolstered the field of genetic counseling, which helped prospective parents make reproductive decisions. In the early years of genetic counseling, many counselors were quite directive, believing it was their duty to instruct parents whether they *should* have children.[46] By the end of the 1950s, however, standard practice dictated that counselors did not have the right to tell a couple not to have children. In the aftermath of the Holocaust, scientists in the field of genetics needed to distance themselves from their eugenic forebears and establish their work as an independent and respectable scientific pursuit. To legitimize their investigations to a public still wary of eugenics, genetic scientists and population scientists narrowed their focus to the goals of improving society's understanding of the human species, improving future children, and diagnosing and treating disease.[47]

By the early 1960s, molecular biologists began to see that there might be a possibility for chemically altering the human genome. They suggested, rather than the slow process of breeding, a new technique of "splicing" or "surgically repairing" genes that would be far more efficient.[48] With the possibility of "genetic therapy" on the horizon, defining the "ideal genetic man" became pressing, but many scientists continued to believe that debating such ends was not in their interest. Instead, some suggested that the ends of genetic research should be decided by "an enlightened and broadly based public opinion."[49] Because of the advancing techniques in in vitro fertilization (IVF) and popular books written by scientists to help lay people better understand genetic science, public attention to scientific endeavors intensified. The public outcry against IVF and other genetic technologies, however, caused many scientists to reconsider their openness to public opinion. By the end of the 1960s, the public tide had turned against much of the work done in reproductive and genetic science, particularly in response to advances in IVF and its implications for human genetic engineering, which Aldous Huxley had fictionalized in his famous novel *Brave New World*. In response, genetic scientists, many of whom were still concerned with promoting human control over evolution, began to demand "scientific freedom" from public input.

Unimpeded for decades and shocked by the counterculture that challenged science in the midst of its success, laboratory-based science went on the offensive, asking the government to shift important conversations away from direct public input. Geneticists such as H. Bentley Glass argued that the public had no role in controlling scientific research, writing, "[Science] requires fearlessness in the defense of intellectual freedom, for science cannot prosper where there is constraint upon daring thinking, where society dictates what experiments may be conducted, or where the statement of one's conclusions may lead to loss of livelihood, imprisonment or even death. . . . No doors must be barred to its inquiries, except by reason of its own limitations."[50] Today, many prominent scientists continue to argue that the public should not have a role in the regulation of genetic technologies. Many assume the opponents of genetic engineering are trying to impose their religion on the rest of society.[51]

RELIGIOUS RESPONSES TO GENETIC TECHNOLOGIES

Roman Catholic Responses

In response to advances in science and the counterculture movement, Catholics and Protestants found themselves embroiled in new political controversies. Around the time that scientists were beginning to better understand DNA, genetics research was still nascent and only had the potential to create genetic technologies that could alter human DNA. Roman Catholic theologians, however, were generally quicker than their Protestant counterparts to consider the ramifications of these technologies. The Roman Catholic magisterium praised the potential of genetic research to yield new medicines and technologies to relieve suffering, while at the same time cautioning about its potential to create immoral technologies. Although many Catholics remained divided over the use of hormonal birth control to regulate pregnancy, the magisterium has held fast to its teachings on sexual ethics, even while remaining cautiously open to the rising field of genetics.

Just six months after James Watson and Francis Crick published their findings on the double-helix structure of DNA in 1953, Pope Pius XII gave the first documented religious response to the breakthrough. In an address to the First International Symposium of Genetic Medicine, Pius XII acknowledged the potential benefits and perils of genetic research. Interestingly, Pius XII applauded the aims of eugenics while condemning its means. "The fundamental tendency of genetics and eugenics is to influence the transmission of hereditary factors in order to promote what is good and eliminate what is injurious. This fundamental tendency is irreproachable from the moral viewpoint. But certain methods used to attain this end, and certain protective measures, are morally questionable, as is also, in fact, a misplaced esteem for the ends to which genetics and eugenics tend."[52] Like Pius XI, Pius XII was most concerned with eugenic sterilization, which he believed violated the integrity and natural purpose of human bodies.

The magisterium continued to affirm the potential goods of science, without condoning technologies aimed at preventing procreation. The Second Vatican Council document *Gaudium et spes*, for example, "affirms the legitimate autonomy of human culture and especially of the sciences."[53] *Gaudium et spes* recognizes the importance of the sciences for solving particular problems that cannot be solved through religion alone. Yet that science must not violate the dignity of the human person. "All things are endowed with their own stability, truth, goodness, proper laws, and order. Man must respect these as he isolates them by the appropriate methods of the individual science or arts."[54] To be moral, science should work in conformity with God's order of nature and should not seek to circumvent the goods of nature (e.g., procreation).

The magisterium's sexual ethic continues to place limits on medical technologies that interfere with procreation. Although many expected that the church would lift its ban on hormonal birth control in the 1960s, Pope Paul VI overruled the majority recommendation of the commission established to consider the matter, claiming that the unitive and procreative acts must be held in unity in every conjugal act. In *Humanae vitae* he speaks of "man's stupendous progress in the domination and rational organization of the forces of nature, such that he tends to extend this domination to his own total being: to the body, to psychical life, to social life and even to the laws which regulate the transmission of life."[55] He goes on to note that some technologies, such as contraceptives, go against natural law because they dominate humans rather than serving their natural ends.[56] As more concrete genetic technologies developed, this logic was extended to genetic research using embryos as well as to concern over the risks and benefits of gene therapy, which I examine in chapter 6.

Conservative Protestant Responses

Less than fifty years after liberal Protestants were first taken to task for their disreputable cultural alliances with eugenicists, new shifts in America's political landscape pulled them squarely back into the center of scientific controversy. The cultural revolution of the 1960s and early '70s brought a reshaping of culture, and by the 1980s the American religious landscape began to resemble that of the 1920s in its religious divides and debates. Mainline Protestant leaders, who had mostly retained their ethically centered theologies and moved toward the moderate left in politics by the 1980s, struggled to find relevancy in modern culture once again. Fundamentalism, which was considered extinct by many following the Scopes trial, was resurrected in the 1970s and 1980s through the Moral Majority and the Religious Right. Once again, many "fundamentalistic evangelical Protestants" contended that America was essentially a Christian nation that had forsaken its Christian heritage.[57] Landmark decisions in *Roe v. Wade* (1973), *Engel v. Vitale* (1962), *Abington School District v. Schemp* (1963), and *Bob Jones University v. United States* (1983), as well as the election of the "born-again" Ronald Reagan, helped to reignite the passions of fundamentalism. Once again, many in the movement questioned the science of evolution.

In 1981, religious and scientific leaders were called together to debate the teaching of evolution and creation science in schools. In *McLean v. Arkansas Board of Education* (1981) various parents, religious groups, and scientists filed a lawsuit arguing against the constitutionality of the Arkansas state law known as the Balanced Treatment for Creation-Science and Evolution Science Act (Act 590), which mandated the teaching of "creation science." As was the case in the Scopes trial, religious leaders and scientists occupied both sides of the debate. In *McLean*, unlike the Scopes trial, however, fundamentalists who supported teaching creation science in schools did not do so primarily as a reaction to liberal Protestantism or as a reaction against urban, university-educated elite society. According to Langdon Gilkey, who served as a member of the American Civil Liberties Union (a plaintiff in the case), the religious reaction against evolutionary science was a reaction against the overreach of science itself:

> In a scientific culture the step for natural science from regarding science as the most immediately useful and so the paradigmatic form of knowing (which it is) to regarding it as the *only* form of knowledge is a short but fatal step. . . . "Science tells us that Genesis is wrong"—with each such statement by the biology teacher in class, repeated at home that night to father and mother, two new creationists are generated! Creationism is not a reaction to Protestant liberalism as was the older fundamentalism. It is a reaction to the establishment of modern science insofar as science has claimed to provide a total explanation of our existence and of the world in which we exist.[58]

As the natural sciences began to claim sole access to truth, even religious truth, creationism was revived. Science has helped to generate strong reactions against those who wish to preserve religious doctrine within a culture they see as dominated by science. As the domain of science becomes even more extensive in society, the religious reaction against evolutionary science continues to grow. Today, science is one of the only university disciplines taught without substantial reference to its own history, so it functions as if it exists apart from its given cultural and historical matrixes. Without acknowledgment of its own situatedness and limitations, science helped breed another strong reaction from religious fundamentalists to the teaching of evolution, which helped to grant legitimacy to the myth that religion and science are, and have always been, in conflict.

Despite new discoveries in the biological and social sciences, in 2012 more people believed "God created humans in present form within the last ten thousand years" than in 1982.[59] Today's "creationists," much like those in the 1920s, continue to promote a scientific worldview that is out of sync with contemporary scientific methods and assertions. Along with their scientific and liberal counterparts, however, creationists still promote a worldview where science is centralized. Ironically, although creationists are often considered "antiscience," their propensity to treat science as a methodological norm mirrors the efforts of liberals to do the same. The difference is that creationists view Genesis as a superior scientific text to *On the Origin of Species*. As I show in the next chapter, the desire to merge science (or natural philosophy and natural history) with theology dates back to the seventeenth century, when thinkers concerned with the natural world attempted to use science to validate biblical stories that they believed were literal, historical events. It was only later that the "historical" nature of biblical stories was contested and "religion" and "science" came to be understood as distinct conceptual objects. Today, science still has the power to sanctify and lend credibility to biblical beliefs for both fundamentalists and liberals. But unlike William Jennings Bryan, who claimed he was "more interested in the Rock of Ages than in the age of rocks," creationists today seem very interested in determining the age of rocks.[60]

Liberal Protestant Responses

The response of many liberal Protestants to the new, politically active Religious Right (and its antievolution stance) was as virulent as it had been to the rising movement of fundamentalism in the 1920s. Less critical of the advancing encroachments of science in culture, and wanting to distance themselves from what they believed were the decidedly "antiscience" expressions of fundamentalism, liberal theologians wished to appear proscience in the public eye. In what can only be described as a radical reluctance to distance himself from eugenics (or an exercise in historical amnesia), liberal theologian and early bioethicist Joseph Fletcher declared, "It is impossible to see how the principle of social justice . . . can be satisfied if the community may not defend itself and is forced to permit the continued procreation of feeble-minded or hereditarily diseased children."[61] Enthralled by advances in genetic technology, Fletcher later wrote, "Genetics is the real frontier, revealing exciting possibilities of quality control for our children."[62] Although there were liberal Protestants who resisted Fletcher's myopic protechnological thinking, few theologians explicitly acknowledge their tradition's complicity in the eugenics movement or the necessary limits of scientific thinking. To date, only two denominations, the United Methodist Church and the United Church of Christ, have apologized for their role in the eugenics movement.[63] Instead, theologians and denominational committees struggle to find their unique voice in bioethics debates.

In 1982, three mainline Protestant churches—the United Church of Christ, the United Methodist Church, and the Episcopal Church— issued statements assessing genetic engineering. Although these three denominations do not share a common theology, the formal resolutions and positions statements they published from the 1980s onward reach similar ethical conclusions concerning the proper use of genetic technologies. Statements issued by the three denominations share certain elements that might loosely be identified with the liberal Protestant tradition's affirmation of the goods of science, desire to work cooperatively with secular institutions, and need to respond theologically to modern culture. First, all three churches applaud the good intentions of genetic engineering itself, which has the potential to lessen human suffering by eradicating disease. The UMC, for example, affirms the potential within genetic engineering for the relief of suffering and the healing of creation.[64] The Episcopal Church declares genetic engineering should be encouraged when it is thought to reduce human suffering, and they later add, "The genetic testing of children can be an important part of parental responsibility."[65]

Second, all three documents support the necessity of working cooperatively with secular institutions, such as the scientific community and the government, to ensure that the application of genetic technologies is carried out morally. None of the churches advocate that they should act as a moral authority in deciding the morality of biotechnologies; rather, they want moral evaluations to be worked out concomitantly with the government or to be taken up primarily through governmental organizations. The churches also implore their own clergy and laity to become more educated on genetic matters to help in the process of moral evaluation with laity considering genetic engineering for themselves or their children.[66] Finally, all three denominations express worry that genetic information could be used as a way to discriminate against people in matters of employment and health insurance.[67]

In terms of theology, all three documents limit their theological assessments of genetic engineering almost entirely to an affirmation of the goodness of creation and humanity's responsibility to be good stewards and intelligent cocreators. Between its four resolutions that mention genetics, the Episcopal Church makes only one theological reference, which reads, "DNA is a great gift of God, lying at the center of life and directing our development, growth and functioning."[68] Likewise, among the United Church of Christ resolutions on genetic engineering, only one document references a "biblical and theological rationale" for its position. The UCC cites Bernhard Häring—"As co-creator and co-revealer with God, man has to take into his hands to transform it [nature] in accordance with his goal to grow in his capacity to reciprocate love and to discern what enhances human dignity and what blocks it"[69]—and then expresses the need for wisdom (citing Prov. 8:12 TEV and Prov. 2:6–7 RSV) to moderate scientific knowledge.[70]

The Methodist Church provides the most thorough theological grounding for its position on genetic engineering, citing creation's relationship to its Creator, the call to stewardship, the potential for scientific idolatry, human dignity in Christ, and God's sovereignty.[71] Within this analysis, however, the UMC makes some surprising claims about genetics that verge on genetic essentialism, or the belief that the essence of human beings can be reduced to their genes. For instance, in "New Developments in Genetic Science," the UMC states, "In spite of the rapid growth in genetic research, many people tend to see genetics merely as an extension of the changes in medical, agricultural, and other technologies. In fact, genetic science crosses new frontiers as it explores the essence of life."[72] The UMC also declares genetic science might prompt Christians to reexamine traditional church doctrines. It remains unclear, however, how genetic science might challenge the classical Christian doctrines of free will, sin, personhood, or the human telos or whether scientific discovery ought to shape Christian concepts quite so directly. As I show in later chapters, these traditional Christian teachings might best serve as a critique against the ever-increasing encroachment of science upon the religious domain. Rather than "reevaluate" traditional Christian teachings, Protestants should rearticulate these teachings in light of advancements in genetic science and technologies.

The statements produced by these church denominations provide little theological analysis. In trying to speak to both the advancements of genetic science and the theology of their respective denominations, the documents actually fail to engage either a robust scientific or theological discourse. The classic Christian doctrines of sin, grace, redemption, salvation, and reconciliation are either ignored or outright questioned. Churches should hardly be expected to recount an entire systematic theology to evaluate genetic engineering (particularly within such pithy documents), but an affirmation of humanity's "cocreator" status and the need to use technology wisely fails to answer the more complex questions presented by genetic engineering and risks falling into the naive optimism displayed by nineteenth- and early twentieth-century liberal Protestants. Beyond the question of whether the notion of our "cocreatorship" is theologically productive (and there are many, including myself, who believe it is not), questions about the moral (dis)order of nature, the status of suffering and disease in God's redemptive plan, and the ultimate purpose of the human body are all relevant to assessing genetic technologies. Until Protestant theologians are able to give an account of the moral order of nature, or what the term *natural* even means, they cannot begin to parse out what in nature is in need of redemption or remediation.

Genetic technologies present complex ethical questions that Christians must engage. Protestants' ability to do so, however, is suspect. Over forty years ago, theologian James Gustafson remarked that Roman Catholic moral theologians have been more successful in relating their theological bioethics to their constituency.[73] This should be surprising to liberal Protestants who believe liberal theology is uniquely suited to engage and evaluate modern science because this is "the birthright of liberal Christianity."[74] Unfortunately, many Protestants seem unable to supply a theological analysis of genetic engineering that the bioethics community, or their own church communities, can consistently and seriously implement. Given the history and theological commitments of liberal Protestants, this is a particularly damning evaluation. To be relevant to modern Christians and modern society, Protestants must attune themselves to cultural phenomena affecting their communities.

Little has changed in Protestant and Roman Catholic approaches to genetic science in the past forty years. Mainline Protestants continue to favor evolutionary understandings of life's origin, to accept stem cell research, and to endorse genetic testing.[75] Among the religious, they are the least likely to believe that their scientific beliefs conflict with their religious beliefs.[76] Catholics tend to reject the use of human embryos for genetic therapies and are wary of genetic screenings because they are linked to abortion. Most evangelicals have not seriously engaged medical technologies beyond their prohibition against abortion and the use of embryos in medical research.[77] Many evangelical Christians are convinced that their prolife political agenda is a faithful response to their biblical interpretation, but it is unclear how helpful an entirely "biblical theology" will be for answering the difficult questions present in contemporary biotechnological and biomedical dilemmas.

Without a theology of nature, liberal Protestants lacked the critical edge necessary to assess eugenics in the twentieth century and are likely unable to do so easily in the twenty-first century. As the church statements previously mentioned reveal, for many Protestants, genetic engineering can only conjure up their theological commitments to end suffering and promote social justice. By aligning themselves with a medico-scientific project, liberal Protestants have not been able to develop the theology necessary to resist a eugenic future.

WHEREAS CONSERVATIVE PROTESTANTS have often been far too critical of scientific advancements, liberal Protestants have been far too concerned with defending science against conservative fundamentalists and have failed to examine how their own understanding of the human person or the good life might differ from that promoted by the genetic sciences. Lacking a clear theology of nature, twentieth- and twenty-first-century Protestants have had few theological resources to draw upon when they ethically evaluate genetic technologies. In this situation, the possible dissimilarities between the Christian message and genetic determinism have been obscured. Protestants must learn to appreciate how a robust metaphysics sustains a religion in secular culture (as it does for Roman Catholicism), and they must heed the warnings from neo-orthodox theologians, who remind liberals that "accommodation" and "translation" can easily make theology redundant and vapid. Protestants must move back toward their theological roots if they hope to avoid lapsing into complete irrelevancy. To do theological bioethics well, Protestants must employ a particular theological method to engage the natural world, but they must also draw on their tradition's theological language, ideas, and symbols.

Before detailing a more constructive theological response to the use of genetic technologies, however, chapter 2 takes a step back, examining how religion and science came to be understood as separate and potentially even incompatible disciplines. Ironically, it was the merger of theology and natural philosophy by the seventeenth century that helped to set the stage for the evacuation of theology from modern science. Once theology and natural philosophy were placed onto the same explanatory territory, the two disciplines eventually came to be seen as competitive, rather than complementary, as they had been for centuries. Reforms in both theology and natural philosophy helped to separate God from nature as well as to diminish the importance of metaphysics in the scientific enterprise. Without a robust metaphysics, Protestants have struggled to understand how God interacts with nature and whether God directly causes all natural phenomena, including genetic disabilities. An understanding of the theological and metaphysical roots of early modern science will make clearer why metaphysics remains an essential tool for theological engagement with nature as well as the implicit metaphysical assumptions that linger in modern medicine.

CHAPTER TWO

Theological Influences on the Scientific Revolution

In the twenty-first century, the conflict myth, which maintains that science and religion have always been separate and competing disciplines, remains a powerful narrative in the West. At the same time, it is not unusual for scientists, including geneticists, to use quasi-religious language when discussing their projects. After the first working draft of the human genome was completed in 2000, Dr. Francis Collins, former director of the National Human Genome Research Institute, reflected, "It is humbling for me and awe inspiring to realize that we have caught the first glimpse of our own instruction book, previously known only to God."[1] Collins may or may not have meant to equate mapping the human genome with divine revelation, yet there remains an implied sacred significance given to human DNA by many scientists. Metaphors about the sacred power of DNA abound. DNA is commonly referred to as "the code of codes,"[2] "the essence of mankind,"[3] the "fate" of mankind,[4] "the holy grail,"[5] and even "the gospel documents of all life."[6] Such metaphors suggest genes are the key to understanding human identity and destiny—categories that were once reserved for theological explication.

Such theological rhetoric may seem odd coming from a group that purports to bracket theological and metaphysical concerns when carrying out their scientific pursuits, but it is neither unprecedented in the history of science nor a departure from the moral or theological foundations of the Scientific Revolution. As much as modern science attempts to break itself off from the robust cosmological traditions in which it originated, it has yet to do so completely. The routine practices of scientists do not need to account for larger metaphysical or theological concerns, but it is difficult to avoid moral, metaphysical, or theological language when presenting the investigations and discoveries of science to the public, particularly in societies that invest considerable time and resources in those scientific endeavors. In other words, when promoting the usefulness of science, it is difficult, if not impossible, to separate science as a realm of knowledge from science as a value-laden and metaphysically driven enterprise.

Modern science, including genetic science, cannot fully escape metaphysics or theology, even as many of its popularizers attempt to replace religion with science. The quasi-religious language used by many geneticists and biologists mirrors the speech of secular theologians in the sixteenth and seventeenth centuries, who looked to bring together natural philosophy, natural history, and theology in unprecedented ways. Understanding the theological and metaphysical roots of early modern science will help to illuminate the ersatz theologies embedded within contemporary genetics. In other words, it is not simply that scientists use religious language to cater to a religious public; rather, modern science functions as a moral and metaphysical project that is deeply indebted to its theological forebears.

This chapter explores the historical relationship between (what we now call) religion and science from the ancient to early modern period, paying particular attention to reforms in natural philosophy and theology that led to the Scientific Revolution. I provide this history to show that modern science (against its frequent protestations to the contrary) has an implicit metaphysics that Christians should critically assess rather than naively adopt. For this reason, my investigation of the historical relationship between science and theology will not be exhaustive; rather, I selectively highlight moments in this history (1) to show that the conflict thesis is mistaken; (2) to present the alternative ways Christians, particularly Protestants, have understood God's relationship to nature; and (3) to show how this history continues to shape the metaphysics of modern science. To better understand the influence of theology on early modern science, I first provide a brief history of how Christian theologians understood the enterprise of natural philosophy, beginning with the early church, the medieval era, and the Reformation. Next, I show how theology and natural philosophy came together in the sixteenth century and the influence this relationship had on the Scientific Revolution and the rise of experimentalism. In no small part because of a changing understanding of how God interacts with nature, natural philosophers eventually came to bracket the study of nature's formal and final causes, resulting in the stigmatization of metaphysics. Finally, I explore how science attempted to break away from theology and write religion out of the history of the rise of modern science. By following scientists in abandoning metaphysics and natural theology, many theologians have failed to adequately explain how God relates to nature and what difference this would make for the ethical evaluation of genetic technologies that aim to alter nature. Adopting the metaphysics of modern science uncritically has led many to collapse God's intentions for nature with scientific progress. It is no wonder, then, that many saw eugenics as soteriological; science could carry out God's commands by eliminating qualities injurious to human flourishing.

Precursors to Early Modern Science

Augustine

Whereas it is now commonplace for many to distinguish religion from science by claiming that religion is chiefly concerned with moral virtue and science with uncovering facts about the material world, the church fathers resisted limiting Christianity to morality. For many of the church fathers, including Augustine of Hippo, the material world mediated God's grace, so understanding the material world helped humans to know God and what God desired for them. Thus the material and the spiritual, as well as the physical and the metaphysical, were never truly separate. Particularly in a fallen world that requires God's continual grace, Christians needed to understand how God interacts with the world, particularly in material practices that confer grace, such as the Eucharist.

Christians were not alone in considering how the natural world related to the supernatural. The Patristics debated what insights they could incorporate from classical philosophy, and Augustine helped to ensure that Christianity robustly engaged — and at times adopted — what he believed to be important insights from ancient metaphysics, natural theology, and ethics.[7] Later, Augustine went so far as to claim that Christianity was the final form of philosophy and could answer the questions of classical metaphysics.[8] Augustine allowed for a unity of philosophy and theology, seeing metaphysics as the science of God, which became the predominant understanding of metaphysics before the thirteenth century.[9]

While laying out a Christian metaphysics, however, many early Christians generally disregarded questions posed by natural philosophy. Before the thirteenth century, many believed scripture was the superior way to understand the natural world. If some historical or natural event was not explained by scripture, it was not overly important to explain it using other means. In *Enchiridion*, Augustine cautions, "For the Christian, it is enough to believe that the cause of all created things, whether in heaven or on earth, whether visible or invisible, is nothing other than the goodness of the Creator."[10] In *On Christian Doctrine*, he again cautions, "Although the course of the moon . . . is known to many . . . knowledge of this kind in itself, although it is not allied with any superstition, is of very little use in the treatment of the Divine Scriptures and even impedes it through fruitless study; and since it is associated with the most pernicious error of vain prediction it is more appropriate and virtuous to condemn it."[11] Being overly concerned with the physical world in itself could be seen as idolatrous, not least because, after the Fall, the natural world had lost its similitude to God.

Of course, early Christians were still interested in how God relates to the physical world, even if they were cautious not to be overly concerned with the physical world in and of itself. Rather than explain the mechanics of the physical world, many early Christians believed that when creating the world, God had infused nature with signs and symbols that would point people to the divine. God related to the world symbolically, and natural objects could, therefore, point to higher moral and divine truths.[12] Just as early Christians attempted to find historical events and persons in the Old Testament that anticipated God's participation in the world through Christ, so too did they look within nature to find God's symbolic presence.[13] In early Christian thought, God was not understood solely as the initiator of a causal series of events that gave way to nature, nor was God opposed to natural causation. Instead, God actively and continually participated in nature in such a way that God's causal activity was analogously related to natural causation without being identical to it.[14] As I will show, confusion over nature and supernature has made this distinction unclear to modern Christians, who often speak as though God battles against natural phenomena (such as disease and disability) for the benefit of humankind. The modern notion that God is in competition with nature has helped to further the understanding that certain natural states or events are clearly evil or against God's intention for creation and that science can carry out God's plan to cure the natural world of such evils.

Medieval Thinkers

Although figures such as Augustine set the stage for when and how Christians should engage natural philosophy, the early medieval period ushered in a highly systematic approach to relating natural philosophy to theology. Against Augustine, many theologians in this era attempted to show how the careful investigation of nature could reveal the mind of God and show human beings how to live an ethical life. Whereas today many Protestants have attempted to separate metaphysics from ethics, this would have been inconceivable for most medieval theologians. Medieval thinkers offer to contemporary Christians ways to understand the coherency of what we now call "science" and "religion" as well as a way to conceive of God and nature as noncompetitive. Aquinas in particular was tremendously influential in shaping the Christian medieval conception of the relationship between theology and metaphysics.

The renewal of Christians' attention to the natural world in the twelfth and thirteenth centuries was due in part to the recovery and translation of ancient texts. Whereas earlier Christians believed it was important to identify the spiritual truths signified within natural things, between the thirteenth and sixteenth centuries scholastics, aided by Aristotelian thought, began to treat the relationships between physical things as important in their own right, which encouraged systematic investigation of the natural world and elevated the place of natural philosophy within religious thought. Natural entities and objects not only were seen as pointing to spiritual truths in and of themselves but came to be seen as part of an endless chain of resemblances. The horizontal relations between objects also contained spiritual truths to be discovered. According to the historian Stephen Gaukroger, many scholastics elevated the status of these ancient writers and began to systematically investigate nature through their writings. Reading nature through ancient texts often encouraged the idea that nature could be read as a book. Interpreting the book of nature required methods similar to scriptural interpretation.[15]

Aristotle's four causes, material, formal, efficient, and final, had the greatest influence on the growing medieval interest in the natural world. Aristotle's philosophy helped explain why objects moved by describing the physical properties of objects (material cause), the design of an object (formal cause), the agent or source of the object's change or stasis (efficient cause), and the purpose for which the object was made (final cause). For Aristotle, there was an intimate connection between how bodies moved through space (physics) and the cause and destination of that movement (metaphysics). Motion is the means of perfection of things within nature, so everything innately moves toward its natural place. "Everything moved must be moved by something. For if it has not the source of motion in itself it is evident that it is moved by something other than itself, for there must be something else that moves it."[16] Aristotle explained motion as beginning in an unmoved mover; all of nature thus moves as a result of its cause.

Aristotle's causal theory also applied analogously to ethics because humans move toward their telos, or their perfection, within nature. Humans move toward their good through the practice of their virtues.

Medieval Christians held to the ancient Greek notion that the human mind participated in the intelligibility of the cosmos and thus could form true and universal concepts of the divine nature of "intelligible forms" within material existence. Among Aristotle's four causes, medieval natural philosophers elevated formal and final causes—the pure potentiality of matter (the material cause) was understood to become a particular thing only because of the archetypal idea that in-forms it (formal cause) and its purpose (final cause). Whereas few modern natural scientists believe nature communicates anything on its own, in the medieval mind even efficient causality was understood as communicating the depth of a being and being itself.[17]

Using Aristotle, Aquinas and others developed systems where Aristotle's metaphysics was the bridge between philosophy and theology. In opposition to earlier Christian theologians such as Augustine, Aquinas believed that a thirst for knowledge about the physical world was ordained by God, was nonidolatrous, and could even serve as a remedy for sin.[18] Aquinas thus encourages Christians to investigate the natural world through his belief that the mind is ordered to satisfy this desire and that the knowledge we acquire through sensory objects can contribute to our natural good.[19] Christians can come to know the natural law, the precepts of the eternal law that govern human behavior, through their God-given reason. I discuss natural law in detail in later chapters, but for now it is important to note that Aquinas believed humans can grasp the tenets of natural law by rationally understanding nature. In other words, understanding nature, including human nature, helps humans to know God and know how to act.

For Aquinas, Christ's humanity reveals the deep structures of human nature by elevating archetypal humanity into the divine realm, and by analogy, theology can begin to understand the creaturely realm, including the order of creation, through divine revelation. Medieval scholastics debated whether Aristotelian natural philosophy could ultimately be reconciled with Christian doctrine, particularly because Aristotle supposed nature to be an independent autonomous realm, whereas Christian theology believed God to be an *ex nihilo* Creator who continued to sustain the world. Nevertheless, Aquinas's appropriation of Aristotle shaped the nature, methods, and solutions to natural philosophy well into the sixteenth century.[20] In particular, Aquinas's natural law theory remains important in philosophy and theology today.

Aquinas's careful synthesis appropriated Aristotle's philosophy without damage to the integrity of his theological enterprise. Later scholastics, however, were not as careful in keeping the synthetic ties between philosophy and theology together. Whereas Aquinas believed the telos of the intellectual life was mystical union with God, this telos became somewhat lost in the highly rationalistic theology of the scholastics.[21] Knowledge became valued in its own right, rather than being valued for its ability to bring one closer to God. Once philosophy — detached from its theological grounding and ordering — became its own discipline for scholastics, it took its own autonomous path to truth. Concepts became valued instrumentally without reference to their theological framing.[22] In opposition to Aquinas's synthesis, theology became reliant upon philosophy for its inner justification, and spirituality became increasingly thought of, in the words of theologian Larry Chapp, as part of the "interior realm of affective dispositions."[23] Mystical theology was thus forced out of public theological debates and became relegated to the private sphere. Eventually, religious feelings became associated with the moral life rather than the intellectual life, and by some accounts Christianity "degenerate[d] into the bourgeois domestication of good deeds."[24] The split between monastic and academic theology helped to lay the foundation for the expulsion of metaphysics from most of Christian ethics.

Meanwhile, later scholastics, such as John Duns Scotus and William of Ockham, began to move away from the notion of universal intelligible forms, instead emphasizing how the human mind can know things in their particularity and through direct sensual perception. These scholastics believed God creates unique individuals out of God's sovereign will and not through any constrained pattern or form.[25] Nominalism—the idea that universals or abstract objects do not exist—began to replace earlier notions of universal intelligible forms. Universal concepts were relegated to the names (*nomina*) given to similar objects for utilitarian classification. Voluntarist theologies, which assert that God has infinite power to do whatever God wants and for whatever reason, evolved out of nominalism as a result of nominalism's emphasis on God's utterly unique acts of creation.

In the thirteenth century, theological debates concerning God's absolute and ordained power were renewed as theologians considered whether God could have fashioned the world in a different manner, according to different laws. After rigorous debate concerning God's ability to create many alternative worlds, in 1277 the Vatican declared God could have created the world in any way God pleased. The differentiation between God's absolute (*potentia absoluta*) and ordained (*potentia ordinata*) power dates back to the Patristic era, when theologians questioned whether God was able to arrange the world in a way other than the way the world as we know it is arranged. God's absolute power denotes God's power in itself, without reference to the way God's power is ordered in creation. God's ordained power, on the other hand, refers to the way God has actually ordered the natural world.[26] The Vatican's declaration gave further credence to nominalist ideas that only particulars, not universals, exist and that they are held in existence through God's continual activity.[27] Within nominalism and voluntarism, the ability to relate the world to God, or the ability to link the providence of God with the intelligibility of the world, was diminished because it eliminated the analogical link between God and the world provided within the idea of intelligible forms. As a result, God became more distant and inscrutable because God was free to change the order of nature at any time, and reasoning alone could not determine the order of nature. At the same time, voluntarism and nominalism allowed thinkers to speculate about alternative constructions of the universe, which, in the work of mathematicians such as Galileo, would allow room to reconsider medieval models of the universe.[28] Bracketing God's absolute power, later thinkers also began to investigate the laws of nature set out by God, which they believed could reveal the mind of God.

In the medieval period, one can see how Christians justified their investigations of the natural world as well as the use of non-Christian natural philosophy. The natural world had its own integrity and could communicate its depth of being to humans. For many, the natural world held important truths concerning God and the goods of human life. Understanding nature and the natural law, therefore, could bring one closer to God. Metaphysics and ethics, in other words, were intimately related. This tight connection, however, began to fall apart once Christians began to view philosophy as an independent field that did not require a theological ground. As I show in later chapters, a Christian metaphysics must rely upon certain theological precepts to function as authentically Christian. Likewise, Christian bioethics requires an explanation of how God participates in the natural world and what difference this makes for our evaluations of biotechnologies. If God's actions and the order of nature are inscrutable, then it will be difficult to assess the moral use of biomedicine, including genetic technologies. If, on the other hand, God continues to participate in nature in discernable ways, then we can begin to understand how God relates to human bodies and what God desires for human life.

The Reformers

Major theological reforms in the sixteenth and seventeenth centuries ushered in yet another way for Christians to understand God's relationship to nature and theology's relationship with natural philosophy. Reforms in natural philosophy during this time period were heavily influenced by the Reformation. Nature came to be seen less as analogously related to God and more as literally revealing God's actions in history. God's relationship to the natural world became one of direct causation, making nature more passive and dependent upon God's direct activity than it had been conceived of previously. Perhaps most importantly, however, the reformers' insistence upon the devastating effects of the Fall on humans' reason and will undercut Aquinas's assertion that humans could rationally discern the goods of human life. The result was that the tie between metaphysics and ethics further unraveled. Nature could no longer teach humans what was good or fulfill their spiritual needs, but it could serve human's physical needs if it was harnessed properly.

As mentioned in the previous chapter, when allegorical approaches to reading nature and scripture were replaced by more literal readings by reformers, scripture itself came to be seen as supplying historical and geographical information that could be useful to natural history and philosophy. Of course, Protestants were not the first to suggest scripture could be read literally. Augustine elevated the literal reading of scripture, while retaining other modes of interpretation, such as allegorical readings, which could stand alongside literal interpretations. The medieval *Quadriga*, or fourfold sense of interpretation of scripture and nature, also gave primacy to literal readings but made room for *allegoria* (past- or future-oriented), *anagogia* (allegorical or spiritual), and *analogia* (moral) interpretations. As described in chapter 1, in an attempt to make the Bible more understandable to the laity, reformers highlighted literal interpretations of scripture. The Protestant emphasis on literal interpretations undercut the medieval orderings of nature focused on similitude, which would help usher in taxonomies based upon mathematics and mechanisms. Protestant literalism later gave rise to the idea that biblical events and persons could be empirically investigated.

The Protestant emphasis on *sola scriptura*, *sola gratia*, *sola fide* also encouraged the idea that laypersons could secure knowledge about God without the assistance of the priestly hierarchy. Lay or secular theology encouraged a focus on the natural world and on human labor as containing inherent value. Protestant reformers helped to strip away the intermediaries between God and creation, which made God simultaneously more transcendent and unknowable, as well as more intimately involved in nature.[29] The focus on God's transcendence, power, and lawfulness helped to reinforce the idea that nature was passive and dependent upon God's will. During this time, reformers in natural philosophy also sought a way to read nature nonallegorically. As I will show, natural philosophers in physics and astronomy retained the notion that nature could reveal God, but instead of looking for symbols, they read the world mathematically. Searching the cosmos revealed God's geometry.

The Protestant insistence that theology go back to the original sources (the early church) uncorrupted by the Roman Church mirrored the reforms in natural philosophy that attempted to (at least initially) correct errors in earlier interpretations of Aristotle. Later, Francis Bacon along with other natural philosophers would challenge the use of Aristotle as pagan philosophy.[30] Influenced by Calvin's insistence on the devastating effects of the Fall on human cognition, Bacon argued that Aristotle did not adequately account for the impact of the Fall on humans' mental faculties and thus was inconsistent with Christian anthropology. Similarly, medical reforms were taking place in an effort to rid Galenic medicine of the influences of Aristotle.[31] Even though many natural philosophers attempted to rescue Aristotle from his more vociferous critics, the Aristotelian synthesis between metaphysics and ethics began to unravel in the late medieval period.[32]

New articulations of God's relationship to nature also brought about a shift in what was understood to be the purpose of nature. For early and medieval Christians, nature was understood to serve both physical and spiritual needs, which were found through nature's symbolic function. In the sixteenth century, however, the practical utility of nature began to supersede its symbolic function. Devoid of symbolic importance, natural objects needed a different kind of utility. If God created the world with a purpose other than contemplation, then perhaps purpose could be found in discovering the function of things within God's creation. Once an object's purpose was discovered, it could be put to its proper use, as God intended it. Natural philosophy thus took on a soteriological function. As I show in the next section, the search for nature's utility would help to collapse the distinction between efficient and final causality, and eventually Aristotle's four causes merged into a single, univocal cause, which flattened the scope of meaning and causation.

Today, the biomedical sciences maintain this focus on nature's utility. Nature is investigated so that scientists can help cure illness and other maladies. Nature has become a neutral object to be mined for its usefulness to human beings. Of course, since what constitutes the good life is no longer agreed upon, "usefulness" has become an ambiguous moral category. At the same time, a focus on utility does not mean that modern science no longer has a metaphysics. As I will show, modern metaphysics has maintained a focus on material and efficient causality, while dropping formal and final causality from its agenda.

CHANGES IN SIXTEENTH- AND SEVENTEENTH-CENTURY NATURAL PHILOSOPHY

Science eventually distanced itself from an explicit theological rationale, but many influential natural philosophers in the sixteenth and seventeenth centuries continued to have strong theological motivations that drove their work. The Protestant Reformation and Counter-Reformation ushered in major cultural and political changes in Europe by moving monastic culture into the sensibilities of the laity, which resulted in an intensely religious climate in the sixteenth and seventeenth centuries.[33] Reforms in natural philosophy were affected by and in some cases the result of theological reforms. In the seventeenth century, many natural philosophers saw their work as a kind of secular theology—secular because the thinkers that carried it out had no formal theological training and because they were concerned with earthly matters. In the seventeenth century, according to historian Amos Funkenstein, scientist, philosopher, and theologian were seen for the first time as almost one occupation.[34] It would be too much to say that Christianity alone birthed modern science, but it did affect the motivations of natural philosophers, as well as the methods they used to study nature. Highlighting the theological and metaphysical concerns of seventeenth-century natural philosophers will make more apparent why it remains difficult to evacuate all metaphysical and theological concerns from science.

As Aristotelian natural philosophy was abandoned, various programs worked to replace it, including practical mathematics, mechanism, and experimentalism, all of which were deeply influenced by religious concerns.[35] As I show in the next chapter, mechanism and experimentalism are particularly important for understanding the nature and function of genetic science in the twentieth and twenty-first centuries. Although natural philosophy was mostly concerned with what we would now call physics, reforms in natural philosophy helped to bring about important components of modern science, including the scientific method. The new natural philosophy of the seventeenth century would also greatly alter the way nature was understood and investigated, as well as how modern people relate to nature, including their own bodies.

Practical Mathematics and Mechanism

The exact start of the Scientific Revolution is debated among historians, but many agree changes in practical mathematics, including astronomy, led the way. Reforms were made possible in part by a breakdown in the Aristotelian prohibition against what we would now call the unity of the sciences. Aristotle believed it was a category mistake to use the methods of one discipline for another. Advances in the practical-mathematical disciplines such as astronomy, however, undermined the traditional separation of sciences Aristotle had prescribed.[36] Already by the fourteenth century, mathematical considerations were being taken up in physics, partly because of a breakdown in the barriers that separated the disciplines in the medieval university and the rise of competing peripatetic programs.[37] By the seventeenth century, the use of mathematics in physics was seen as a virtue, which ushered in a new ideal of a unified system of knowledge.[38] Whereas earlier Christians believed God and nature worked equivocally, the nominalist emphasis on unequivocation and the Protestant emphasis on *sola scriptura* encouraged a belief in the direct presence of God in nature. God's direct interaction in nature was no longer seen as miraculous but as necessary for ordinary operations within nature, which were increasingly seen as mechanical. God directly willed each and every action in nature; therefore, even naturally evil events were divinely ordained for the good of creation as a whole. As I will later show, many theologians today maintain this understanding of natural evil when explaining the presence of disabilities.

The rejection of Aristotelianism also led to reforms in matter theory in the seventeenth century. For Plato and Aristotle, natural philosophy was the search for the essential principles that govern entities. Aristotle restricted natural philosophy to the explanation of natural phenomena using a theory of essences. As with mathematics, there was no room for mechanics in Aristotle's natural philosophy.[39] The new approach in mathematical physics sought to reduce natural phenomena to the motion of geometrical bodies, but within this program an explanation of matter that could account for motion was still important. In the seventeenth century, natural philosophers such as Gassendi, Hobbes, and Descartes continued to view natural philosophy as matter theory but rethought matter in terms of mechanics.[40] Mechanist natural philosophy studied all natural and unnatural phenomena by using a corpuscularian theory, a mechanistic understanding that views all things through their simplest entities. Mechanist philosophers attempted to describe foundational microcorpuscularian explanations as first principles to account for macroscopic phenomena, subverting Aristotle's first principles.[41] Mechanical philosophy thus began to change the scope and nature of metaphysics within natural philosophy. Whereas metaphysics once served as the foundational understanding of the essential nature of entities or beings, metaphysics began to be understood as externally validating principles in natural philosophy.

Mechanist philosophy also helped to collapse the distinction between causes and expel teleological causes from natural philosophy. As historian Amos Funkenstein describes, debates concerning God's absolute and ordained power were reinvigorated by seventeenth-century natural philosophers, many of whom were more concerned with distinguishing between divine and human knowledge as it related to divine and human power.[42] A century before, Calvin's focus on God's sovereignty and the Fall of humanity helped to lay the groundwork for this new understanding of God's activity in the world and humans' ability to understand God. Calvin believed God laid down laws for nature according to divine will rather than reason. Following Calvin's logic, reformed theologians, such as Malebranche, came to see God's knowledge as active. In other words, God knows through doing. God created the world from nothing (*ex nihilo*); therefore, God knows beings by virtue of the act of creation as well as natural causes and forces by acting upon them.[43] The implication is that God causes all entities as well as all interactions between those entities. Nature, therefore, is merely passive, waiting to be acted upon by God. Divine causation thus replaces other forms of causation, and God's will is understood as the singular force in the universe. Only God can know things in their actuality; humans can know only ideas. This understanding of God's will forced natural philosophers to bracket the idea of God's absolute power because it was inscrutable. They instead focused on God's ordering of nature, which could tell them something about the divine order but not about the purpose of natural objects.

Bracketing God's absolute power, Descartes and others focused on the immutable laws of nature as a mirror for God's own immutability when developing their mechanical philosophy.[44] God's infinite unknowable will meant the human mind could never truly understand the cause or finality of natural phenomena, but by understanding the dynamic principles of the universe, mechanical philosophers could come close to knowing mechanisms of the universe the way that God knows them.[45] Natural philosophy, for Descartes, was thus limited to how phenomena occur according to the laws of mechanics.

Unable to know the cause or finality of natural phenomena, mechanists generally disregarded the Aristotelian emphasis on teleology. There was little need for teleological explanation in corpuscularian theories, which were chiefly concerned with describing motion and collision. Any goal-directedness of entities was placed in the realm of the divine. For example, Descartes continued to believe God directed certain activities such as fetal development and the formation of the earth, but he did not believe natural philosophy should attempt to account for God's goal-directedness.[46] Without a doctrine of forms, it was no longer important for natural philosophy to explain how objects or creatures move toward their natural state. The intrinsic goal-directedness of life, therefore, was dropped from mechanistic natural philosophy. Both Bacon and Descartes attempted to rid natural philosophy of final causes, believing fallen humans could not know them. Descartes believed the search for final causes was useless in physics, and Bacon went further by declaring that final causes corrupted the advancement of the sciences.[47] Thus the metaphysics of natural philosophy was reduced to that of material and efficient causation.

Without an internal meaning, natural objects lost their intrinsic causal powers as well. Instead, the laws of nature were needed to help explain the operations of the natural world. In Descartes's work, those laws were set by divine volition. Later, Newtonians would also presume that the regularities of nature were due to the direct activity of God.[48] Naturalism and supernaturalism began to collapse in on each other; causal explanations came to be seen as exclusively divine or natural, and eventually as natural only. Aristotle's four causes merged into a single, univocal cause, which flattened the scope of meaning and causation and enabled natural philosophy (what would become modern science) and theology to be understood within the same explanatory territory (which would become the grounds upon which religion and science were seen as competitors for explaining nature).[49] Thus the search for efficient causes took on a new importance and became somewhat conflated with the search for purposes. In searching for meaning in physical objects, the natural philosopher looked within rather than beyond those objects. If they had a purpose in God's creation, the natural philosopher could not know it. Experimentation, dissection, and magnification, therefore, became important tools in the practice of new natural philosophy.[50]

Mechanist philosophy was successful in unifying various disciplines that would have never been crossed under Aristotle. Already by the 1660s, however, the mechanist program was beginning to unravel. Descartes himself had already begun to see how a mechanist understanding of the world could not account for all phenomena. Gravity, electricity, magnetism, and chemical reactions were difficult to explain using mechanism alone.[51] To account for certain phenomena, corpuscularianism needed to be suspended. When phenomena could not be explained in corpuscularian terms, philosophers began to rely on horizontal (rather than vertical) explanation.[52] In other words, one did not need to explain larger phenomena by basic properties; instead, one could explain natural phenomena by finding relationships between things that were alike. Natural philosophers such as Robert Boyle (1627–91) did not do away with vertical causes but did believe horizontal causes could explain phenomena in their own right. By the time of Newton, a new explanatory pluralism emerged that was less concerned with fundamental microscopic matter than with the relationships between entities.[53] Mechanist philosophy ultimately failed and was severed from matter theory because foundational or vertical explanation could not organize or explain all phenomena. Instead, natural philosophers began to look for correlations rather than causal connections between things. Eventually, the new natural philosophy that emerged rejected foundationalist, speculative approaches in favor of experimental ones. The rise of experimentalism led many to believe that metaphysics was no longer necessary for natural philosophy. One did not need a grand theory of how everything was connected to understand something important about natural objects and other phenomena. Experimentalism, however, maintains its reliance upon material and efficient causation as its reigning metaphysics.

Experimentalism

What we now consider the scientific method gained prominence in the mid-seventeenth century, most notably in the English Royal Society. Today, few people doubt that experimentalism is the best way to study nature or carry out the scientific enterprise. Experimental methods were not immediately popular in the seventeenth century, however, and natural philosophers who promoted experimentalism needed theology, moral postures, and political maneuvering to secure the acceptability of their methods. As the leader of the Royal Society, Robert Boyle was instrumental in promoting the value of experimental practices in natural philosophy. Unlike mechanism, experimental philosophy did not have a conception of the unity of natural philosophy; instead, it offered methodological rules and patterns of inquiry.[54] Boyle used experiments to focus and unify heterogeneous phenomena rather than first looking to a fundamental grounded matter theory or a foundationalist perspective. Boyle's proposal to bracket metaphysics and causal explanations and rely instead upon reproducible empirical observation of an experiment was a break with hundreds of years of natural philosophy.

Boyle's avoidance of metaphysical foundations was heavily criticized in the mid-seventeenth century. Thomas Hobbes (1588–1679), in particular, was fearful that Boyle's experimental method could not produce certain knowledge, because any explanation of the natural world demanded metaphysical language.[55] As a geometer and civic philosopher, Hobbes prioritized the manmade component of knowledge. Knowledge needed to be demonstrable to be certain, meaning one could completely explain or understand only things that were made and could be shown to have efficacy when applied to the world.[56] Moreover, for Hobbes, sensory impressions, or empiricism, could not be given epistemological authority. The knowledge produced from the senses, which could be called factual knowledge, was valuable to overall knowledge but could not produce moral certainty or universal assent.[57] Against Hobbes's objections, Boyle's new experimentalism would come to replace the traditional ways of doing natural philosophy, which later became stigmatized as "metaphysics."[58] Today, Hobbes's work in natural philosophy has nearly been forgotten.

In the 1660s and 1670s, the English Royal Society fought a fierce battle to establish the experimental method as a legitimate enterprise, but it was not immediately popular in Restoration England. Faced with criticism from certain natural philosophers, Boyle sought ways to establish experimentalism as a credible enterprise taken up by serious, objective, moral, and honest men. As a result, a community of experimentalists was formed with rules for its internal and external discourse as well as its social relations. New "social and discursive conventions" needed to be accepted before experimental knowledge was established as the surest way to gain knowledge.[59] In their classic text *The Leviathan and the Air-Pump*, Shapin and Schaffer describe the material, literary, and social technologies that needed to be established to legitimate Boyle's experimental program.[60] Material technologies, such as the air pump, tested a hypothesis; literary technologies allowed the results to be made known and reproduced by others; and social technologies bounded how new experimentalists were to deal with one another to establish themselves as a moral community. The emphasis on the need for witnesses to experiments cohered nicely with the Protestant preference for the testimony of direct witnesses over the scholastic tradition of interpolations of generations of theologians.[61] Modesty displayed through publishing experimental failures, essays that made only modest as opposed to systematic claims, and plain unadorned writing helped to establish the enterprise as socially acceptable.[62] Experimentalists also sought to make their work relevant to the public by solving everyday problems encountered by citizens. Physicists could help create more effective weapons, chemists more reliable ales, and physicians more effective treatments.[63] The usefulness of nature (through manipulation) became the way natural philosophy understood nature and promoted their work to the public. Nature was valuable insofar as it had potential for human use, rather than having its own internal integrity or telos. In other words, the meaning of nature was reduced to how it could be used.

In the realm of medicine, Boyle rejected the popular notion that illness had to do with the imbalance of humors. Instead, he considered illness a phenomenon in its own right that was separate from the ill person. The generalizability of illness led to the idea that cures might be sought in medicines that could be prescribed to a variety of people with the same illness.[64] Explaining the action of medicines, therefore, became the work of natural philosophical inquiry. Boyle also positioned medicine as a religious endeavor and advocated that drug discoveries be shared freely as a way to extend Christian charity.[65]

Whereas Hobbes extended his natural philosophy into civic philosophy, Boyle encouraged the Royal Society to stay out of politics and particular religious debates, which he believed bred division. Boyle wanted to secure a space that would be insulated from the major political fights of the day and avoided meddling in the affairs of church and state.[66] What experimentalism provided was a way to understand the natural world that could avoid religious controversies and civil differences.[67] This is not to say Boyle believed natural philosophy had nothing to do with religion. In fact, Boyle believed the natural philosopher could act as a Christian apologist and contribute to the practice of religion and the moral order, even while avoiding sectarian disputes.[68] The Royal Society presented themselves as a godly community, and Boyle made frequent use of religious language to describe their work: laboratories were given a sacred status, experimental trials were performed on Sundays, and theologians were encouraged to come to the laboratory to help convince people of the God's power in nature.[69] Members of the society believed their role, in part, was to "convince men there is a God," and Boyle began calling experimental philosophers "priests of nature."[70] This presentation proved to be powerful in establishing the legitimacy of experimentalism. The bounded nature and rules of the society ensured that intense internal disputes between the experimentalists did not occur and their political and religious differences were muted. The experimentalists created respectable, nondisruptive spaces that did not infringe upon the political and religious establishment of Restoration England.

As part of their work as Christian apologists, the Royal Society attempted to bring together natural philosophy and theology. Focusing on the laws of nature as divine volitions, natural philosophers collapsed natural and supernatural causation and came to see their work as the study of God's direct activity in nature. Peter Harrison refers to the work of seventeenth-century natural philosophers as "physico-theology."[71] The result of the physico-theological program was a new natural theology that defended and promoted Christian theology through an understanding of causal mechanisms and empirical investigation. Natural theology came to be seen as a way of supporting theological doctrines on the basis of reason alone.[72] Boyle, unlike Aquinas, did not believe theology and natural philosophy could be bridged by metaphysics; instead, he believed one could triangulate natural philosophy and revelation to converge on the truth. Within experimentalism, theology and natural philosophy were equal partners in the search for truth. The desire to do both theology and natural philosophy at once put theology and natural philosophy on the same explanatory plane. Having allowed natural philosophy to function somewhat independently for centuries, however, theology was not up to the challenge of explaining nature as well as natural philosophy could. Eventually, this would mean that theology became useless in the scientific enterprise.

How Theology and Natural Science Begin to Break Apart

The split between science and religion was perhaps not inevitable. The "crises of faith" in the nineteenth century had as much to do with political events and disputes within Christianity as with the rise of science.[73] Yet it is not difficult to see why natural philosophers were able to carry out their project without explicit reference to God. By rendering God utterly transcendent, they made God's being unnecessary to explicate within the order of nature. Once the natural and supernatural were placed in a zero-sum equation, it became unnecessary to reference God or other theological language explicitly when carrying out natural philosophy. By the end of the seventeenth century, explicit theological justifications for reforms in natural philosophy were unaccounted for in descriptions of the scientific method.[74] The rise of Deism in the 1680s, for example, showed an extreme version of a natural theology devoid of classic Christian notions of creation.[75] Whereas for Aquinas God's "motionless motion" provided the ontological basis and goal of all motion, natural scientists in the eighteenth century had an easier time discarding Descartes's theological voluntarism while maintaining his materialist ontology, leading some historians to conclude, "Descartes simply exalted these sublime matters of faith into irrelevance."[76] Similarly, Newton's emphasis on divine volition eventually rendered God incidental to understanding the cosmos.

The alliances made between natural philosophers and theologians, which positioned them as part of the same enterprise, would later put them into competition. A few philosophers, such as Baruch Spinoza (1632–77), went so far as to show that mechanist natural philosophy could supplant Judeo-Christian teachings concerning the world and humanity's place within it and could even inculcate piety better than Christianity.[77] Whereas physico-theologians tried to use natural philosophy to prove events in scripture, later thinkers, such as Spinoza, saw scripture and natural philosophy as opposed.[78] Spinoza's attempts to rid natural philosophy of religion were not initially successful; instead, between the seventeenth and nineteenth centuries thinkers tried once again to separate theology from natural philosophy to preserve the integrity of each arena. Immanuel Kant helped to separate the realms of theology and natural philosophy by positing that religion offers moral insight whereas natural philosophy works to discover facts about the physical world. Certain Enlightenment thinkers after

Kant shared his distaste for the explicit use of theology in natural philosophy. The result was that natural theology was severely diminished within both natural philosophy and theology.

The early modern era's absorption of natural theology, which argued God from nature, into natural philosophy, which described nature more generally, meant it came to be seen as less essential within theology. As described in chapter 1, Protestants' interest in historical-critical methods favored an attention to history over natural science. Natural theology itself suffered as a result of its merger with natural philosophy. To enter into the partnership with natural philosophy, natural theology needed to be reduced to its cognitive content. When compared to advances in natural philosophy, however, natural theology was found to be lacking. The questions posed by natural philosophy increasingly gained prominence in Western society, and by the mid-nineteenth century those questions, along with the answers found in the natural sciences, came to displace those of theological inquiry.[79]

In the second half the nineteenth century, natural philosophy began to coalesce around a common method, a professional identity, and a new nomenclature ("science") rather than a common set of theological beliefs. Religion and science were perceived as distinct conceptual objects and separate disciplines. Once this separation occurred, it was easy for some to anachronistically read back the religion and science division throughout all of Western history. For those invested in promoting the conflict narrative, science is seen to displace religion as the superior, if not sole, explanatory force for the natural world. To combat the conflict myth, some historians of science, such as Stephen Jay Gould, have developed alternative ways of understanding the relationship between religion and science, which allow each discipline to have distinct domains of inquiry.[80] Although scientists, historians, and theologians dispute the most appropriate way to distinguish religion from science, few believe it would benefit either science or religion to once again merge the two enterprises. This is not to suggest, however, that modern theology and science did not co-emerge. Modern science has roots in theological understandings of the world. Post-Enlightenment thinkers, however, were quick to distance themselves from religion after its place as a dominant cultural force in society began to wane. Scientists themselves might still adhere to religious beliefs, but when doing the work of science, few identified their work as apologetics or as serving an explicitly theological purpose.

The break between nature and science, however, was never fully completed. The conflict narrative is entirely mistaken. Rather than breaking away from science, Christianity's transcendent God was collapsed into nature. God's attributes were assigned to nature, and thus the intelligibility and value of nature came from the human confrontation with the empirical world.[81] In American history, nature came to be seen as having its own immanent rationality, which gave humans natural rights and universal moral laws.[82] As we continue to see, and as will become more evident in chapter 3, there remains an implicit, and at times explicit, belief that the technologies of modern science can be used for soteriological ends. The idea that nature is sacred or transcendent frequently emerges in modern culture.

HISTORIANS OF SCIENCE AND RELIGION make it clear that the two fields have never been neatly divided, nor have they always been understood as separate conceptual domains. The conflict myth is an invention of post-Enlightenment philosophy that obscures the important influence theology played in the rise of modern science. Christian theologians have long been interested in how God interacts with nature, and at various points in Western history Christian theology inspired and drove the investigation of the natural world. For many early Christians, God's creation of the world *ex nihilo* meant that the material world was intimately connected to the Creator. Understanding nature, including human nature, helped Christians to know something about God as well as how they ought to relate to other human beings. For medieval thinkers such as Aquinas, metaphysics was the bridge to relating theological claims to the claims of natural philosophy. Changing notions about God in the late medieval and Reformation periods gave rise to new investigations of nature, in which God was collapsed into empirical investigations of the world. Positioning God's will as inscrutable made the investigation of formal and final causes irrelevant within natural philosophy, severely reducing the scope of classic metaphysics and even leading some to believe metaphysics was no longer necessary for natural philosophy or theology. At the same time, by collapsing the natural and supernatural, natural philosophers were able to see their work as kind of theology, in which God could be read literally from the earth. Such thinking created fertile ground for the Scientific Revolution to occur.

Once theology and natural philosophy became the same enterprise, however, theology came to be seen by many as irrelevant within the study of the natural world. Yet the appropriation of religious language by prominent geneticists mentioned at the beginning of this chapter suggests that our secular scientific culture cannot completely dispense with theo-logic. The implicit religion of modern science emerged but is now distinct from classic Christian understandings of the world as God's creation (a point that I will take up explicitly in chapter 4). Yet, as I will show in later chapters, mainline Protestant denominations still attempt to integrate scientific findings into their theological doctrines, and many view genetic technologies as a way of participating in God's redemptive actions on earth. Like sixteenth- and seventeenth-century physico-theologians, many continue to see nature as a passive, neutral realm that can be used for the benefit of humankind. At the same time, the collapse of causes in this era has helped to breed confusion between natural and supernatural causation, which makes discussions concerning the origins and character of disease and disability, as well as the proper use of medicine, particularly difficult to resolve. As I will later show, the confusion between natural and supernatural causation has had lasting impacts on how we discuss the evils of genetic disability.

One can see within the history I have provided several alternatives for how Christians may conceive of God's relationship to nature and theology's relationship to science. With Augustine, they might try to limit which investigations of nature are appropriate for theologians; with Aquinas, they might wish to relate a philosophical metaphysics to their theological understanding; with the reformers, they might seek to restrict what can be known about God from the natural world as a result of humankind's fallenness; or with the physico-theologians, they might wish to merge theology, science, and natural history into a single enterprise. Alternatively, a path might need to be forged that seeks to articulate a Christian metaphysics in light of foundational Christian doctrines.

Chapter 3 shows how theological and metaphysical assumptions of the Scientific Revolution have carried over into the biological and medical sciences. Biology was one of the last scientific fields to do away with the notion of final ends. Even in the late eighteenth and early nineteenth centuries, biologists continued to believe species were moving toward a state of perfection for which they were designed, which necessitated the notion of a designer God. By studying the design of creatures, therefore, biologists believed they could come to know God rationally. The Darwinian revolution helped to transform this thinking, however, by doing away with formal and final causation in biology, as it had been previously dispensed with in physics, astronomy, and other natural sciences. Biologists went even further in expelling traditional Christian notions from science, sometimes claiming to have a superior scientific religion. Modern science and technology provide what classical religion only hoped to offer: access to truth and the means to salvation.

CHAPTER THREE

The Metaphysics and Theology
of Genetic Medicine

After the seventeenth century, it became less popular to explicitly align a theological agenda with the methods and practice of natural philosophy, but this does not mean that religious sensibilities were evacuated from scientific inquiry. Well into the eighteenth century, natural philosophy and natural history were thought to offer a path to renew natural theology. Even when religion and science began to be seen as distinct disciplines in the nineteenth century, scientists did not completely do away with religious language or theological modes of inquiry. In fact, some scientists, particularly evolutionists and eugenicists, saw their work as replacing formal religion. In 1874, the eugenics pioneer Francis Galton (1822–1911) concluded his book *English Men of Science: Their Nature and Nurture* by calling for a new generation of scientists to take up a "scientific priesthood." After bemoaning the fact that educational systems were opposed to science, Galton expressed his hope that educational reforms "will, even in our days, give rise to the establishment of a sort of scientific priesthood throughout the kingdom, whose high duties would have reference to the health and well-being of the nation it its broadest sense."[1] Galton believed the clergy running the education systems were

55

"opposed to science" and "crushed the inquiring spirit, the love of observation, the pursuit of inductive studies, the habit of independent thought."[2] In response, Galton wished to take power away from the clergy and bestow it upon the "friends of science."[3]

Similarly, T. H. Huxley (1825–95), "Darwin's bulldog," sought to disturb traditional religious teachings with science. Huxley applied his science to biblical events and stories but, unlike his seventeenth-century physico-theologian forebears, mostly saw science as discrediting biblical accounts.[4] Huxley was quick to point out that his work was not meant as an attack against the Bible or hatred against Christianity; rather, he intended to treat biblical accounts with the same scrutiny as any other account that could be put to the scientific test, which was already what Protestant theologians were doing with their historical-critical mode of theologizing in the mid- to late-nineteenth century.[5] As described in the previous chapter, the collapse of natural theology and philosophy was crucial for placing religion and science on the same explanatory territory and allowing figures such as Huxley to investigate scripture scientifically. Like Boyle before him, Huxley called his scientific lectures "lay sermons."[6] Other evolutionary theorists, such as Alfred Mathieu Giard (1846–1908), believed science had begun to replace religion in society.[7] Ernst Haeckel (1834–1919), sometimes referred to as "the German Darwin," developed a "religion of science," which he called "monism." Haeckel was vocal in his opposition to orthodox Christianity, and in particular the Catholic Church; he believed that Darwinism was opposed to religious dogmatisms and that it yielded a superior ethic and social philosophy, as well as a "monistic religion of humanity grounded in pantheism."[8] Far from ridding their work of religion, many leading scientists began to take up the language, imagery, and ritual of religion as their own.

One can also find popular scientists today claiming their field has replaced traditional religious beliefs. "New Atheists" such as Sam Harris, Richard Dawkins, and Daniel Dennett are vocal critics of religion, combining their philosophical and scientific insights to attack religion. The neuroscientist Sam Harris has called for a "scientific morality" that does away with all traditional religion.[9] Richard Dawkins similarly believes science can provide the answers to the deep questions about meaning, morality, and life's purpose more adequately than religion.[10] These "New Atheists" eschew religion as irrelevant in contemporary culture while at the same time endowing science with religious significance. Not only is science the only field to provide legitimate knowledge about the natural world, it can also provide answers to what were once considered theological questions, such as "Who are we as humans?" "How do we relate to the rest of the natural order?" and "What is our destiny as a species?"

Most scientists, however, are much more cautious in what questions they believe science is able to answer. The scientific method in the twenty-first century is no longer explicitly connected to a religious or theological agenda. To advance science, most scientists believe they must bracket divine or supernatural concerns when deploying the scientific method. Yet the tendency toward taking up metaphysical and theological questions when speaking to lay audiences might speak to science's continuing indebtedness to its secular theologian forebears. Understanding the theological influences on the formation of early modern science begins to explain why many continue to believe that science, particularly genetic science, is able to provide meaningful information about human identity and human destiny.

Questions concerning the foundations and purpose of human life were once reserved for the realm of theology. As was true in the seventeenth century, such questions are now being taken up by scientists, who function as our contemporary secular theologians. Insofar as the Human Genome Project implicitly or explicitly answers the question "Who are we as human beings?" it is inherently asking philosophical questions. When genetic scientists offer up soteriological solutions to the problems of finitude, they have wandered into the realm of theology. Like the physico-theologians of the seventeenth century, many popular scientists claim their discoveries will answer the fundamental questions of human life and instruct communal living. Scientists today, however, are mostly unwilling to seriously engage theologians to help further their ends.

This chapter explores how developments in biology and genetics helped change the relationship between science and religion, while never fully escaping theology or metaphysics. I begin with reforms to the biological sciences initiated by evolutionists, particularly Charles Darwin (1809–82), and the religious responses to those reforms. Next, I reveal how these reforms made their way into the burgeoning field of genetics. I investigate how lay understandings of genetics fall into a material/spiritual dualism and confusion between divine and natural causation that have bolstered the science/religion conflict narrative. Similarly, some scientific popularizers suffer from the slippage that exists between methodological and ontological naturalism, which can lead to genetic determinism. Ontological naturalism, genetic determinism, and dualism are not foundational or necessary for the scientific method, but their origins can be traced back to an earlier time, described in the previous chapter, when natural and divine causation began to be seen as competing forces.

EVOLUTION AND THE DARWINIAN REVOLUTION

Darwin's impact on biological understanding cannot be overstated. Just as the Scientific Revolution led to significant reforms in natural philosophy and helped to transform its relationship with theology, Darwin's work led to important changes in how biological organisms, including humans, were investigated and understood. In contrast to popular mythology, Darwin's theories were not immediately offensive to most Christians, nor were they instantly or uncritically accepted as superior to other evolutionary theories.[11] Robust objections to evolution began long after Darwin's *The Descent of Man*, and initially had as much to do with a clash of scientific worldviews as they did with a confrontation between science and religion. Evolution seemed to run against a literal-historical interpretation of Genesis, but it also did not appear to depend on fact and demonstration. Darwin's variational evolutionary theory was debated for eighty years after *On the Origin of Species* (1859) was published, even though evolutionary theory itself had been readily accepted in the scientific community.[12] Darwin's theories would, however, come to be seen as the foundation of evolutionary biology. Darwin's methods of "observation, comparison and classification, as well as the testing of competing historical narratives," helped to establish new methods for evolutionary biology not premised on the experimental methods that had revolutionized natural philosophy two centuries earlier.[13] Unlike other natural sciences, evolutionary biology is a historical science, which does not rely solely on laws and experiments but instead hypothesizes about the historical circumstances that led to current natural conditions and then looks to empirical evidence to verify those proposals.[14] The content of his theories as well as the methods used to advance them has led some historians to argue that Darwin did more to change modern thought than any other scientific reformer or Enlightenment thinker.[15]

Darwin was not the first thinker to advance a theory of evolution. What separated him from his predecessors most distinctly was his theory of natural selection. In contrast to earlier theories, Darwin's evolutionary biology proposed a vertical evolutionary chain where all living things traced their descent to a single origin, rather than a horizontal relationship in which species were fixed and moving toward greater perfection. Darwin's theory of gradual natural selection also proposed a new mechanism of evolution that broke with earlier notions. Charles-Georges Le Roy (1723–89), Marquis de Condorcet (1743–94), and Jean-Baptiste Lamarck (1744–1829), for example, believed that traits acquired in life could be passed on to the next generation.[16] As was typical in both natural history and natural theology of the time, Le Roy and Condorcet believed animals were destined toward particular ends and, therefore, new species could not arise from older ones. Lamarck, on the other hand, proposed an idea of unlimited change, which gave rise to the great diversity of living creatures in the world.[17] (In *On the Origin of Species*, Darwin also accepted the inheritance of acquired traits as one possible source of variation within natural selection.) Lamarck, unlike Darwin, however, did not offer an explanation as to the mechanism by which creatures passed on characteristics to their progeny.[18] Although it would take some time to understand genetic inheritance, Darwin did propose that small, material particles or "gemmules" might be responsible for passing on traits from one generation to the next.[19]

Darwin's theory of natural selection made it possible to understand organisms in an entirely new way, not simply as individual entities, but as artifacts of a common history or ancestry. For Darwin, a "species" is a group of interbreeding individuals with a common ancestor, not a type or a form. Whereas evolutionary theorists such as Lamarck focused on the changes undergone by a single organism, Darwin focused on the changes undergone by a lineage. Any one individual of a species was a mere instantiation or accident in the animal's time line.[20] This move helped to historicize species. Just as Newton helped to make change, rather than stability, the defining feature of objects in physics, Darwin helped to make change the most important feature of biology. Modern science after Newton became much more interested in the relations between things than things in themselves. For Newton, this meant a focus on forces rather than motion per se. For evolutionary biology, the emphasis on relationships rather than organisms has led to a focus on the evolutionary process itself and its mechanisms rather than on life or living things per se.[21] Species in modern evolutionary biology thus have no ontological identity apart from their history. As mere products of history, organisms become indistinguishable from artifacts. Before Darwin, many biologists believed organisms maintained themselves through change and were irreducible to the sum of their elements, whereas artifacts had parts essentially external to each other without intrinsic unity beyond the mind of their maker.[22] Darwin, however, positioned organisms as artifacts or the "summing up of many contrivances" that were "built up" from natural selection.[23] Darwin's theories, therefore, made it possible to conceptually reduce organisms to the sum of their parts.

Darwin also helped to rid biology of teleology. As noted in the previous chapter, teleological explanations had been rejected by many natural philosophers, but explanations for biological phenomena continued to invoke teleology in the eighteenth and nineteenth centuries. Other evolutionary theories in Darwin's time, such as orthogenesis, used teleology to describe species.[24] In opposition to teleological theories, Darwin did not posit a direction in which organisms were headed. Instead, he made use of chance as the first step of natural selection. Rather than relying upon universal laws, evolutionary biology now understands the regularities in nature as probabilistic.[25] Within Darwin's theory, there is no need for a cosmic teleology, which presumes that the natural world moves toward greater perfection. Natural selection allows for local progress, but *progress* itself is an ambiguous term that relates more to the organism's fitness for the environment than to a "perfection" of form.

In addition to doing away with direct teleological explanations for organisms, Darwin also bracketed any reference to God in his theory, which broke with other popular interpretations of evolution during Darwin's time. The work of William Paley (1743–1805), for example, was quite popular in Britain in the late eighteenth century. In the tradition of the natural theologians of the seventeenth century, Paley sought to describe God by investigating the natural world. Like earlier physico-theologians, Paley believed empirical study of the natural world could reveal the character of God. Unlike earlier thinkers, however, Paley believed natural theology was the basis for accepting revelation, rather than knowledge alongside revelation.[26] Paley's *Natural Theology* argues that if objects have a purpose, then they have been designed, which implies a designer. Paley believed God designed objects with a purpose so that God could be known: "It is only by the display of contrivance, that the existence, the agency, and the wisdom of the Deity, *could* be testified to his rational creatures."[27] In other words, God works through natural laws and with design so that God can be known rationally. As humans come to understand natural laws, their understanding of God changes.

In rebuking Paley, Darwin may have misread him as describing the *origins* of complexity, rather than the *purpose* of complexity.[28] Paley's "watchmaker" God, who was somewhat juxtaposed to the world in order to be understood by rational creatures, was easy for Darwin to discard in favor of "natural explanations" for the central problem of adaptation. Rather than base his understanding of natural selection on a theological understanding of God's relationship to the world, Darwin practiced what Connor Cunningham has called "methodological naturalism," which brackets questions of the supernatural to describe natural explanations on their own terms.[29] Paley's somewhat distant designer God (like Descartes's voluntarist God) was easily removed from direct explication by Darwin, who opted instead for "natural selection" as nature's designer. Darwin understood the world materialistically, without reference to a creator or designer God. Whereas physico-theologians in the seventeenth century sought to know God by the design of the world and the laws of nature, Darwin's theories did not directly comment on God as either the originator of the natural world or its culmination.

Darwin's Legacy in Christianity

The coherence of Darwin's theories of evolution and orthodox Christianity has been debated since Darwin first published his work. Darwin concluded *On the Origin of Species* (1859) with the Genesis metaphor of the breath of life and reference to the Creator, which he later regretted because he was not prepared to align his scientific findings with a particular theology. Unlike biologists in the eighteenth and early nineteenth centuries who sought to defend particular religious values they saw as under assault from rival cosmologies, in the latter half of the nineteenth century a shift toward neutrality began to take over.[30] Speculations about the meanings and purpose of life were increasingly seen as beyond the purview of science, but this did not end the debate concerning Darwin's relationship with Christianity. People continue to debate whether Darwin's theories helped or undermined orthodox Christianity.[31]

Shortly after Darwin rose to popularity, Christians and non-Christians alike debated what effect his theories had on Christian doctrine. For some scientists, Darwin's theories ushered in a new era of religion centered on science and nature. As previously mentioned, Galton proposed practical Darwinism as an alternative religion, and Haeckel hoped for a time when churches would be replaced by monists who cherished nature and science.[32] Wilhelm Boelsche (1861–1939) also believed Darwinism had created a "Second Reformation," offering a Third Testament of science that transcended the Old and New Testaments.[33] Although Darwin attempted to bracket the supernatural in favor of natural explanations for evolution, his interpreters debated whether Darwin was implicitly attacking the Christian faith. Catholic and Protestant commentators considered whether the Christian doctrine of creation required the belief that all species were created independently of one another.[34] They also debated whether Darwin's theory of evolution meant that natural morality could exist apart from religion. Others worried that Darwin's emphasis on chance in natural selection undermined God's providence. Several Catholic and Protestant theologians, on the other hand, advocated for the compatibility of Darwinism and Christianity, and some even believed that Darwin's theories enriched their religious beliefs and helped to explain biblical doctrines such as original sin, God's immanence, and the problem of suffering.[35] William James even argued that Darwinism helped to jettison the God of physico-theology, who James believed was too intellectually posited and prevented people from experiencing life and moral courage.[36] For James and others, scientific naturalism did not drive out religion but helped to purify it.

Darwin did not set out to attack the idea of God or disprove God's existence and, therefore, should not be seen as the enemy of orthodox Christian theology. Many Christians in the nineteenth century did not find Darwin's theories threatening because, following an older Christian tradition, they believed God was beyond the known universe. In *Confessions*, Augustine responds to the question "What was God doing before He made heaven and earth?" with "He was preparing hell . . . for those who pry into mysteries."[37] Although this was a somewhat crude response, Augustine cautioned against speculating as to what was "before" creation. For Augustine, theology was not about our physical origins but about our ontological ones. Darwin's explanation for our natural origins is a problem for Christians only if they read the Bible as a modern history and science book. Likewise, Darwin's methodological naturalism is a problem for Christians only if they believe that matter is opposed to spirit, or that God cannot work through natural means.

The theological shifts and scientific methods that emerged in the sixteenth and seventeenth centuries might have contributed to the particular way modern people dichotomize the natural and supernatural or spirit and nature. The debates concerning Darwin's threat to Christianity reveal the tendency of modern people to see conflict between both matter and spirit and divine and natural causation. Christians have long struggled with the tension between nature and supernature, especially when considering how God's grace becomes manifest in the natural world, but the idea that God and nature are in conflict has become particularly popular in modernity. If divine and natural causation are understood as opposing forces, then the chance element of natural selection might undermine God's providential plan or design for creation. Chance and design cannot coexist. Similarly, if divine and natural causation are opposed, then material nature is seen as opposed to God's divine presence. Some of Darwin's defenders, such as Haeckel, believed Darwin's theories promoted a monistic religion that could replace the dualisms present in Christianity (e.g., matter/spirit, nature/supernature).[38] As I explore in the next chapter, however, orthodox Christianity presumes that God is not opposed to nature or matter. The spirit/matter dualism that was rejected by theologians such as Augustine has crept back into modern thinking. If anything, Darwin and Darwinism have helped to expose this tendency of modern people, including modern Christians, to see God merely in the gaps of scientific knowledge, as if scientific explanation and divine causation were in competition.

Christians should not understand the theory of natural selection as an attack upon their faith, but they should resist positing Darwinism as a first philosophy. Whereas methodological naturalism has become a requirement in modern science, ontological naturalism assumes the natural is all there is and ever could be.[39] Ontological naturalism rules out the existence of divine or supernatural forces, even forces that act with, rather than against, nature. Whereas methodological naturalism is agnostic about the existence of God or divine activity, ontological naturalism presumes that there is no God. In the Scientific Revolution, science (natural philosophy and history) was understood as the handmaid of theology, helping to confirm the truths of the Bible and Christian doctrine, but within ontological naturalism, philosophy and theology become handmaidens of science.[40] Ontological naturalism can easily lead to "scientism," which seeks to make natural science the *only* source of real knowledge. Within scientism, there is no room for independent (or even complementary) philosophies or theologies alongside science, because scientism makes science a first philosophy—the only begetter of truth.

Ontological naturalism and scientism do not cohere with the scientific method. The scientific method has certain limitations that restrict what kinds of truths science is able to offer. According to the philosopher of science Karl Popper, science is a system of hypotheses that must always be fallibilistic, or subject to correction.[41] Science itself is built on faith in its methods; we must believe in the efficacy of reason and the ability of the scientific method to accurately describe reality. In the seventeenth century this was widely debated, but today most people take for granted that the scientific method provides real (and useful) facts about the material world. Many have forgotten the hard-fought battles that ensured the success of the scientific method (the empirical method and the importance of prediction). Although it has certain belief structures and metaphysical assumptions, the scientific method has its own internally placed limitations. Under its own canons, the sciences are limited to explaining finite, material, and objective causes. Science thus can ask about *proximate* origins, but it cannot ask about *ultimate* origins. Science should function nontheistically, using methodological naturalism, and thus should have nothing to say about the question of God's existence, divine activity, or the telos of human life. Certain scientists today, however, claim an understanding of the meaning of human nature and the divine (or lack thereof) based on their own scientific discoveries. When scientific explanation attempts to supersede all other metaphysical and religious accounts of the universe, it must be called to account, and alternatives must be offered.

Christians should also resist making Darwinism or any evolutionary theory into the basis for their moral system or theology. In the nineteenth century, many thinkers began to use evolutionary theories as a justification for particular moral and political systems. The historian Leslie Jones contends, "Individualism and socialism, militarism and pacifism, pro-natalism and neo-Malthusianism, organized religion and agnosticism, all have had their Darwinian exegetes."[42]

Many of the so-called Social Darwinists of the nineteenth century, including the grandfather of Social Darwinism, Herbert Spencer (1820–1903), developed their theories of social evolution before Darwin published his works but found in Darwin an ally to promote their ideas for social reform. Once Darwin's theories became more universally accepted, they were used to justify systems and ideologies that in retrospect many find repugnant. Christians should be careful not to base their foundational doctrines or moral systems on scientific theories, which are all too easily co-opted to justify a range of ideologies. As the old saying goes: the theology that marries the science of today will be the widow of tomorrow. This is not to say that Christians should ignore scientific findings altogether; often scientific findings can reveal heresies within contemporary Christian thought, as was true of Darwinism. Instead, Christians should not allow particular, fallibilistic, scientific theories to alter their foundational principles and doctrines.

From Darwin to the Genome

Discoveries in the life sciences, including geology, paleoanthropology, and genetics, helped to prove many of Darwin's central ideas correct. The discovery of genes was particularly useful in explaining how certain characteristics are passed down to progeny. Genetics is not the core of evolutionary theory, nor is all evolutionary change internal to the organism, but genes did help to explain the mechanism behind inherited traits.[43] Although today genetics and Darwinism go hand in hand, they developed somewhat independently. Many trace the birth of genetics to Austrian monk Gregor Mendel's work *Experiments in Plant Hybridization*, in 1865. Mendel's experimental work on peas established laws of hybridity. Mendel's work, however, went fairly unacknowledged until it was rediscovered in the early twentieth century by botanists Hugo de Vries, Carl Correns, and Erich von Tschermak and biologist William Bateson. Bateson coined the term *genetics* to describe heredity, and by 1906 genetics had already become a discipline with an international meeting devoted to it.[44] These early scientists connected their work to Darwin's theories.

De Vries, for example, initially named hereditary particle "pangenes" after Darwin's theory of "pangenesis," in which he described how cells in organisms shed minute particles (gemmules), which are collected in the gonads and transmitted to offspring.[45] Chromosomal theories, which had already begun in the late nineteenth century, were fused with Mendelian theories to help explain the mechanistic foundation for Mendel's theories of inheritance and gave genetics a material basis (though not necessarily the material nature of the gene or their mode of action) and spatial significance (genes being located on chromosomes).[46]

Major breakthroughs in genetic research came when deoxyribonucleic acid (DNA) was discovered to be the material basis of chromosomes and genes. Already by the 1940s, genes were understood to be units of heredity, but there was question as to what genes themselves were made of. In 1944, a group of researchers discovered that DNA was the chemical basis for heritable transformation in bacteria.[47] In the early 1950s, Rosalind Elsie Franklin, an X-ray diffraction expert, first noted the double-helical structure of DNA, which was later confirmed by Francis Crick and James Watson (who were given access to Rosalind's images and reports without her permission or knowledge and then downplayed Franklin's role to take credit for her discovery).[48] This discovery allowed researchers to understand how genetic information is stored and replicated and how it carries biological information. Frederick Sanger developed techniques to sequence DNA in the 1970s, and these became automated in the 1980s.[49]

With these essential discoveries in place, researchers were set to begin sequencing the entire human genome. In America, the Department of Energy and the National Institutes of Health were given congressional funding to explore the human genome, which gave birth to the Human Genome Project (HGP) in 1990. The HGP was a thirteen-year-long, publicly funded project aiming to sequence DNA base pairs that make up the human genome, locate all genes in humans, and sequence the human genome (along with other organisms).[50] Additionally, the project planned to make its findings public by recruiting public and private researchers, as well as a group of international researchers (International Human Genome Sequencing Consortium) who openly published their sequencing information. Three percent of funds were set aside to study the consequences of genomic research for society through a program known as Ethical, Legal, and Social Implications (ELSI), which continues to be funded today.[51] Finishing ahead of schedule, the HGP was heralded by many as a huge success and well worth its publicly funded expense of $3 billion.[52] New promising branches of medical science, including genomic medicine, have been established as a result of the HGP. Precision medicine, neurogenetics, and pharmacogenomics all use a patient's genetic information to find the most appropriate and effective therapies for groups of patients who share similar genetic profiles.

Although the HGP has been foundational for various advancements in the medical sciences, many of the early promises of the HGP have yet to be fulfilled, largely because many early researchers overpredicted the power of genes. When the project was completed, many believed new treatments for common diseases such as cancer, Alzheimer's, and heart disease would soon follow. President Clinton announced that the HGP would "revolutionize the diagnosis, prevention and treatment of most, if not all, human diseases."[53] Francis Collins boldly predicted that researchers would discover the genetic diagnosis of most diseases within ten years of the completion of the Human Genome Project and that new treatments would be found five years after that. "Over the longer term, perhaps in another 15 or 20 years, you will see a complete transformation in therapeutic medicine."[54] Curative treatments for most common diseases have remained elusive, however. It turns out that the genetics of most diseases are far more complicated than researchers initially presumed. Very few diseases arise from a single-point mutation. In many areas of medicine, taking a family history continues to be more predictive than genome sequencing.[55] In 2010, Harold Varmus, the director of the National Cancer Institute, controversially declared, "Genomics is a way to do science, not medicine."[56] Although basic scientists have learned a tremendous amount about biology as a result of the HGP, including the surprising fact that humans have far fewer genes than initially predicted, direct medical benefits have lagged behind.[57]

Today, whole-genome sequencing is far less expensive than it was ten years ago, and there are now more than two thousand genetic tests for human conditions, which help physicians diagnose disease and understand a patient's genetic risks for disease.[58] Pharmacogenomic tests, which use both genome sequencing and population data, allow physicians to identify whether drugs for cancer, heart disease, AIDS, and other diseases will be effective and which treatments will pose the fewest side effects for patients. As of today, only a few large-scale studies have shown improved outcomes for patients using "genotype-guided" dosing alone, and many now believe more complex information needs to be taken into account.[59] The most promising outcomes appear to be in cancer therapies. For cancer, precision medicine, which "takes into account individual variability in genes, environment, and lifestyle for each person," allows physicians to more accurately predict what therapies might be most effective in groups of people who share certain genetic factors.[60] Still, relatively few effective therapies are based on precision medicine, and the therapies that do exist remain expensive.[61] It is difficult to use genomic information to make accurate predictions concerning whether or for how long a therapy will be able to target an individual cancer as well as what genotype may evolve to resist that therapy.[62] Cancers evolve both deterministically (as prescribed in Darwinian selection), and randomly (through genetic mutation and genetic drift), making cancer a moving target.

Predicting genetic risk for disease also comes with its own complications. Initially, many presumed the HGP would allow us to take charge of our future by preventing diseases for which we have a genetic risk. In perhaps what is one of the more immoderate expressions of this future hope, in a speech at Robert Morris College, Bill Clinton stated,

> The Human Genome Project . . . will one day in the not-too-distant future enable every set of parents that has a little baby to get a map of the genetic structure of their child. So if their child has a predisposition to a certain kind of problem, or even to heart disease or stroke in their early 40s, they will be able to plan that child's life, that child's upbringing, to minimize the possibility of the child developing that illness or that predisposition, to organize the diet plan, the exercise plan, the medical treatment, that would enable untold numbers of people to have far more full lives than would have been the case before.[63]

Clinton's hope to control the minutiae of our children's lives has not yet been realized, although opportunities for "risk management" based on one's genetic profile have increased. Discovering a BRCA gene mutation now prompts physicians to offer prophylactic mastectomy or at least suggest extra monitoring techniques. Persons who are likely to develop heart disease due to an inherited genetic condition are counseled to begin changing their lifestyles. Studies show, however, that knowing one's genetic risk rarely changes behavior,[64] and some of the diseases assessed, such as late-onset Alzheimer's and Parkinson's disease, do not yet have effective treatments or cures, so the benefit of knowing one's risk profile for them is less obvious.[65] Moreover, few diseases have a strong enough genetic component to make sequencing an effective way to assess individual risk.[66] Whole-genome sequencing has also enabled researchers to develop blood tests to discover certain chromosomal and genetic defects prenatally, but because these anomalies generally have no cure, abortion remains the only "therapeutic" option.

Incredible insights have been gained through the HGP in biology and medicine, even if genomic medicine is only in the early stages. Gene interaction is more complex than initially presumed because genes are far less determinative than some had imagined. Many researchers predict that great strides in genomic medicine will be made once these genetic and environmental complexities are better understood. As with the failure of older mechanistic theories, reductionism cannot adequately account for natural processes, nor can it provide meaningful insight into complex human behaviors. Most geneticists and molecular biologists recognize that genes cannot possibly live up to the significant role they were given in the HGP. Molecular biology has now challenged the idea of atomistic explanations that could separate the gene from its context into a discrete entity.

The classic genotype/phenotype divide no longer holds; only rarely does a gene cause certain phenotypic effects in a one-to-one relationship. It turns out that the connection between genotype and phenotype is heterogeneous. Different genotypes can produce the same phenotypic trait, and different phenotypes can arise from the same genotype. Moreover, the position of genes changes the effects of genes, as can environment. Scientists drastically overestimated the number of genes in the human genome because they did not initially understand the multifactorial nature of gene expression. Some geneticists now believe genes are the products of evolution and not their producers. Peter Beurton writes, "Genes are the product of evolutionary dynamics going on in populations and are brought into being by downward causation."[67] Biology tried to replicate physics in making the gene like the atom, but this project failed because genes are not directly correlated to an organism's characteristics; rather, genes respond to nature. We now know that the external environment can "act as a mutating agent on the genotype, as a paragenetic agent on the formation of the phenotype . . . and as a selective agent on the phenotype."[68] The more we learn about genes, the more it appears that genes are complex and interactional, not discrete entities that "code for" characteristics. Deterministic thinking, however, has not been eradicated.

Many in the West have become enamored with genetic determinism because certain voices in the biological and genetic sciences, particularly ultra-Darwinists and certain sociobiologists and evolutionary biologists, have confused ontological naturalism with methodological naturalism. Richard Dawkins, for example, often speaks about animals as if they were merely the hosts of genes. According to Dawkins, "We are all survival machines of the same kind of replicator — but there are many different ways of making a living in the world, and the replicators have built a vast range of machines to exploit them. A monkey is a machine that preserves genes up trees, a fish is a machine that preserves genes in the water."[69] For Dawkins, it is DNA that matters most in the natural world. All of visible nature "is in aid of one thing and one thing only, the spread of DNA. This is not a metaphor, it is the plain truth. It couldn't be any plainer if it were raining floppy disks."[70] Dawkins offers a kind of mechanistic microcorpuscularian theory for biology, using genes as the fundamental explanation for all of life. The problem with understanding genes as the fundamental units of life is not only that this thinking overdetermines genes (simply saying genes replicate says nothing about what they select for) but also that it sets up (mortal) organisms as disposable tools of (immortal) DNA.

Dawkins and other ultra-Darwinists offer deterministic theories that not only are misleading and antievolutionary (because genes cannot be tied to behavior without the influence of the environment) but can become dangerous when they are used as a justification for certain human behaviors. Some scholars have suggested that after World War II it was no longer "politically tolerable" to claim that human behavior or intelligence was inherited,[71] but by the late 1980s scientists once again were boldly claiming that genetic inheritance played a large role in human behavior. Contemporary genetic science is thought to have unshackled itself from the inherent racist, classist, and anti-immigrant beliefs and policies of the eugenics movement. Prominent evolutionary biologists and geneticists, however, continue to claim that intelligence is heritable and tied to race, that the welfare state is "unnatural," that genetics account for male (over female) success in politics, business, and science, and that territoriality, tribalism, xenophobia, genocide, violence, and rape are part of the human genetic constitution.[72] In the 1980s, the British philosopher Mary Midgley referred to sociobiology as the "biology of Thatcherism" because it reads all of daily life through a Darwinian lens of competition, arriving at the conclusion that capitalism is itself a kind of biological imperative.[73]

Evelyn Fox Keller believes this newer resurgence of genetic determinism was a result of the optimism associated with molecular biology and its rapid rise within the life sciences.[74] A new optimism about the malleability of nature through molecular biology, combined with the promise of individual choice in medicine, allowed for a new public acceptance of genetic determinism, albeit a presumably "softer" determinism than evidenced previously. Much of sociobiology and evolutionary psychology, however, has been criticized by geneticists and biologists for its ontological naturalism. Evolutionary biologists have accused sociobiologists of combining "vulgar Mendelism, vulgar Darwinism, and vulgar reductionism in the service of the status quo."[75] Sociobiology was not well received by other scientific disciplines and eventually matured into the discipline of evolutionary psychology. Both disciplines, however, tend to argue that everything about the human person, including our relationships with one another, is merely a by-product of genes, which are of primary importance.

Of course, many scientists realize the fallacy of reducing human life to biology or genetic determinism, particularly since the completion of the HGP. The flood of data that came from mapping the genome created at least as many questions as answers regarding the causal mechanisms of genes and the potential for genetic therapies. As Linda and Edward McCabe recount, "Many of us in the genetics community sincerely believed that DNA analysis would provide us with a molecular crystal ball that would allow us to know quite accurately the clinical futures of our individual patients."[76] As it turned out, translating "the book of life" into meaningful explanatory causes was far more difficult than first imagined. Still, many scientists continue to speak publicly as if genes were an essential, or perhaps the most essential, determinant of human identity and can be used to determine the fate of an individual. Evelyn Fox Keller explains, "Most responsible advocates are of course careful to acknowledge the role of both nature and nurture, but rhetorically, as well as in scientific practice, it is 'nature' that emerges as the decisive victor."[77] Given the philosophical history that animates contemporary medico-scientific projects, it may be that genetic research is susceptible to a kind of unconscious deterministic thinking.

Epigenetics has been proposed as the antidote to the problem of genetic determinism. Against the claim that human fate can be determined through genes, epigenetics, the study of heritable changes in gene activity not caused by changes in DNA sequences, is promised to provide the "revolution" in our scientific and philosophical understanding of human identity, health, and disease that the genetics revolution has failed to produce.[78] Epigenetics challenges the nature/nurture distinction and genetic determinism by suggesting that human behaviors may affect gene expression and may be passed on to future generations. Steve Talbott explains that while the "genomic revolution" never came to fruition, the idea that "context matters" is creating a "revolutionary adventure" for scientists.[79] "It means reversing one of the most deeply engrained habits within science—the habit of explaining the whole as the result of its part."[80] Research into epigenetics promises to create a "new paradigm" in evolutionary science and health care. The imperative now is to fund epigenetic research. In 2008, the NIH gave $190 million to research mapping the epigenome, and the costs of finishing are projected to be far more than the costs of the HGP.[81]

Although epigenetics acknowledges that explaining human identity and fate is more complex than originally thought, a lingering ontological reductionism remains. Perhaps we cannot reduce human identity and health to genes, but scientists continue to explain all of human health and identity materially, as the result of environment on gene expression. The search for precise explanatory models grounded in the mechanistic understanding of being continues. The human being is still nominal, the sum of parts, and there is no part of the human being that lies beyond science's domain. Likewise, our technological imperative remains, and scientists are now investigating how they can harness the power of epigenetics for good.[82] Drug therapies, workout routines, diet plans, emotional therapies, and even pastoral care plans have been developed based on epigenetic findings.[83] In the end, the most profound change epigenetics may herald is the scrutiny we direct toward those who engage in "unhealthy" behaviors. Now we know bad behaviors can affect not only our own destiny but also that of our great-grandchildren.

HGP's Animating Metaphysics

In principle, outright genetic determinism is now largely shunned in the scientific community, and many have pushed back against the ontological naturalism exhibited by certain ultra-Darwinists. At the same time, it is difficult to rid the life sciences of reductionist thinking altogether. As Cunningham describes, methodological naturalism can easily become ontological naturalism when the limits of scientific inquiry are not recognized or when science is believed not to have a metaphysics. It is entirely appropriate for scientists to bracket metaphysical concerns when investigating genes, but it would be wrong to presume such metaphysical presumptions do not exist. The life sciences need a unifying metaphysics to justify their investigation of the natural world as well as the methods used to make truth claims about nature. As with previous generations of scientists, metaphysical assumptions often have moral implications. It would seem there continues to be a need for the life sciences to have a unifying narrative that can speak to a moral vision of the future. Genetic science cannot claim to be useful without some understanding of the question: "Useful for what?" Truth and goodness remain connected in any notion of social utility. Far from being a completely objective and value-neutral activity, genetic research contains certain assumptions about human nature because it is embedded within a theophilosophical tradition that understands nature, including human nature, and scientific progress in particular ways.

Although most practitioners of science recognize that the inherent limitations of the scientific method restrict what they are able to say about the existence of mysterious or divine forces, some influential thinkers have attempted to reclaim what was seemingly lost from ancient and medieval cosmological traditions. James Watson, for example, illustrates the link between modern metaphysics and genetics research in his book *DNA: The Secret of Life*. Watson claims that the double helix brought the Enlightenment's revolution in materialist thinking into the cell. The double helix, for Watson, definitively answers the question of what it is to be human. He writes, "Our discovery put an end to a debate as old as the human species: Does life have some magical, mystical essence, or is it, like any chemical reaction carried out in a science class, the product of normal physical and chemical processes? Is there something divine at the heart of a cell that brings it to life? The double helix answered that question with a definitive No."[84] As the title of his book implies, Watson sees within DNA the answer to one of the eternal questions that has plagued humankind for centuries: Who are we? DNA, "the human instruction book," contains the secrets of life and legitimates the disposal of divine providence. The scientific materialism animating the HGP thus affirms empirical science's nonteleological character; we do not need final causes to explain the phenomenon of human existence. Genetic mapping is thus ideal for helping to explain human nature in nonteleological forms, because it is the simplest and most fundamental material of our bodies. The discovery of our most basic material elements completes our quest for our human "essence." For Watson, the human being is left with no remainder; materiality is the whole story.

Is it even possible to describe human nature through materiality alone? It is certainly appropriate for scientists to bracket the inward dimensions of life when studying the external, but to claim that the material is all there is begs the question of what counts as "matter" and how it could possibly account for life, death, consciousness, existence, desire, free will, pain, and so on.[85] Moreover, materialism alone cannot account for the real differences between things—for that we need a metaphysics. Not only this, but the sciences themselves cannot come together if biologists or geneticists insist upon materialism as an ultimate category, since matter now only plays a minor role in explaining the physical world within physics. Naturalism itself needs a metaphysics to make sense of reality.

As I will show in subsequent chapters, the other problem with scientific materialism and naturalism is that they do not allow for mystery, excess, or meaning in human life. Even though scientists now admit that understanding human nature is more difficult than once presumed, there is still an implicit assumption that eventually all things can be known. Modern ways of "knowing" involve mastery and control. It is rarely enough to *know* something about the natural world, we must be able to *use* that knowledge. Useful knowledge has become a moral requirement in much of modern natural science. As briefly alluded to in chapter 2, utility has become an important part of how we investigate nature. Francis Bacon epitomized this epistemological shift when he famously stated, "Truth is power." For Bacon, truth was no longer the grasp of being itself but rather utility. Truth, in other words, had to prove itself through results. Having bracketed the study of final, teleological ends, Bacon and subsequent thinkers were left to work out the material cause of existence, which needed to be efficiently manipulated to achieve the ends of the human and, by analogy, the ends of God.

Unlike the rest of the natural order, human beings were granted a will that set them *against* nature. "Nature" was understood as outside human life, but with the potential to improve the conditions of human life if manipulated properly. Bacon understood these "improvements" to include "the prolongation of life, the restitution of youth in some degree, the retardation of age, the curing of disease counted incurable, and the mitigation of pain."[86] For Bacon and his fellow Calvinists, divine grace alone (not human effort) granted salvation, so Bacon believed human effort ought to be directed not toward moral perfection but toward service to one's neighbor. Service to one's neighbor required an instrumental approach to nature. According to Gerald McKenny, "In this spirit Bacon praised the mechanical arts and disparaged speculative science for doing nothing 'to relieve and benefit the condition of man.'"[87] From the belief that God gave nature for the preservation and enhancement of human life came a requirement that all scientific endeavors prioritize technological improvement of the human condition. Similarly, for Descartes, the most important reason for mastery over nature was the good of health, "to show that the decay of the body does not imply the destruction of the mind," and "to give mortals the hope of an after-life."[88] Humans now seek to master themselves through their own genetic codes so that we can fix those aspects of human life that we do not find acceptable, including disease and disability. This thinking has made it difficult for modern people to tolerate the ambiguity or seeming randomness of life. Instead, we seek to know, master, and control human life.

Building on the insights gained in the Scientific Revolution and the decentralizing of Christianity in intellectual culture, Enlightenment thinkers sought to manipulate nature to maximize choice and eradicate suffering. According to Gerald McKenny, the result is that modern medical enterprise elevates the place of health in a morally worthy life in such a way that the relief of suffering and the expansion of choice are primary. Nature has become "a neutral instrument that is brought into the realm of human ends by technology, and the body as object of spiritual and moral practices is replaced by the body as object of the practice of technological control."[89] From the modern scientific perspective, there is little need to constrain genetic research, since self-transcendence is already contained within the idea of what it means to be human. For medicine to be moral it must free human beings from their subjection to fate or necessity. Slowly but surely, health has become an end in itself rather than a condition or component of the virtuous life.[90] Any attempt to limit medical progress or what can be done to the body is now seen as backward or even cruel.

The HGP offers itself up as a thoroughly modern technological medicine, manipulating "natural" materials (genes) to maximize our freedom of choice (through preventative techniques) and limit our suffering—or at least what is presumed to be suffering when people have genetic abnormalities. Modern genetic medicine took up natural science's metaphysics—its ontological reductionism and technological imperative—to establish itself as a legitimate scientific endeavor. According to Jeffrey Bishop, "Medicine's metaphysical stance . . . is a metaphysics of material and efficient causation, concerned with the empirical realm of matter, effects, and the rational working out of their causes for the purposes of finding ways to control the material of bodies; that is to say, medicine's metaphysics of causation is one of material and efficient causation at the expense of final causes or purposes. Among Aristotle's four causes, early modern science—including medical science—historically repudiated or, at the very least, minimized formal and final causation and elevated material and efficient causation."[91] No longer able to rely upon a consensus about the purposes, or "whys," of the human being, medicine instead relegated itself to manipulating organisms to relieve human suffering. Today, there are few limits placed on medical technology because it is seen as the primary good, and access to the goods of medicine is understood as a matter of justice.

Whereas theological and philosophical understandings of the world once dominated Western thought, natural science now plays a significant part in how modern people understand the natural world, including the human body. Natural science has superseded theology as the "queen" of the sciences and has made itself central to the daily aspects of Western life. Whereas empirical science was once practiced and understood only by society's educated elite, it now permeates a much larger sector of the public life. Today, scientists have become our society's experts in matters of medicine, technology, social policy, economics, defense, and education. Science has established itself as necessary in nearly all aspects of our life, and, with some notable exceptions, our society supports, funds, and reveres science. Even those religious traditions that reject certain scientific theories such as Darwinian evolution use alternative scientific theories to establish their own beliefs about life's origins.

The Human Genome Project helped to amplify the seeming importance and usefulness of genetic science in American culture. Nobel laureate Walter Gilbert, who was an early proponent of the HGP, is apparently fond of introducing his public lectures on gene sequencing by pulling out a CD and saying, "Here is a human being; it's me!"[92] For Gilbert, "The information carried on the DNA, that genetic information passed down from our parents, is the *most fundamental property of the body*."[93] According to Gilbert, we now understand the internal mechanisms of the human body—the most fundamental part of our bodies—as never before. Just over two decades ago, Gilbert assumed that one result of mapping the human genome would be "a change in our philosophical understanding of ourselves."[94] Of course, Gilbert's materialist and reductionist thinking is not necessarily shared by all genetic scientists today. Still, it is hard to deny that many high-profile scientists have taken up questions once reserved for philosophy and theology. Once again, we are seeing a merger of the disciplines, but philosophers and theologians themselves are rarely called upon to enter into scientific discussions. The exclusion of such voices can be dangerous when scientists confuse what one can measure with ontological reality and omit any possibility for mystery, meaning, or excess. Rather than meaning, it would seem modern science offers a promised triumphalism. Combining ontological reductionism with a technological imperative, genetic research has become akin to a form of salvation in the hands of technical reason and the power of modern science because it espouses an eschatological hope of escaping finitude and living a perfected life within a perfected (and perfectly controlled) society.

Clearly, the American eugenics movement displayed just this sort of soteriological scientific triumphalism. Through their understanding that genes influence personal traits and behaviors, eugenicists offered a utilitarian vision of the world where the population could be controlled and enhanced through selective breeding. Eugenicists understood the world as inherently flawed but controllable. Bad genes (already a philosophically loaded concept) create inherently defective people who lack the ability to improve upon the human race and the natural world, which leads to bad societies. Eugenic science's triumphalist understanding was predicated on the causal belief that desirable genetic traits result in social harmony. Eugenics thus had a soteriological character, promising to create the perfect society through good reproductive practices. Theologians easily complemented this logic by equating the perfect eugenic society with God's Kingdom on earth. For some theologians, bad genes were seen as a result of a fallen state, which could be corrected through the work of well-meaning Christians. Christians could usher in the Kingdom of God by correcting their own failed communities. Thus communal "well-being" demanded hereditary control.

While no longer advocating eugenics, many Christians continue to struggle with the moral dimensions of genetic technologies because they have virtually abandoned the study of nature and metaphysics. As was the case in the 1920s, religious people who support the theories of evolutionary biology are also more likely to favor the programs of genetic science.[95] Over the past century, genetic science has provided substantial confirmation of Darwin's evolutionary theory. As will become evident in later chapters, the centralizing of science in both liberal and conservative theologies has led to a sidelining of the Bible's spiritual and moral teachings, particularly as they relate to our care of persons whose bodies radically fail to measure up to medicine's ideal genetic (wo)man. Whereas William Jennings Bryan was chiefly concerned with what Darwin's "brutish" theory would mean for the care of the "imbecile," the maimed, the sick, the poor, and the helpless, few theologians today (liberal or conservative) seem overly concerned with how our general understanding of "the human genome" might affect the poor and vulnerable.[96] That the government is not forcing sterilization does not make the range of services from "family balancing" to "preimplantation genetic diagnosis (PGD)" any less eugenic. Unlike classical eugenics, however, gene therapy today promises to relocate the site of control of our genes from governmental institutions to individual choice. Of course, as geneticist Richard Lewontin writes, "The ideology of biological determinism on which eugenics was based has persisted and . . . eugenics in the social sense has been revivified. This has been in part a consequence of the mere existence of the Genome Project, with its accompanying public relations and the heavy public expenditure it will require. These alone validate its determinist *Weltanschauung*. The publishers declare the glory of DNA and the media showeth forth its handiwork."[97] A new, softer eugenics might easily attract Protestants who refuse to be accountable for their tradition's past grievances. Contemporary geneticists rarely propose massive government control over society's genetic makeup, but genetic science still attempts to save humanity from the burdens of bad genes.

In the next chapter, I show how a robust doctrine of creation may correct some of the reductionism and instrumentalization of nature that can infect our understanding of genetics. Chapter 4 offers a theological rejoinder to the metaphysics discussed in this chapter. A Christian understanding of creation is not incompatible with a secular scientific investigation of the world, nor is it incompatible with the development and use of medical technologies that manipulate human DNA. By beginning with the assumption that God is the Creator and primary cause of a universe that is essentially good, however, Christians may find deeper cosmological significance to the existence of genetic anomalies. Chapter 4 explores an alternative metaphysical account of nature that is informed by the Christian understanding of creation and what difference this might make in understanding genetic disabilities.

CHAPTER FOUR

Natural Theology and Genetic Ontology

The ersatz theologies of some contemporary scientific popularizers, such as those described in the previous chapter, can be questioned from within the classic Christian tradition. To appreciate what is distinct about the Christian conception of the natural world, we must first understand God's creative activity. As a matter of faith, Christians believe that God is the cause of all things and that creation receives its meaning and orientation from God. "Creation," therefore, is a religious notion that orients the Christian understanding of nature. Of course, a Christian understanding of the metaphysics of creation will demand a faithful investigation of nature that cannot help but engage the natural and medico-sciences. After all, God grants the world its autonomy, making it possible to study the operations of nature apart from direct revelation. Theologians must not, however, confuse the truth of scientific discovery with the truth of revelation. To know the world scientifically, we must objectify it; to know God, we must be grasped by something we cannot contain.[1]

The natural and medical sciences may be a helpful *ancilla theologiae nova* in discerning how Christians should understand genetic disabilities, but they must be considered a supportive dialogue partner in theology's task and not its leader. In part because of the changing metaphysics of modern science, scientists in the twenty-first century no longer entertain questions about *why* birth defects or genetic disabilities happen, only *how* they happen. Theologians, however, still have something at stake in explaining God's participation in the natural order and the generation of new life. Christian theology teaches that God's creation is good, but genetic disorders complicate our vision of the "natural," the "good," and the "disordered."

Historically, Christians have prioritized the "healing of the sick" in their missionary and evangelical efforts, but not every instance of exceptional physical or mental variation has been considered diseased or disordered. Indeed, the nature of illness as well as what we consider to be a disability has changed considerably over time. Augustine, for example, believed monsters, including conjoined twins, were part of God's marvelous variety and played an essential part in representing a universe that was harmonious, well created, and mysterious.[2] Today, however, genetic abnormalities that negatively affect "normal human functioning," as described in evolutionary biology, are nearly always considered "problems" to be fixed or prevented. Thus people who have genetic or congenital "defects" are seen primarily as bodies to be cured or prevented. In response, many modern theologians have been concerned with problems in theodicy, or explaining why God lets "evil" natural occurrences happen, without first interrogating what they mean by natural evil.

A doctrine of creation is essential for understanding the Christian orientation toward genetic disability. The Christian claim that creation is good is at tension with the assertion that the Fall has rendered the world corrupt and deformed. Discerning whether certain genetic disabilities fall within the realm of the goodness of nature or natural evil will help shape how Christians approach conceptualizing and ameliorating genetic conditions. I begin by exploring the metaphysical foundations of the Christian account of the cosmos and how it has been influenced by modern science. Here I rely heavily upon the liberal theologian Paul Tillich, who, among twentieth-century Protestant theologians, has one of the clearest articulations of the relationship between metaphysics and theology, and on Thomas Aquinas, whose understanding of metaphysics continues to be influential in theology today, particularly within Roman Catholicism. Next, I interrogate the modern conception of nature and explore how the doctrine of creation supplements, and at times undermines, a mechanistic understanding of nature. Finally, I address the particular problem of natural evil and how this concept might be understood in light of human variation and abnormality. It is far from obvious that genetic disabilities are best understood as a kind of "natural evil" that must be overcome or prevented. Such thinking led to the eugenics movement and continues to inform many secular as well as religious projects today.

Metaphysics

Theology has ceded cosmology to the sciences for far too long. The principle of "nonoverlapping magisteria," made popular by Stephen Gould, has become fashionable in many theological circles,[3] but the quest to isolate science from religion completely is a difficult if not impossible task. Theological understandings have shifted as we have discovered new facts about the natural world and new methods for investigating the world. As described in the previous chapters, the theological beliefs of the scientists who brought about the Scientific Revolution influenced how they understood their task. Today, many natural scientists retain an overarching notion of how the natural world should be conceived of and related to. Many popular scientists wax poetic about the majesty of nature and the processes of evolution (a single episode of *Cosmos: A Spacetime Odyssey* uses dozens of competing metaphors to describe the formation of our universe), others view nature as hostile and distant,[4] while still others maintain that the natural world exalts human beings.[5] Even within the scientific community, researchers critique one another's dominant metaphors and underlying metaphysics. Mary Midgley, for example, critiques certain sociobiologists' understanding of genes, noting, "Metaphors did not bother them, so long as they were metaphors expressing the familiar clichés of Enlightenment individualism."[6] Most scientists cannot help but use metaphors to describe the natural world, but talk of "selfish genes" is more than a language game. The use of metaphors reveals as well as shapes the way modern people conceptualize the world and its value. Persons who value market capitalism and individualism are likely to find credence in the selfish gene theory because it highlights the importance of egoism and competition. Persons who believe in the Gaia theory, which suggests that life on earth is a harmonious self-maintaining system, on the other hand, have de-emphasized the importance of individual genes in the development of organisms.[7] Clearly, it is difficult to describe the natural world without importing some of our human values; therefore, maintaining strict boundaries between disciplines such as natural science, ethics, philosophy, and theology can be difficult. Since moral values and metaphysical commitments are always being imported into science, the question is *which* values and commitments are being implicitly supported.

The boundaries between science and theology remain amorphous, but both disciplines retain a metaphysics that acts as a bridge between them. Any metaphysical understanding of the world will affect what comes to be valued or devalued within the natural world. In other words, how we understand the organisms or processes within the natural world will necessarily influence what we appreciate in the world. Those who believe the world is merely a series of physical forces, measurable material, and evolving species may come to understand the cosmos as essentially pointless.[8] If, however, we understand the cosmos as a sacred realm, teeming with potency and participating in the divine, we may find divine meaning and purpose in even the lowest individual organism or most mundane physical process.

The separation between theology and the sciences has led many Christians, particularly Protestants, to neglect a rich theological account of the natural world. Without a metaphysical account of the natural world, Christians have allowed the natural sciences to explain the natural order and the medical sciences to define health and illness. The medical sciences rely upon the biological sciences to help determine "normal human functioning."[9] Evolutionary biology explains the nature, origins, and capacities of human beings and implicitly informs us what physical attributes, behaviors, or attitudes are unnatural or deficient expressions of the human species. Hence, the Christian mission to heal the sick will necessarily rely upon the natural and medical sciences to help Christians understand the nature of health and disease. This is not to suggest Christians should develop wholly alternative understandings of nature that ignore dominant scientific paradigms and consensuses; rather, Christians should interrogate the metaphysics of contemporary science and how the sciences have come to shape what they believe to be natural, naturally deficient, or naturally evil. To understand the proper role of genetic medicine in their lives, Christians must first understand how the sciences have shaped their view of nature and natural human functioning in such a way that certain natural variations are considered "diseases," "disorders," or "disabilities." If God interacts with the material world in any fundamental way, then accounting for God's relationship with creation will help Christians understand nature, including human nature, as well as what is good or evil within nature.

Any attempt to describe God's relationship to the world will necessarily use metaphysical language, because metaphysics is the field of inquiry that deals with the fundamental nature of being and the world that encompasses it. Whatever the sciences are able to say about the nature of human beings, they will never be able to fully describe the human because humans cannot be reduced to their materiality. Human beings will always exceed their psychological, biological, and neurophysiological attributes because they are connected to the primal cause of all things. Designed and destined for God, human beings have a telos that reaches beyond their material being. In Philip Clayton's words we are "always open toward a *telos* that science alone cannot predict. . . . That *telos* is also implicit in the beginning: the One toward whom we strive is also the One from whom we spring; and to understand the One who created us is to understand our final culmination."[10] In other words, to understand creation is to understand something of God as well as human destiny. Understanding God as the Creator and Redeemer is foundational for Christian doctrine. The God who saves is also the God who created all life. As I will detail in the next section, to account for God's activity in creation, we must begin to give a metaphysical account of the world that reflects the

Christian doctrine of the Trinitarian God who creates and meets the world in the Incarnation.

Most Protestants in the nineteenth and twentieth centuries rejected metaphysical and ontological language in favor of biblical and more personal descriptions of God, such as Father and Judge. God is not merely a powerfully personal God, however; God is also the ground of all being. Christians must affirm God as the unconditioned source of all existence if they wish to make God's promise of victory over death intelligible. God is not only our personal Father but also the one who infinitely transcends creation in power and glory. Some notable Protestant theologians have observed the problems inherent within the Protestant neglect of the natural world and metaphysics. The theologian Wolfhart Pannenberg, for example, describes how, since Ritschl, Christian theology has closed itself off from metaphysics in an attempt to purify itself from the metaphysical influences of the so-called Hellenization of Christianity, which contaminated the Christian doctrines of God, the world, and humanity.[11] Amid the liberal theological quest for the "historical Jesus," theologians such as Adolph von Harnack viewed the Hellenization of Christianity as an estrangement from the original, simple gospel of Jesus.[12] Pannenberg rebuts this thinking, noting: "Theological discourse about God requires a relationship to metaphysical reflection if its claim to truth is to be valid. For talk of God is dependent on a concept of the world, which can be established only through metaphysical reflection. . . . Unfortunately, theologians today rarely concede this dependence upon metaphysics. Nevertheless, the dependence is only too clear: a theological doctrine of God that lacks metaphysics as its discussion partner falls into either a kerygmatic subjectivism or a thoroughgoing demythologization—and frequently into both at the same time!"[13] For Pannenberg, metaphysics must be paired with a religious tradition to explicate an understanding of God. Without metaphysics, nothing meaningful can be said about the finite world (including human beings), much less the infinite God.

There is no easy separation between the metaphysician and the theologian. Religious questions concerning God as Creator, Sustainer, and Redeemer are the same questions about being and reality that metaphysics addresses. If Christians believe God creates and pre-serves all life, then this affirmation will necessarily color their meta-physical understanding of the world. At the same time, Christian theology must move past purely metaphysical questions and seek God as its primary goal. Paul Tillich acknowledges that both the metaphysician and the theologian are concerned with ultimate reality and being but that they do so from different perspectives. Philosophy deals with the structure of being itself, whereas theology deals with the meaning of being for humans. The philosopher must be detached from her object, and while she may have passion for the objective truth, the theologian accepts the truth as saving and personal. The philosopher looks for the universal *logos* in which everything has a common basis, but the theologian looks toward the particular Logos "who became flesh" and is manifest in particular historical events.[14] Knowledge of this Logos comes not through rationality but through "the church, its traditions and its present reality."[15] Finally, whereas the philosopher deals with categories of being in relation to their material structure, the theologian looks upon that same content and relates it to God. The philosopher discusses causality as it appears in physics, and time as primarily historical and biological, whereas the theologian discusses causality as it relates to a *prima causa* and time in relation to eternity.[16]

Not only can a metaphysical account of the world help Christians to reconceive creation's relation to God, it can also help ground Christian ethics. Although liberal theologians like Ritschl discarded meta-physics in favor of a more ethically oriented theology, formulating a coherent metaphysics can actually enhance rather than diminish a Christian social ethic. Within his systematic theology, Paul Tillich at-tempts to provide a liberal Protestant metaphysics that bears directly upon ethics. Much like Aquinas, Tillich regarded God as "being-itself," which he believed was a nonsymbolic statement.[17] Finite beings have a double relationship with God as the infinite power of being: humans participate in God's being, and at the same time God lies beyond all finite beings.[18] Tillich believed finite things could point to God, so he understood his metaphysical task as studying and tracing the movements of the Unconditional within culture. The task of the

theologian-metaphysician is to trace our "meaning-giving orientation" through both the theoretical and the practical spheres. By deal-
ing with both the theoretical and practical simultaneously, Tillich
refused to separate his metaphysics from his ethics. "Every proposition of a creative metaphysics is an expression of an ethos; every ethos
expresses a metaphysics."[19] Tillich's metaphysics is thus defined from
"both the ontological and the social-ethical side."[20] Ethics and metaphysics share a concern with the Unconditional, that which seems
beyond all conditions.[21] For Tillich, all things, including human and
nonhuman nature, are connected through the ground of all being
(God). Therefore, Tillich's social-ethical critique of culture was predicated on his understanding of the uniting feature of all of creation. In
other words, to know how we ought to interact with others and with
nature, we must first know how everything is essentially connected.

Tillich's metaphysical propositions may be enhanced in combina-
tion with the insights of Roman Catholic thought. Unlike many of
their Protestant counterparts, most Roman Catholic theologians believe metaphysical speculation is important for Christian theology,
particularly when they engage the sciences. As suggested in chapter 1,
Roman Catholics have made ready use of their moral theology to
critically engage the medical sciences. Although many Protestants
will not agree with the Catholic judgments on certain medical technologies or services, or the Catholic emphasis on natural law arguments (which I will describe in more detail in subsequent chapters),
they should take note of how the Catholic engagement with metaphysics, particularly in the Thomistic tradition, has led them to more
definitive moral conclusions on medical technologies when compared
to liberal Protestants. To understand where they converge with and
depart from Thomistic metaphysics, as well as how to move from
metaphysics to ethical evaluations of medical technologies, Protestants must first consider how Aquinas understood creation and divine
action. Unlike many early modern theologians, Aquinas was able to
keep nature and supernature as well as primary and secondarily causality separate, ensuring that God could not be collapsed into nature
or understood as in competition with nature. Aquinas's distinctions
remain helpful for modern Christians who wish to understand how
God is related to genetic disability.

PRIMARY AND SECONDARY CAUSALITY

Roman Catholic theologians, particularly those in the Thomistic tradition, approach the study of the natural world with a metaphysical apparatus in mind. Particularly useful for all Christian thought is Thomas Aquinas's emphasis on God's unique being and divine action. Aquinas drew heavily upon Aristotle's understanding of causation, modifying it when it contradicted the Christian message. In particular, Aquinas parted ways with Aristotle by distinguishing the Creator God as the Pure Act of existence. Aquinas differentiated God and the world through his understanding of God's unique existence, which is indistinguishable from God's essence. Aquinas writes, "God alone is Being by virtue of his own essence, since his essence is his existence; whereas every creature has being by participation, so that its essence is not its existence."[22] God's action cannot be distinct from God's being because God's being is one with God's existence. God's being is distinct from that of creatures, however, and since action follows from being, God's action is also different from that of creatures.

According to Aquinas, we cannot know God's essence, but we can know something of God through God's creation because God is the cause of the being of things (the effects of the cause). God's action in the creation and preservation of the world can be mapped onto Aristotle's four causes. God brings all of creation into existence and hence is its efficient cause. Because God created *ex nihilo*, God is also the material cause of creation, and because God created according to God's wisdom, God is also creation's formal cause. Finally, all of creation is oriented toward God as its end, and so God is also creation's final cause.[23] In other words, God makes the world, orders the world, and guides the world toward Godself. It can be said that God causes all actions in the created world, because God gives creation its being and thereby its power to act. Furthermore, God sustains all of creation in every moment and preserves creation's power to act.

Being the source and telos of all of creation does not mean, however, that nature does not have its own internal causes or that human beings do not have genuine freedom. God is the primary cause of all that happens (whether through necessity, change, contingency, or freedom) without depriving events of their contingent or indeterminate character.[24] To explain why God's actions are not in competition with nature, Aquinas distinguishes primary causality from secondary causality. God is the universal cause of all things and so is understood as their primary cause. Secondary causes, on the other hand, are the processes of change and becoming, which are particular by nature. Creation is not a mere (Neoplatonic) emanation from God; rather, creation is distinct from God, because God sets creation free. At the same time, secondary causes cannot be understood without recourse to the universal cause, because creatures have their being through participation.

In terms of the cause of effects in the natural world, God is the "principal cause" and secondary agents cooperate in producing effects through God's power as "instrumental causes."[25] Effects in the natural world thus have dual agency, because the powers of nature are insufficient to produce their own effects and require God as a primary cause.[26] Just as a person causes the knife to cut by applying pressure to the knife, so God moves things in nature to act according to their nature. According to Aquinas, both agents are said to produce the effect immediately: "Just as the lowest agent is found immediately active, so also is the power of the primary agent found immediate in the reduction of the effect."[27] This does not mean that effects are attributed partly to God and partly to the secondary agent; instead, both contribute wholly to the effect in different ways.[28]

Aquinas characterizes nature as participatory; creation exists contingently and, therefore, participates in God's being. Creatures are metaphysically participatory beings. Finite creatures depend upon some ground of existence other than themselves, something infinite as their cause.[29] Because we are created by God, however, and share in God's likeness, all creatures share a form of identity with the infinite.[30] All creatures participate in God, who gives the creature its being, but each does so in its own way, in freedom, according to its nature.[31] For this reason, we can say that God and nature are not in competition. God's universality does not exclude or repress the existence of something else. Nor can it be said that God cooperates with nature, because

God is not *a* being but the ground of being. God's creative causality is distinct from the causality of nature. Creatures are totally dependent upon God for their being while also being free. In our freedom, God's omnipotence is revealed. The goal of human life is to use one's freedom to surrender to God, who is our true fulfillment and telos. Ours is a dependent freedom. God wills our dependent freedom to be united with God's absolute freedom, but creatures are given the deliberative will to resist God's grace.[32]

Distinguishing between primary and secondary causation is one of the more difficult metaphysical tasks in Christian theology. Historically, when theologians have considered divine agency in the created world, they have attempted to avoid both conservationalism, which denies divine involvement in secondary causes, and occasionalism, which sees God as the sufficient cause of all secondary effects. In modernity, speaking about God's action in the world is made more difficult because we have lost the important distinction between primary and secondary causality. Theologian David Bentley Hart asserts that theologians of the sixteenth and seventeenth centuries (certainly the reformers but also some Catholics) are partly (if not mostly) to blame for the collapse between primary and secondary causality. The changing understanding of causality in the late sixteenth century, influenced by mechanical philosophy, undermined the idea of created freedom.[33] During this period, efficient causality, as I have tried to show in previous chapters, became the cause par excellence. Rather than affirming that God's creative activity was outside of the regular causality of the finite world, theologians grounded God's transcendence in efficient causes, albeit supreme efficient causality. The problem with this kind of thinking, as will soon become evident, is that it allows for God to be associated with evil, perhaps even the author of evil. If God predetermines all things, then creatures do not have true freedom and God becomes the author of evil insofar as God wills that evil to occur for the greater good.[34]

The problem in modernity is that we have forgotten that the comparison with our freedom and God's freedom, natural causality and divine causality, is only one of analogy. We do not have access to God's kind of creating, but many have mistakenly come to think of divine and secondary causality as equivalent, rather than of different kinds. The result is that in modernity theologians came to think of God as either determined or determining. As they favored determining, God became the God of absolute will and irresistible causal power within Voluntarism in the late Middle Ages. Modern science after Newton reduced the ancient and medieval understanding of causality to the efficient causality of physical force. Modern thinkers are thus tempted to understand God's action as a force alongside other natural forces. God's actions are seen as univocal because we have lost any notion of secondary causality. Hence, when God acts in the world, the modern mind tends to think God must disrupt nature and causality. Within this understanding of God's causality, God can intervene in nature as a lawbreaker, bind Godself to the initial act of creation, or refuse to intervene in the natural course of events implemented in creation. All of these solutions, however, assume that God's mode of causation is limited to efficient causality or identical to creaturely causality. A univocal God must either limit Godself or sneak around to avoid detection by the empirical sciences. Neither of these descriptions, however, sounds much like the classic Christian God.

The God of modernity is one of pure sovereignty so that all that happens in nature is subject to God's divine will. Aquinas, however, allowed for a distinction between what God wills according to God's nature and what God does not will but permits.[35] Unless we have a doctrine of divine permission, God's primary causality will be understood as the only determining cause in nature. God does not will evil in the world, even for the sake of redemption; rather, God wills good for creation, and it will come to pass despite creation's rebellion against God. This is what Christians mean by "providence."[36] The importance of divine permission will become evident in the discussion of natural evil below.

Aquinas's careful distinction between primary and secondary causality rebuffs the metaphysics of modern science and helps contemporary theologians understand how to characterize God's involvement in nature, including things that are seen as naturally defective or deficient. A genetic anomaly, under Aquinas's understanding of causality, therefore, can be caused both by a gene mutation and by a divine act. Rethinking God in this way can help Christians escape the dichotomy of thinking of genetic disabilities as either willed by God or caused by nature working against God. In the later discussion of theodicy, it will be clear that some theodicies that attempt to make sense of the sufferings caused by natural events focus on God's primary activity while neglecting secondary causation. If God is the ground of all being and the primary cause of all acts, then genetic and chromosomal disabilities can be at once caused by God and indeterminate. Yet, as I will show, this distinction does not yet tell us whether any genetic disability is willed by God or simply permitted. For this, we will need to understand how the anomaly contributes to or restricts human flourishing.

What Is Nature?

Along with a shift in the understanding of causality in modern science came a confusion over the terms *nature* and *natural*. Before the modern era, it was reasonable to believe that nature was the source of "compelling moral truths," but modern people tend to understand nature as passive and directionless. According to Hart, as nature came to be understood as the artifice of a transcendent God, natural theologians began to search for evidence of a craftsman God who could be known through his handiwork.[37] Sometimes lovely, sometimes terrifying, nature today is a sheer fact, unmoved by any transcendent will or intelligence. Within such a world God is understood as a "wise and powerful engineer."[38]

Whereas the distinction between nature and artifact was clear in Aristotle's metaphysics, without a clear and consistent metaphysics, defining nature has become increasingly difficult in modernity. Nature is a plastic concept because the modern era lacks a universally agreed-upon metaphysics that can explain what is intrinsically true about nature. Alister McGrath argues, "Without an ontological foundation, 'nature' is simply one person's construction and projection, and what is 'natural' a restatement of that person's own moral vision, which has been read into—and not out of—an ethically philosophical amorphous world."[39] Is nature "out there" with no regard for any individual life, or is nature a harmonious and delicate balance promoting life? Certainly, there is no longer a consensus that nature is sacred and worthy of respect. Without an explicit unifying metaphysics, nature simply becomes a material or ethical well of resources to draw upon without reference to its own integrity.

In modernity, distinguishing nature from human art and culture (as well as the nonhuman from the human) has been an important task for scientists, philosophers, and politicians alike. There is a common belief that science discovers things about the world, whereas philosophy, theology, and politics construct meaning and order within the world. We must, therefore, not confuse scientific truths with politics or faith lest we confuse "fact" for "belief." Moreover, the blameworthiness of certain actions can be delineated by whether they were caused by nature or by human interference. A death that is the result of a hurricane and a death that is the result of murder are both tragic, but the latter calls out for justice more readily because of its human cause. This tidy division, however, between nature and culture and the human and nonhuman is increasingly difficult to maintain. Debates over global warming, genetically modified crops, vaccines, artificial intelligence, gene editing, and chimera research reveal that the nature/culture and human/nonhuman divides are not as clear as some modern philosophers have proposed.

The rise of modern science and the rejection of Aristotelian metaphysics contributed to a new understanding of the nature/culture divide. For Aristotle, nature could be distinguished from artifice by its inner principle of motion and rest. Nature "has in itself a source of motion and of rest in respect of place or of increase and diminution or of alteration."[40] Animals are distinguished from plants because they have locomotion or kinesis, which allows the animal to move from one place to another, whereas plants have only the power of growth. Animals move toward that which they desire. An outside object or end stimulates that desire and the animal is internally driven to move.[41] Artifacts, on the other hand, do not have any innate impulse to change or move.

With the rise of mechanical philosophy came a new understanding of nature as well as new methods of studying nature. In particular, the Aristotelian concept of "final cause" was radically transformed, and by some accounts eliminated, during the early modern period. In medieval philosophy, the questions of *why* events happened (final cause) superseded the immediate *how* (material and efficient cause).[42] In the new mechanical philosophy, there remained a place for God's providential activity and the belief that God's existence was demonstrable from the design of nature (the argument from design), but the search for immanent final causes within nature (what Aristotle called the actualization of forms) was abandoned. The concept of nature itself thus changed significantly during this time because philosophers no longer explained natural objects primarily by their ends. Instead, the focus on material and efficient causation led many early modern philosophers to believe they could study matter and motion directly without the need to explain why objects moved or the perfection of their form. By empirically observing nature, philosophers could discover impartial, timeless facts about the natural world. Boyle, for example, believed he could discover nature's secrets through careful empirical examination. Even while creating what we would now call scientific laboratories to run experiments in, Boyle and his contemporaries were not *creating* nature, they were merely discovering what had always existed, albeit in an artificial space.

Society, on the other hand, was understood to be an artificial human construction, created to help humans escape from the state of nature. Even before Darwin's *On the Origin of Species*, many had come to believe nature was brutish, particularly with regard to individual animals. In Hobbes's *Leviathan*, the "state of nature" or the "war of all against all" must be overcome by government. Nature, which is seen as foreign to human beings, is remote and hostile to them. Without sovereign rule, nature would not allow for human flourishing. Whereas Aristotle believed humans were by nature political animals, early modern philosophers attempted to divide non-human nature from the human political/social realm.[43]

To study nature, however, early modern philosophers needed to construct it. In *We Have Never Been Modern*, Bruno Latour explains how the modern divide between nature and culture has never held up. Boyle's study of nature required that he artificially (re)construct natural laws in the laboratory. The air pump was designed to replicate natural conditions but was itself a fabrication. For Hobbes, on the other hand, the Leviathan was a manmade construction, but it also transcended the individual humans who created it.[44] Both Boyle's laboratory and Hobbes's society were hybrids, rather than pure nature or culture. Boyle and the Royal Society attempted to speak of nature apart from human influence by way of the experimental method. Hobbes, on the other hand, thought that he could describe the social and political spheres independent of the material, nonhuman world. Boyle and Hobbes thus worked together to purify the concepts of nature and society (nonhuman and human). The modern constitution keeps us thinking that science and medicine should be free of politics and religion (though they are certainly influenced by these spheres in American politics). To describe science as merely producing facts about the natural world obscures both the triumphs of science and the lives of scientists. We construct nature, and our politics is constructed in science and technology.[45] There is no pure nature apart from human beings, nor is there pure society apart from the natural world. Science is sponsored by governments and increasingly private industry and raises ethical and religious questions about who we are and what we should and should not create. This does not mean that science is pure ideology; certainly there is objectivity in science. But to ignore the social dimensions of science risks bolstering conspiracy theories about science's alliance with political agendas or profit motives (as is often claimed among "antivaxxers").

Advances in genetic engineering in the twenty-first century have created a new set of hybrids to consider. The lines between nature and culture are continually blurred as scientists further manipulate what were once considered "essential" natural properties such as genes. Cautions against scientists "playing God," which were popular during the rise of bioethics in the 1960s and '70s, were an attempt to draw lines between what humans should and should not change in nature. While less common today, the charge of "playing God" sometimes resurfaces in debates around synthetic biology. The "playing God" debates, however, have mostly fallen away in science and bioethics, in favor of questions concerning how to distribute the goods of science and medicine justly. Bacon's charge that natural philosophers drop (immanent) final causes from their metaphysics and instead use their scientific knowledge to alleviate the ills of the human condition has come to fruition in the medico-sciences. Today, "discovering" nature is only the first step toward changing nature, particularly when parts of nature are seen as "defective" and the cause of suffering. Thomists can object to certain medical practices as abrogating nature only because they have a natural theology that includes a teleology. Some actions, according to Thomistic natural law, violate the natural ends of human beings and are thus illicit, which is why many Roman Catholics rejected eugenic sterilization. Without a robust concept of final causes, however, there is little room to argue that certain actions "violate" nature.

Disability scholars have brought to light the hybrid nature of "disability" as well. *Disability* itself is a difficult term to define, in part because there is considerable controversy over how to conceptualize disability as a category. As I will explain further in chapter 7, the medical model of disability presumes disability to be an objective natural category, where disability is an obvious problem with the individual body that results in a "negative departure from normal functioning."[46] The social model of disability, on the other hand, sees disability primarily or exclusively as a social construction, made possible by the architecture, attitudes, and social norms of modern societies. Although certain natural or physical characteristics might fall under the category of disability, what unifies the concept of disability rests on social features and not natural characteristics. Many contemporary disability scholars acknowledge, however, that disability is neither a wholly natural nor wholly social category but rather a construction of both, a hybrid.

Nature through the Doctrine of Creation

Christians often speak of the natural world as "creation," rather than "nature." Creation is a religious concept that is bound up with the notion of a Creator God. For Aquinas, *creation* is a word of faith that connects the material world with its invisible meaning and orientation in God.[47] *Creation* ought to frame Christian theologico-metaphysics. Of course, Christians do not simply give an alternative philosophical account of metaphysics called "Christian metaphysics." Neither scripture nor the creedal tradition will supply Christians with a singular metaphysical account of the world, which is why theologians such as Aquinas needed to draw upon the metaphysics of philosophers and modify them when they contradicted the gospel message. A Christian conception of nature will have metaphysical implications, but it will primarily be a reflection of the doctrine of God, which relies upon biblical revelation and the history of the Christian tradition. By first understanding something about God, Christians can begin to make sense of God's creation and God's relationship with creation. God's Trinitarian nature as revealed in the Incarnation, therefore, will inform how Christians understand "nature" as God's creation.

God's revelation in Christ creates the necessary bridge for Christians to begin speaking of God's nature as revealed in creation. Christians know God and God's intentions for the world through Christ, who is God incarnate. Thus the Christian understanding of creation will need to involve God's unique relationship to the world through Christ. The Incarnation reveals God to humanity, and Christ's role in creation reveals God's relationship with humanity. Christology, therefore, reveals the full meaning and destiny of nature. Perhaps the clearest biblical passage about Christ's role in creation comes from the Gospel of John: "In the beginning was the Word, and the Word was with God, and the Word was God. He was in the beginning with God. All things came into being through him, and without him not one thing came into being. What has come into being in him was life, and the life was the light of all people. The light shines in the darkness, and the darkness did not overcome it" (John 1:1–5 NRSV). We learn from John's first verses that God is the sole Creator and that God does not create alone, but with the Word who *is* God and is *with* God. John's Prologue suggests that through the Incarnation God reveals God's eternal union with the world. In opposition to ancient Greek philosophy, the Incarnation reveals a new kind of intimacy between God and the world. God is neither purely other than the world (as in Deism) nor the same as the world (as in pantheism); God is simultaneously other and "not-other."[48] In Christ, it is disclosed that God can be so immanent that God assumes human nature without losing God's divinity.

If God created *all things* through Christ, then there is reason to believe God created the world from nothing. Although a number of contemporary theologians claim that the doctrine of *creatio ex nihilo* "imposes a dubious metaphysics upon biblical theologies of creation," such criticisms often misrepresent God's relationship to the world as one of brute force and power.[49] Early Christians debated whether God created from nothing or from the preexisting chaos, and today many contend that "creation from nothing" is not a clear biblical teaching. By the fourth century, however, *creatio ex nihilo* became the dominant teaching among Christian theologians. The Fourth Lateran Council (1215) formally declared, "We firmly believe and simply confess that there is only one true God . . . the Creator of all things visible and invisible, spiritual and corporeal; who from the very beginning of time by His omnipotent power created out of nothing [*de nihilo condidit*] both the spiritual being and the corporeal."[50] The ancient Greeks had generally affirmed that nothing comes from nothing, so the Christian belief that God created from nothing was a radical departure from Platonist metaphysics. For early Christian writers such as Theophilus and Irenaeus, creation from nothing establishes God's transcendence from the world and God's immanent engagement with the world. God's intimacy, as expressed in Christ, allows *creatio ex nihilo* to function both Christologically and soteriologically. Only a God who exists outside the world can save the world, but only a God who loves and communes with the world would desire to do so. Theophilus and Irenaeus agree that God made the world so that God might be known by human beings; therefore, God must be present within the created order so God can be known.

We cannot know God in God's essence, but we can know something about God through God's creation and through scripture. According to Ian McFarland, there are three things we can positively and substantially know about God, which are essential for laying out a Christian theology of creation: (1) God is living, (2) God is productive, and (3) God is present.[51] To say that God is *living* is to assert that God is dynamic and not static. God is One in three Persons, so God is inherently relational. In the Trinity, God's nature is simultaneously possessed and given away. The Father donates his being without remainder to the Son, and the Son is himself through the act of self-donation from the Father, which he offers back to the Father.[52] The Spirit, in turn, functions as the "we" of the Father and Son.[53] For the sake of God's creation, the Father sends the Son, the Son reveals the Father (John 1:18) and glorifies the Father (John 13:31–32; 14:13, 17:1), and the Father in turn glorifies the Son (John 8:54; Acts 3:13). The Spirit bears witness to the Son and glorifies the Son and witnesses to the Father's faithfulness (Heb. 10:15–17). God's relationship to Godself affirms that God is plural and irreducibly diverse, so God's love is not envious or threatened by otherness.[54] God did not create in isolation, but in relationship already marked by diversity and otherness.

Through the biblical language of God's "begetting" the Son (Acts 13:33; Heb. 1:4; 5:5) and of the Spirit "proceeding" from the Father (John 14:26), we can also gather that God is *productive*. God's productivity is not the same as God's creation. God does not create God in Trinity; rather, God's productivity is the basis for the affirmation of God's freedom within Godself. In the Godhead, persons must let the other be in infinite freedom and self-donation; therefore, the Trinity is characterized by freedom and relationship. In the Trinity, God has space for the Other without collapsing all persons of the Trinity. God's allowance of Otherness within Godself creates the conditions by which the world can exist in its own right, while at the same time being preserved by God. Creation's being participates in the divine life without being reduced to God. Just as the members of the Trinity are irreducible to one another—transcending each other even while indwelling one another (perichoresis)—our union with God comes not in spite of our difference from God but in and through it.[55] Our relatedness to God through the act of being relates us and binds us to the cosmos.

Finally, God is *present* in Godself as the Trinity. In other words, God's hypostases are not opposed to one another but mutually present to one another in relationship. Jesus is the Word of God, a complete expression of the Father's being, and communicates the

Father's being (Col.1:27; 2:2; 4:3). The Spirit then prevents the Father and Son from collapsing into one another by recognizing a "second difference within the Godhead, which secures the integrity of the first since the Spirit's role is precisely that of confessing the Son as the Father's only-begotten (John 15:26)."[56] The Spirit affirms the Word's oneness with the Father and difference from the Father by bearing witness to the Son's distinctiveness (John 4:2–3).[57] God's presence with creation is thus already characteristic of Godself. God's presence to Godself is self-giving and loving; therefore, God's omnipresence in creation is not an occasion for terror but is reflective of God's own goodness, and therefore, God's omnipresence is good news for creation.[58] God's openness to creation is a reflection of God's openness to Godself, so God can be with creation without obliterating creation. Just as God is one (*ousia*) yet irreducible in God's persons (*hypostasis*), so creation can exist as other than God without being fully separated from God.

The *Who* of creation explains its fundamental character in relation to its Creator. It is fitting for the God who is living, productive, and present to create. Creation does not add anything to God, but the act of creation is consistent with the character of God described above. God did not create the world out of necessity, because God's infinite freedom and superabundant fullness did not have any lack that needed to be filled by creation. Because God did not create out of any need but from God's excess, creation must be understood as a gift that is not deserved. Augustine asserts that God created freely — "He did not create under stress of any compulsion" — but that, at the same time, God did not create arbitrarily. God's actions must be actions of volition and not spontaneous spasms.[59] God's goodness, therefore, does not merely spill over into creation by accident of God's superabundance; rather, God's generosity in creation is *bonum diffusivum sui*, God loves the world not because it is good but because God is good, and God's goodness is diffusive, it spreads and is communicated throughout creation.

Understanding God as Creator in relation to the creation, as opposed to a general and contested understanding of "nature," can begin to help Christians parse out what is to be valued and devalued within the natural world. Whereas evolutionary fitness is the subtle telos of evolutionary biological thinking, the telos of creation is eternal life with God in Christ. What constitutes a "fit" life in biological terms, or "quality of life" in medicine, therefore, may differ from the Christian understanding of the "good life." Christians should be cautious, therefore, when conflating scientific interpretations of the meaning of the body with theological ones.

Nature Good and Evil

Of course, the Christian affirmation that the world is "good" as proclaimed in the Genesis narrative is in tension with the suffering experienced by postlapsarian creatures. For all that was gained in the proposition of *creatio ex nihilo*, the problem of evil remains. If God created out of primordial chaos, as some early Christian theologians and modern process theologians claim, then evil can be both real and outside God. If God is the universal cause of being and all things fall within God's providence, however, then the existence of evil is more difficult to explain. Creaturely experiences of evil and suffering suggest that, while creation is good, it is not yet perfected. Evil intrudes upon the goodness of the world. God can and will conquer evil, but evil stands against God's purposes for the world in the here and now. But what exactly is evil? And how can we know that some human conditions are a product of evil (by divine permission) and not of God's goodness (divine will)? Science has generally removed the problem of evil by removing divine influence from the natural sciences, but if Christians believe that God continues to create and care for creation then they must account for God's allowance of suffering and evil within the world.

Natural Diversity in God's Creation

First, it is important for Christians to keep in mind that variation and diversity within the world are not evil but divinely intended. God's own multiplicity helps to make sense of the diversity of creation. Not only did God create a plurality of creatures, God also created a rich diversity of creatures to reflect God. Aquinas writes, "[God] brought into existence so that his goodness might be communicated to creatures and reenacted through them. And because it was not possible for his goodness to be represented through any single creature, he produced many different ones, so that what was wanting in one expression of the divine goodness might be supplied by another; for goodness, which in God is single and united, in creatures is multiple and divided. Hence the whole universe shares and represents his goodness less incompletely than any one creature by itself."[60] Finite creatures can represent the goodness of God only partially. God made a diverse set of creatures to represent God's own rich diversity. Creatures reflect God's multiple perfections by way of their own multiplicity.[61] Although some Christians worried that Darwin's theory of evolution undermined the Christian belief that God created all creatures in the beginning of time, the creation of new beings does not contradict God's action in creation for two reasons. First, God did not create all things at one point in time. The Genesis story is not a natural history. Second, novelty is not opposed to God. Creation shows that God creates things that are other than God. Augustine taught that novelty in the course of natural history was a product of "seeds in a sense of future realities, destined to germinate in suitable places from hidden obscurity into the manifest light of day through the course of the ages."[62] Creation is not limited to the reproduction of existing forms; it can also give rise to new kinds of beings.[63] Novelty and diversity are parts of God's good creation, a manifestation of God's goodness when viewed as a harmonious whole.

Individual human diversity can also be understood as good on its own terms. Whereas from an evolutionary perspective, individual members of a species merely represent one example of a type, the Christian tradition demands that we see each life as deeply related to God and so more than its antecedences and more than itself.[64] Each life is novel and cannot be replicated or replaced. Creaturely uniqueness cannot be captured in the reconfiguration of genes given to us by our parents. All creatures, therefore, are ontologically original, and all life carries within itself a deep interior metaphysical relation to its origin. Augustine writes,

> I have counted and found that Scripture tells us seven times that you saw that what you had made was good, and when you looked for the eighth time and saw the whole of your creation, we are told that you found it not only good but very good, for you saw all at once as one whole. Each separate work was good, but when they were all seen as one, they were not merely good: they were very good. The same can be said of every material thing which has beauty. For a thing which consists of several parts, each beautiful in itself, is far more beautiful than the individual parts which, properly combined and arranged, compose the whole, even though each part, taken separately, is itself a thing of beauty.[65]

It is clear from Augustine that the diversity of creation is good when seen as a harmonious whole, but also each individual creature is good and beautiful in itself.

The goodness of creation as individual and as a whole makes the scientific taxonomies somewhat arbitrary. When Jesus, as a Jewish man, declares all foods clean (Mark 7:19; Acts 10:15), he signals that no classificatory scheme, even the ones initiated through God's people, can be considered absolute.[66] Clearly, the classification of organisms is important in different fields for effective research, but Christians should be cautious when categorizing humans into distinct types, because such classifications often have implicit values buried within. Historically, Christians have established or supported classificatory schemes that place some races above others, one sex above the other, and some physical and mental abilities above others.[67] Christians seem to forget that all beings are part of God's good creation, that God's special relationship with humanity does not come at the expense of other living things, and that all "types" of people are equal in the eyes of God. God created everything, including monsters (Job 10:15; Ps. 104:26).

Although it would be callous to assume that all genetic disabilities are divinely intentioned and therefore not to be interfered with, modern scientists and theologians alike have a history of inappropriately attributing human differences to evil and tying scientific intervention to redemption. In the nineteenth century, for example, Scottish geologist and evangelical Hugh Miller attributed racial difference to the Fall, writing, "The further we remove in any direction from the Adamic center, the more animalized and sunk do we find the various tribes or races."[68] Aesthetically repulsed by other ethnic groups, such as the Hottentots (Khoi) of Southwest Africa and the "flat-headed" Fuegians, Miller declared that the world could be improved by man so as to be "more pleasing both to his sense of the aesthetic and to his more material senses also."[69] Most contemporary geneticists have disentangled racism from the study of evolution and human genetics,[70] but past attitudes toward human diversity should caution those who too easily equate genetic difference with a defect to be cured. As I discuss in later chapters, medicine's general orientation toward the "victims" of genetic disability has at times put it at odds with members of the disability community who wish to celebrate rather than obliterate disability.

Evil and Theodicy

The blanket assertion that all of creation is good and all diversity part of God's providential plan is not likely to satisfy the parent who grieves over a suffering child. On the contrary, Christians today generally view physical suffering caused by disease or genetic mutations to be evil and, therefore, opposed to God's plan for creation. When confronting genetic disability, especially those disabilities that cause physical suffering, Christians are forced to ask how God's good creation can produce so much pain and suffering in the world.

The general framing of God's relationship to disability and suffering may influence the patient's and medical practitioner's basic orientation toward genetic disability. If genetic disability is framed as good and divinely preordained, then there may be little incentive to "cure" genetic disability. On the other hand, if those with genetic disabilities are posited as "victims" of "evil," then curing genetic disabilities may be a Christian duty. For example, in responding to the question of whether nature is ever evil, Leo Ten Kate contends,

For me, as a clinical geneticist, the victims of nature are the infants who are born severely malformed or seemingly healthy but with a genetic constitution that manifests itself in death, disease, and handicap within weeks, months, years. The victims are these children, but also their parents, who could not know that they were at risk, and the other family members who now fear that they will be at risk too. Ask them whether nature is ever evil. They will tell you. It is not the point of view of the philosopher, the scientist, the historian, or the conservationist that is relevant.[71]

Ten Kate's is a common view among clinical geneticists who see their patients (and apparently all of their patient's relations) primarily as *victims* of evolution and genetics. The response to genetic disability, therefore, is to cure at nearly any cost. The mitigation of disability is an irresistible goal in biomedicine when genetic disabilities are viewed as evil. It is not self-evident, however, that most parents who have children with genetic disabilities consider their child's condition evil, or that theirs would be the only perspective on evil that should matter. We ought to be extremely cautious with labeling certain conditions as inherently "good" or "evil," even if we are speaking metaphysically. Good and evil come with inherent value judgments that may color the way we know and attend to other human beings. The rush to call genetic disabilities "evil" and the backlash this has received from members of the disability community demand that we carefully attend to what exactly we mean by evil and how we ought to go about solving the "problem" of evil.

Discussions concerning evil in theology often fall under the category of theodicy. Theodicy is the theological effort to explain God's indefatigable goodness alongside the reality of evil in the world. If God creates from nothing and, as described above, is causally connected to all actions in the world, how can any deviation from God's will be possible? Somehow Christians must be able to say that God is omnipotent (creating the world from nothing), God is good, and evil is real (it is not an illusion).[72] Classically, evil has been divided into at least two types: moral evil and natural evil. Moral evil is caused by the human will misapplied (also known as sin), whereas natural evil is generally understood as brought about through "natural" processes, such as diseases or earthquakes. In both instances, God is thought to permit evil. Such divine permission allows Christians to say that God does not commit evil, while also maintaining that God can redeem all things.

One way that Christians have attempted to hold together God's omnipotence, goodness, and evil is by explaining why some events or occurrences that appear evil are actually good. There are at least three popular theodicies of natural evil that attempt to make sense of illness or disability as an experience of evil. Broadly speaking, theologians primarily talk about natural evil as (1) serving a larger purpose, (2) soul-making, and (3) necessary for the goods of freedom. First, there are those who believe that illness and disability are necessary for God's will to be carried out in the world. Skeptical theists generally believe humans lack the cognitive resources to discern God's will for creation, so while particular natural events appear evil, we cannot know the larger purpose for these events. Likewise, apophatic theologians remind us that the inner workings of God are unknowable and mysterious. God does not answer our questions about suffering and evil but confronts us in mystery, as is clear in the story of Job. Theologians who engage the biological sciences are likely to see that some events that may appear to be harmful or even catastrophic to humans can actually help the earth become more productive.[73] Although it may be hard to discern the good in genetic disease, particularly when it causes suffering, Christians are called to trust that God has a plan for all things.

Alternatively, some theologians contend that God permits natural evil because it helps humans cultivate virtue. The highest forms of moral goodness are not born from comfort but forged through difficulty. "We boast in our sufferings, knowing that suffering produces endurance, and endurance produces character, and character produces hope, and hope does not disappoint us, because God's love has been poured into our hearts through the Holy Spirit that has been given to us" (Rom. 5:3–5 NRSV). Human beings are *becoming* who they are meant to be, and suffering may help them become stronger and more empathetic. Suffering, even suffering born of illness, can provide opportunities to cultivate or exercise virtues such as courage, wisdom, or humility.[74] Christians can gain greater trust and hope in God through their illness and by allowing others to take care of them, which might also create opportunities for others to cultivate their own virtues.

Finally, other theologians argue that natural evil is necessary for the goods of freedom and inherently tied to God's orderliness as displayed in natural laws.[75] Natural laws create the conditions for natural evil to occur; living cells under certain conditions can grow into malignant cancers, and pressure systems can bring forth tornadoes and hurricanes.[76] Without the laws of nature, the world would be supremely chaotic and impossible to understand scientifically. Moreover, if natural laws did not exist and the causality of one's actions could not be reasonably predicted, then morality itself would be difficult to discern, because the consequences of actions are generally discerned from experience.[77] Embodiedness, diversity, and finitude are all goods of creation, but they imply the risk of harm and suffering. The laws of nature allow for both beauty and horror within the created order. To be human is to be finite and vulnerable and subject to all manner of illness and bodily infirmity. This precariousness is not necessarily wholly bad. Tillich writes, "Evil in the divine order is not only a mystery; it is also a revelation. . . . He who can become sick is greater than he who cannot."[78] We can receive God's grace when we are most vulnerable. God permits natural evil because it is the only way to preserve creaturely freedom and to show God's power.

It is not difficult to see how these theodicies fall short. The answer to the death of a small child caused by Tay-Sachs disease cannot simply be that God had a larger purpose in mind, that God's will is a mystery, or that this is the cost of creaturely freedom. The goods that can come from illness or disability do not necessarily justify the suffering they have caused or excuse God from directing them to happen. Deferring justice or goodness to the afterlife also risks trivializing the suffering that can accompany embodied hardship.[79] A rush to theodicy might relieve God from the responsibility of creating evil, but it can also silence the laments of those who suffer. Although we should not assume that every particular genetic variation (a genetic disease, disorder, or otherwise) is cause for suffering and lament, we ought not to prevent anyone from crying out to God when they are in despair. Moreover, it would be wrong to assume that God demands the suffering and death of small children in order to carry out God's purpose in history. To suggest as much would be to ignore the important distinction between God's permission and will and between secondary and primary causation. If we view all natural events as divinely willed, then we have a determinist God and not a providential one. Again, it is important to remember that there is a difference between what God permits and what God intends in creation. God's permission of evil does not make it any less terrible for creation. Christians are scripturally permitted to hate suffering and evil, while at the same time believing that God will rescue us from the absurdity of sin and the sting of death.

To respond to suffering with mystery also fails to provide guidance on how Christians ought to respond to disease and disability. If, for example, Tay-Sachs is part of God's mysterious plan, and one assumes God's plan is always for the ultimate good, then it would be wrong to try to prevent or cure Tay-Sachs. Likewise, "soul-making" suffering can make people more virtuous, but this realization is pastorally insensitive if taken prescriptively. Disease can call forth a virtuous response, but few patients or their family members would likely be comforted by a minister who demanded they become more virtuous as a response to their suffering. Writer Ellen Painter Dollar, who lives with *osteogenesis imperfecta*, notes,

> I believe [illness, disability, and disease] are bad things and that we are allowed to name them as bad things. This does *not* mean, however, that we have license to try to fix what is wrong at all costs or that we can't learn valuable lessons, find meaning, and come to know God and ourselves better as a result of suffering. There is a huge difference between saying that my bone disorder was *intended* to reveal God's truth or teach me something I need to know and saying that by bone disorder *ended up* revealing God's truth or teaching me something I need to know.[80]

Dollar's division between divine intention and redemption recalls Hart's caution against confusing divine will and permission. God can redeem all things, create hope where there is hopelessness, and provide grace in the midst of suffering, but that does not mean that the suffering was divinely intended. Again, if all natural suffering was meant to create more virtuous people, then pain medication would need to be severely limited if not rejected. Similarly, all attempts to justify evil on the basis of freedom cannot adequately account for suffering that results in the loss of freedom. It may be that the orderliness of creation implies the risk of natural evil, but this response would be of little comfort to the parents whose child suffers from a disease of which little is known and that little can be done to cure. Within this scheme, disease demands a medical response that enhances the freedom of individuals in order to justify the presence of natural evil in the world. The demand that we cure all disease and disability to eradicate evil risks becoming a Pelagian quest for perfection, which denies the need for God's grace.

At the same time, all these accounts of evil contain some truth in that they reveal that not all suffering is inherently meaningless or irremediable. The Christian tradition does not demand that we believe God actively wills all tragedies, but it does provide hope that in the end all will be well. After becoming so ill that all those around her believed she was dying, Julian of Norwich was able to declare:

> Deeds are done which appear so evil to us and people suffer such terrible evils that it does not seem as though any good will ever come of them; and we consider this, sorrowing and grieving over it so that we cannot find peace in the blessed contemplation of God as we should do; and this is why: our reasoning powers are so blind now, so humble and so simple, that we cannot know the high, marvelous wisdom, the might and the goodness of the Holy Trinity. And this is what he means where he says, "You shall see for yourself that all manner of things shall be well," as if he said, "Pay attention to this now, faithfully and confidently, and at the end of time you will truly see it in the fullness of joy."[81]

Julian's message is not that the life promised in God will make up for lives irreversibly damaged or tragically lost. Grief and lamentation are proper reactions to loss and are encouraged by scripture.[82] But loss and death are never the final word in the Christian story.

Likewise, some of the most profound Christian texts of love and beauty are born out of suffering. Pain and suffering can only be considered a kind of evil in the medical context, but as disability theologian Sharon Betcher argues, our culture is experiencing "massive levels of chronic pain," and we no longer have the religious resources to tap into that pain to use it as a force for personal or cultural change.[83] Betcher believes our culture's fear of pain has prevented many from becoming alive in the world. Those able to embrace the contingencies of life, even the painful experiences, are better equipped to use this pain as a motivational force for personal and social change.

Defining Evil

The attempt to explain why evil happens or why God permits evil is considered by many to be a modern project, which is inadequate for those who are currently suffering.[84] We may remediate the inadequacies of modern theodicy by looking to older Christian traditions of lament and communal care. Before modernity, few theologians or philosophers, particularly in the Greek, Christian, and Jewish traditions, attempted to justify evil in terms of God's providential design. In fact, some have suggested it was important for early Christians not to explain why evil is needed in the world because this would undermine communal efforts to share and relieve suffering together.[85] For the early church, the "solution" to the problem of evil was Christ's return. It was not until the seventeenth century that new intellectual difficulties arose around the "problem" of evil. According to Kenneth Surin, "It is certainly no exaggeration to say that virtually every contemporary discussion of the theodicy-question is premised, implicitly or explicitly, on an understanding of 'God' overwhelmingly constrained by the principles of *seventeenth and eighteenth century philosophical theism*."[86] In other words, theodicy often focuses on the abstract, ahistorical, idea of God, rather than the personal, active God of Christianity.

With the rise of modern science and technology also came new ways of thinking about suffering, illness, and disability. The imperative that science relieve the human condition likely altered how modern people see the "problem" of suffering—these are no longer normal, taken-for-granted experiences to be endured and shared but problems to be solved. As medicine increases its ability to prevent and correct certain conditions, suffering and anomaly of any kind begin to become intolerable. Perhaps for the first time in history, suffering and evil require technological solutions. Determining how best to respond to a genetic disability, however, requires first considering what we mean by "evil." By unreflectively labeling certain conditions "evil," we risk prescribing a solution to the problem too quickly and ignoring the testimony of persons living with genetic disabilities. There may be good reason to disentangle illness, disability, and suffering from our conception of evil.

Early and medieval theologians were more concerned with explaining what sort of thing (or non-thing) evil is than in solving the problem of evil. If God created the world *ex nihilo*, then creation must be good (because God is good) and, therefore, evil cannot be understood as having its own existence, because God did not create evil. Adhering to the Neoplatonic tradition, Augustine posited that evil does not exist, but rather is a privation of the good.[87] Evil has no ontological status and, therefore, cannot be understood as rivaling God or posing a limit to God's agency.[88] "For evil has no positive nature," Augustine writes, "but the loss of good has received the name 'evil.'"[89] Aquinas holds a similar view, believing that "evil is the absence of good, which is natural and due a thing."[90] For Aquinas, evil is explained by a deficient action of an agent or the unintended effect of a good act.[91] In terms of natural evil, this can mean that evil can occur as result of a defective agent, as when a deficient organ does not produce the good of health, or when a natural process becomes too powerful, such as the winds of a hurricane.

Of course, all of creation is in some sense less good than God, who is infinite goodness, and less good than God intends creation to be at the fulfillment of time, but this does not imply that creation in the here and now is evil. Rather, God has a particular good in mind for each type of creature. "Evil as such is the privation of a particular good," Aquinas writes, "a privation that is associated with a particular good."[92] In the Genesis narrative, it is clear that God found all creatures good, although there were different kinds of creatures. Different types of creatures must, therefore, have different types of goodness. Anything that prevents a creature from fulfilling its particular kind of created goodness, then, is evil.

From this definition of evil, it is easy to see why some theologians have understood disability as a natural evil. When disability itself is viewed as a privation, a lack of some important ability that allows humans to flourish, then it must be considered evil. Aquinas, for example, believed disabilities, or what he called "bodily infirmities" (which is not exactly the same as our modern definition of disability but may be considered an ancestral concept of disability), are a punishment for original sin and prevent full human flourishing.[93] Even after the Fall, creatures have an optimal natural state.[94] Humans have a unique nature as rational animals, which include their being sentient, animate, and corporeal, and they share with other animals the capacity for sense perception. Biological nature was important for Aquinas insofar as capacities are actualized in the lives of creatures, but he did not believe biological nature in and of itself was definitive of human nature, because human nature is teleologically oriented. Aquinas's definition of the human person, therefore, is ontological rather than merely biological. Therefore, Aquinas was able to say that all humans were persons with a human nature, even if they did not exhibit all of the features that he believed were definitive of human nature. For example, not having an actualized physical capacity, such as self-consciousness, does not disqualify an individual from being a person.[95] Personhood was a threshold concept for Aquinas, not a matter of degree. The failure to actualize a particular capacity that is proper to human persons, however, such as sense perception or rationality, does constitute an ontological evil.

For Aquinas, all persons are in some ways impaired as a result of the Fall, so there are no "normal" bodies.[96] All humans share *universal* defects such as pain and hunger,[97] but some humans have *particular* defects such as "leprosy, blindness, fever, and such like things: for these arise from particular corruptions in individual persons" as a result of original sin.[98] "When original justice is lost [at the Fall], the nature of a human body is left to itself, and in this way, even though original sin is equal, the bodies of some are subject to more defects, and of others to fewer, according to the natural diversity of their configuration."[99] The lack of flight for a human, or the lack of sight in a stone, would not be considered a privation because these are not capacities proper to humans or stones.[100] Aquinas notes, "There might also have been bodily disparity [before the Fall]" that contributed to the beauty of the universe, such as differences in strength, height, beauty, and constitution.[101] Arguably, Aquinas even acknowledges there are some bodily configurations that are nonoptimal but still divinely intended by God, and not the result of sin, such as being female.[102] Physical disabilities, however, are not merely different bodily configurations: they represent the person's inability to actualize a definitive capacity of human persons and are thus ontologically evil, because they are a privation of a natural good.

Of course, Aquinas does not believe that disabilities are punishment for an individual's particular sin, but rather for original sin. As such, the punishment of physical impairment can be nonretributive and may even serve a good. Aquinas believes some bodily defects can serve a derivative teleological purpose if they contribute to one's spiritual health. "But it happens sometimes that a human being can suffer loss in some lesser good, so that he may increase in a greater—just as someone might suffer pecuniary loss for the sake of the health of the body, or loss of both of these for the sake of the salvation of his soul and the glory of God. And this loss is not simply speaking evil for a human being, but only qualifiedly so."[103] Bodily infirmities may, for example, contribute to developing the virtues of humility and courage.[104] Moreover, certain impairments may also allow for one to receive gifts of the Holy Spirit. For example, Aquinas believes infants and the persons with intellectual disabilities receive the gift of wisdom in their baptism.[105] One may even argue that a physical and cognitive impairment could be instrumentally good for a person, even if it is not intrinsically good.[106] Because disability can be a nonretributive punishment, then it is appropriate to offer care for persons with disabilities and to remove obstacles that would allow them to flourish.[107] Recognizing a lack in another provides an opportunity for care—a donation of the good by another to the one who is lacking. Caring and receiving care are habits that cultivate virtue, and the presence of a person with disabilities in another's life can be a gift. As a result, Aquinas believed that treating a person with a disability or infirmity with derision was a mortal sin.[108]

OBJECTIONS

Not all disability advocates will be wholly satisfied with Aquinas's understanding of the optimal body, even if his vision of impairment is more generous than some critics have given him credit for.[109] Aquinas may have believed persons with disabilities had full dignity and could contribute to the virtue and gifts of their communities, but for him disability is the lack of a good necessary for full human flourishing and is connected to the disorder of nature initiated after the Fall. As I will show in the next chapter, the association of disability with sin and evil has had a problematic history in the Christian tradition. For many disability theologians, identifying disability with sin, even original sin, is inherently demeaning. Furthermore, although Aquinas does not deny persons with disabilities entry into heaven, he does believe that disabilities, such as blindness or deafness, will not exist in heaven, thus implying that these are conditions antithetical to bodily perfection.[110] I discuss Christian conceptions of the resurrected body in the following chapter, but suffice it to say there are many disability theologians who are wary of this understanding of bodily perfection in the afterlife.

Contemporary theologians who attempt to read Aquinas without an ableist bias do resist pejorative understandings of disability and evil, but there seems to be little room in Aquinas's understanding to see disability as something other than a privation. Understanding disability as a teleological failing does not cohere with how many understand their own disabilities, even with the allowance that disabilities may strengthen virtue and offer opportunities for care. In particular, not all individuals understand their disability as an inherent "absence," "loss," or "lack"; instead, some see their disability as a different form of embodiment, which confers unique goods. Deafness, for some, is not simply a lack of the ability to hear but a unique identity. This is not to suggest that all disabilities should be seen as mere differences,[111] but rather to undermine the idea that disability is *necessarily* or even best understood as an intrinsic lack.

Aquinas's teleological approach to human nature requires a priori judgments about what potentialities are required for flourishing. Like Aristotle, Aquinas believes there is an "objective list" of what constitutes well-being (or flourishing) for humans, within which disability is understood as detracting from full flourishing. Clearly, Aquinas does not have a robust definition of disability or disease, much less one that clearly aligns with our contemporary definitions, but there is a presumption among some Thomists that disabilities are a deviation from God's will for human beings. God permits such privations but does not create them, because God does not create evil. Of course, God can redeem disabilities and even make them positive features within an individual life, but they are not intrinsically good, because they deprive persons of certain goods necessary for human flourishing. Even if Aquinas would allow that some disabilities may be instrumentally good for a person in some circumstances (if, for example, a disability called forth a loving response from the community that increased virtue in the person and those around her), disability would still involve the loss of an intrinsic good.

Yet, if some disabilities or genetic "defects" were seen as an alternative and not necessarily deficient bodily configurations, then there would be room to allow for some forms of disability to be understood as divinely intended and independent of original sin. Disability, after all, can be a *"meaningful and formative aspect of who a person is,"*[112] which should not be understood as deviation from who an individual ideally *should* be. Indeed, there are compelling reasons to assert that at least some disabilities should be viewed as alternative bodily configurations rather than as essential lacks or privations. Disability theologian, Julia Watts Belser, for example, states, "I claim disability as a vibrant part of my own identity, as a meaningful way of naming and celebrating the intricate unfolding of my own skin and soul. . . . I bless God for crafting this holy house of skin and blood: these clear eyes and bony hips, this leg a bit shorter than the next, this hip unwilling to bear weight."[113] Many in the neurodiversity movement similarly believe their bodies and minds are not deficient, even if they fall outside of the cultural understandings of "normal" or "good." There appears to be dispute among scholars as to how best to define disability as a natural category, as well as to conceive of disability in theological anthropology. In response to such a dispute, we must, by Aquinas's own standards, allow them to be opened up to wise investigation.[114] (In the next chapter, I discuss how theologians ought to proceed when ethical matters are in dispute, particularly when nature and scripture are less than clear or even in conflict.)

It is not clear that a list of a priori qualities is the only basis by which we can determine whether a person's embodiment is restricting her flourishing. It may be possible to have a conceptual understanding of human nature and the good life without prescribing what every individual needs to flourish. Surely, most Christians can agree that the goal of human life is friendship with God, but beyond this assertion there is little biblical evidence concerning what physical features, abilities, or capacities a person must possess to commune with God. Surely, God dwells with individual creatures in unique and sometimes unfathomable ways. Presuming we know what constitutes the good for all individuals risks repeating the original sin of desiring to know good and evil. Ian McFarland contends, "A faithful response to the disabled will be the product of engagement with them rather than *a priori* judgments about what it means for them to flourish as human beings."[115] By purporting to know what an individual requires to flourish, we may limit our ability to find the genuine goods that persons bring to the body of Christ. To further assume that all disabilities are "evil" risks presuming God's will for the individual.

Refusing to predetermine what will constitute individual flourishing for any human being does not require us to ignore their suffering or deny them remediation when appropriate. Instead, we ought to discern with individuals what will enable them to flourish and live out their calling. Such an approach allows us to work *with* people rather than *for* them. As I will discuss in later chapters, discerning whether it is appropriate to ameliorate a person's disability ought to be conceptualized as the task of mutual moral discernment, not a battle over good and evil. Because we cannot know God's will, it is best to limit our use of the term *evil*, particularly as it may apply to certain forms of human embodiment. Judging a condition to be evil (even on a metaphysical level) risks prescribing a "solution" to the "problem" too quickly and overlooks the testimony of persons with disabilities who do not wish to have those disabilities ameliorated.

To argue against the association of disability or disease with evil is to suggest, not that such conditions are good, but rather that we should hold off judgment. In general, claims about natural evil are difficult to make with any certainty. Some theologians, such as Calvin, believed the natural order was thoroughly corrupted after the Fall, so that animals began to prey on one another, certain noxious animals (such as caterpillars) came into existence, and disease became prevalent.[116] Yet it may be presumptuous to claim that some parts of nature are clearly the result of the Fall or are divinely intended. To claim to know such a thing (outside of the biblical witness) comes close to saying we know God's will. If we were to define evil as that which is against God's will, it becomes problematic to label certain human conditions as evil definitively.

Rather than answers to the problem of evil, or metaphysical explanations for privation, we need communal practices that allow us to sustain our faith. This is not to suggest that an explanation of evil is irrelevant. Suffering that causes people to lose their faith in God or hope in God's redemption should be counted as an experience of evil.[117] Moreover, there are many Christians who (particularly in times of nonacute suffering) do search for metaphysical meaning related to their illness or physical suffering.[118] In my experience as both a chaplain and clinical ethicist, many hospital patients believe their suffering is divinely intended. Yet to insist that all genetic disabilities are evil does an injustice to many people's lived experience and risks prioritizing arguments and explanations above faithful practices. The "solution" to the problem of evil can itself cause a multitude of evil practices. Many eugenicists and eugenics supporters believed they were doing God's work with regard to natural evil when they forcibly sterilized "unfit" members of the community.

The Christian response to anomaly, illness, and suffering cannot be collapsed into medicine's projects. As genetic technologies proliferate, theologians and bioethicists alike have come to question the moral limits of medicine. The tension between the Christian vision of the good life and scientific understanding of quality of life are revealed in public debates concerning which technologies are enhancements and which are therapies, whether all end-of-life treatments are necessary, and whether genetic engineers are "playing God." Today, Christian theologians should once again consider whether medicine presents itself as the new Pelagianism, allowing human beings to perfect themselves through their own invention. Recognizing that not all instances of bodily diversity represent defects to be overcome may be the first step toward discerning how best to care for those whose body-minds differ from our cultural norms.

SCIENCE, INCLUDING GENETIC SCIENCE, has not completely rid itself of an underlying metaphysics or theology. Past scientific endeavors, such as eugenics, clearly had both a philosophy and a theology. Through their understanding that genes influence personal traits and behaviors, eugenicists offered a utilitarian vision of the world where the population could be controlled and enhanced through selective breeding. As previously described, eugenicists understood the world as inherently flawed but controllable. Defective genes create inherently defective people who lack the ability to improve upon the human race and the natural world, which leads to defective societies. Eugenic science thus had a triumphalist and soteriological understanding of the world predicated on the causal belief that desirable genetic traits resulted in social harmony. Theologians easily complemented this thinking by believing that the science of eugenics participated in the salvation of God's people. For theologians, defective genes could be seen as a result of a fallen state, which could be corrected through the work of well-meaning Christians. As has been shown in this chapter, however, the idea of "defective genes" reflects a particular social and scientific worldview that tends to undervalue diversity and overvalue medical cures. The doctrine of creation, on the other hand, emphasizes the goodness of creation both as a whole and as individual members.

As will become more obvious in the next chapter, to properly understand genetic disease and disability, human nature must be understood in light of God the Creator. Chapter 5 explores how the theology presented in this chapter relates to our conceptions of sin and resurrection. The creation narrative teaches that life is a gift and that all human beings deserve to be treated with dignity, not because of their capacities or abilities, but because of their connection to Christ. Christ's incarnation, along with his status as the image of God, encourages Christians to value their embodiment, finite and limited as it may be.

CHAPTER FIVE

Disability and Personhood

The doctrine of creation grounds Christian ontology and helps us to understand how creation can be both fallen and good. Whereas many theologians have placed all disease and disability into the category of "natural evil," there is reason to believe this category is ill-fitting and perhaps even damaging to people who live with genetic disabilities. The association of disability with evil has led theologians and philosophers to question the personhood of those with genetic disabilities that limit their physical and cognitive abilities. An overvaluation of certain abilities and characteristics has led to the denigration of some persons based on their biology. Some have even gone so far as to argue that certain genetic conditions disqualify humans as persons deserving of dignity and care. At the same time, scientists are developing technologies that alter human genes, causing some to question whether scientists are destroying something essential God has created. Properly relating genes to personhood, therefore, is important for Christians who wish to make sense of their beliefs in light of contemporary genetic science.

When the Human Genome Project began, many denominations started to question how genes related to personhood for the first time. In 1992, the General Board of Church and Society of the United Methodist Church recognized genes as vital to "the sanctity of God's creation."[1] The UMC even went so far as to assert, "Developments in genetic science compel our reevaluation of accepted theological/ ethical issues including determinism versus free will, the nature of sin, just distribution of resources, the status of human beings in relation to other forms of life, and *the meaning of personhood*."[2] In an organizing effort with the Jeremy Rifkin Foundation, the UMC gathered over two hundred American religious leaders to issue "The Joint Appeal against Human and Animal Patenting." Gene patenting is a complicated legal issue worthy of ethical debate, but the reasoning behind the church leaders' statement appeared to have less to do with intellectual property law and more to do the essential nature of genes in God's creation. The statement notes, "We believe that humans and animals are creations of God, not [creations of] humans, and as such should not be patented as human inventions."[3] While astutely acknowledging God's creation of human and nonhuman animals and warning against the commodification of life, the statement seems to imply that genes are integral to—if not central to—animal identity (though surprisingly not plant identity, also presumably created by God). At the time, Richard D. Land, president of the Southern Baptist Convention's Christian Life Commission, observed, "I think we're on the threshold of mind-bending debates about the nature of human life and animal life. We see altering life forms, creating new life forms, as a revolt against the sovereignty of God and an attempt to be God."[4] The religious leaders' intent in the Joint Appeal was to draw attention to a *theological* understanding of life, but their statement offers little specific theological insight. Instead, it appears to confirm the mechanical view of life offered by the medical sciences, rather than the traditional Christian appreciation of the irreducible nature of the human person and the reality of the nonmaterial spirit.

Modern scientific discoveries and church statements call into question precisely what constitutes human identity. As described in chapter 3, since modernity the natural sciences have blurred the lines between nature and artifice, making it difficult to know when we have crossed any moral limits through our alteration of nature, or if such limits even exist. In this chapter, I present an ontology of the human person that is predicated upon a Christian understanding of God the Creator. I argue that defining ontological personhood in relation to

God is essential for determining how Christians should understand personhood and human nature and their relation to genetic disability within human life. To show how a theological account of ontology can influence genetic debates, I first explore why it is necessary to define personhood as an ontological reality granted by God in creation. I then discuss how we ought to understand human nature in relation to fallenness and sin. Finally, I explore how our vision of resurrected bodies within the Kingdom of God can inform our treatment of those living with genetic disabilities in our present communities. Within the classic Creation-Fall-Redemption narrative, I focus on the status of individuals whose body-minds are sometimes seen to disqualify them from moral personhood.

Personhood in Secular and Christian Thought

Defining personhood has had a long history in the West, but determining who counts as a person has been a particularly contentious issue in modern politics. As discussed in chapter 2, in opposition to the ancient world, most contemporary secular philosophical accounts of personhood do not attempt to describe how human nature relates to its telos. Whereas for Aristotle physics and metaphysics were analogous, in contemporary philosophy there is no universally agreed-upon account of formal or final ends that would allow us to derive a purely rational ethic from human nature. Describing the relationship between the human person, human nature, and ethics has become an important but difficult task within a pluralistic society. Within philosophy and law, the criteria for personhood are used to determine who is deserving of rights and protections as well as who can be held responsible for their actions. Moral blame or credit can be awarded only to *persons*. Many of the most contentious issues in bioethics, such as abortion, cloning, stem cell research, and brain death, arise when the individuals involved are considered *persons* by some and *nonpersons* by others.

For many philosophers and bioethicists, personhood is correlated with mental capacities such as rationality and self-awareness. Unfortunately, this means classifications of personhood frequently disqualify people with intellectual disabilities. For example, as one of his

fifteen criteria for "humanhood" Joseph Fletcher proposed those with
an IQ under 40 "might not be persons" and that those with an IQ
below 20 "are definitely not persons."[5] Under Fletcher's rubric, individuals who do not meet the standards of humanhood are not granted
the same moral and legal rights as persons. For example, he believes
physicians are not obligated to maintain life support for nonpersons
as they would persons.[6] Modifying Fletcher's terminology, Peter
Singer argues that personhood is distinct from being a member of
Homo sapiens. Singer maintains human beings are only persons once
they are self-aware, or capable of grasping that they exist over time.[7]
Newborn infants, people in irreversible comas, and the elderly in
states of advanced senility are all *Homo sapiens* but should not be
considered persons.[8] Using this definition of personhood, Singer
believes infanticide can sometimes be justified for "handicapped"
newborns. Singer uses preference utilitarianism to argue that it would
be ethically appropriate to euthanize infants whose lives would contain more suffering than happiness and would threaten the future
happiness of the infant's family.[9]

Singer is right to suggest that care of a disabled infant is a familial
and communal endeavor, but his judgments about "personhood" appear arbitrary and ableist. Within secular philosophical ethics and bioethics, personhood is a foundational concept, but it is rarely convinc-
ingly articulated. The philosopher Daniel Dennett writes, "Human
beings or other entities can only aspire to being approximations of the
idea of [persons], and there can be no way to set a 'passing grade' that
is not arbitrary."[10] Not only is it difficult to define personhood with
a set of universally agreeable criteria, but when personhood is defined
by certain characteristics, qualities, and abilities, those who fail to
meet the standard are seen as essentially flawed or lacking personhood. As alluded to in previous chapters, the ambiguity of personhood has been wielded against vulnerable groups who appear to be
less than persons by virtue of their genetic makeup.

Of course, the ontological status of the human person is set
within contexts where certain qualities and characteristics are valued
over others. Since modernity, Western societies have tended to value
progress and prosperity over other virtuous qualities, and self-

awareness and rationality over other functional capabilities. Within an industrial society, those who cannot work because of mental or physical deficiencies are necessarily ostracized from "normal" society. Hans Reinders explains, "It is not by accident, therefore, that somewhere in the course of the nineteenth century the notion of the 'feeble-minded' emerges to identify those human beings on which society cannot count to participate in its endeavor to be a progressive and prosperous society. Unsurprisingly it is in the same era that we find the emerging concept of intelligence as an intrinsic quality, justifying the invention of a particular category of human beings, which indicates how 'feeble-mindedness' emerged as a conceptual byproduct of the project of modernity."[11] Attempts to profile and categorize human beings reveal our culture's assumptions about what it considers valuable within the human condition. Nearly every current definition of personhood inevitably marginalizes people who fail to meet the standards of normality.

Persons Created in the Image of God

Before delving into how disability affects personhood, we must articulate a Christian ontology capable of responding to the personhood debates. Debates in secular bioethics and philosophy reveal that what constitutes a "person" is highly contested. At the same time, there is general agreement among philosophers, theologians, and bioethicists that *persons* demand some degree of moral respect (even if what counts as respect is also debatable). If a human being is not a person, then society does not owe that individual the same rights and respect as other persons.

Christian theologians, on the other hand, have not always found it necessary to distinguish human beings from persons. Both Augustine and Aquinas believed everyone born of human parentage is a human person and should be afforded full membership into the human community. Aquinas goes on to describe how humans are unique among all beings by their reason and free will. As I will later describe, this does not mean that individuals who cannot use their reason because of a disability are not fully human; it is the capacity for rationality and not its exercise that is essential to human nature. Aquinas's description of human nature, however, has been critiqued by some Protestant disability theologians, including Hans Reinders, who believes that defining human persons in terms of reason renders some individuals with cognitive limitations "defective" and perhaps even subhuman.[12] Before delving into debates concerning reason and personhood, however, I want to articulate a common way in which both Protestants and Roman Catholics ground personhood: the *imago Dei*. Invoking the *imago Dei* will not solve all disputes between theologians on the issue of intellectual disability, but it is worth articulating what it means to be made in the image of God and why it is foundational for Christian anthropology. Properly understanding the *imago Dei* will help reveal how disability is related to our human nature.

The image of God has had an enduring and powerful influence on the Christian tradition, but unfortunately, misunderstandings related to the image of God have diminished the power of this doctrine for Christians. As described by the Christian bioethicist John Kilner, some theologians have mistakenly interpreted the *imago Dei* as separating humans from other animals and have stressed that humans are unique creations because of their capacity for certain abilities, such as the ability to reason, rule over creation, or be in relationship.[13] If we believe that the image of God expresses itself in the ability to perform certain actions (i.e., reason, rule, relate), then humans who do not have these abilities are deemed to be nonpersons or subhuman. Their ability to flourish, therefore, is determined to be limited or nonexistent. To the extent that individuals do not exhibit the capacities or attributes deemed to be uniquely those of "human persons," they do not bear the full image of God and thus warrant less respect or protection than others.

Throughout history, Christians have justified the slaughter, enslavement, and degradation of people by positing that the image of God was not in certain people (because they did not possess the ability to reason, rule, or relate) or that it had been marred or damaged. Unsurprisingly, persons who are intellectually or physically disabled have frequently been denied their *imago Dei* status by Christians.[14]

Joseph Fletcher, for example, believed that it was morally appropriate, and even responsible, to kill children with Down syndrome. In 1968, he wrote:

> People have no reason to feel guilty about putting a Down's syndrome baby away, whether it's "put away" in the sense of hidden in a sanitarium or in a more responsible lethal sense. It is sad; yes. Dreadful. But it carries no guilt. True guilt arises only from an offense against a person, and a Down's is not a person. . . . Guilt over a decision to end an idiocy would be a false guilt. . . . There is far more reason for real guilt in keeping alive a Down's or other kind of idiot, out of a false idea of obligation or duty, while at the same time feeling no obligation at all to save that money and emotion for a living, learning child.[15]

It is unclear whether Fletcher believed that individuals with Down syndrome possess the *imago Dei*, but he certainly believed they did not exhibit proper human attributes and thus should not be afforded the same kinds of care as children who were capable of "learning."

Identifying the *imago Dei* with certain intellectual and physical capacities, however, is theologically mistaken. Rather than arbitrary notions of personhood, Christians ought to turn toward a theology that acknowledges all human beings as persons worthy of dignity and respect because they are created by God. In other words, there is no need to discern which human beings are in fact persons, because all humans are worthy of respect by virtue of their Creator. Being made in God's image is not about displaying or possessing certain attributes, such as rationality or free will. Our whole being is made in God's image, not merely select attributes, even if those attributes appear God-like, such as our ability to love or do justice. Christians, therefore, cannot be reductionist about what makes us persons. What makes us persons worthy of respect has nothing to do with our attributes, our abilities, or even our genes.

After careful examination of the biblical passages that describe the image of God, Kilner determines that all people are made in God's image, a status that can never be damaged or diminished. The biblical understanding of being an "image" involves *connection*, meaning damage to the image damages the original, and *reflection*, meaning the image reflects attributes of the original. Being in the image of God means having a special connection to God and reflecting God's attributes. When discerning which attributes are God-like, we can look to God's image, which is Christ. Whereas Christ *is* the image of God as conveyed in Colossians 1:15 and 2 Corinthians 4:4, people are made *in* (according to) God's image (Gen. 1:26–27; 5:1; 9:6). We are not God, but Christ, as the image of God, is the standard of who people are created to be. Of course, what it means to be like Christ or to reflect Christ's attributes can be debated, but as I will later describe, there is no reason to believe that persons with disabilities are not capable of, or are inherently worse at, reflecting Christ. Even if we believe that disabilities are a result of the Fall, and there is reason to believe this presumption is faulty, sin does not damage God's image in the human person. Humans retain God's image even though they have been damaged by sin; sin damages the person but not God's image (as would be the case if Christ were damaged by sin).[16]

Being made in the image of God, all human beings have a special significance that grants them dignity and equality. The Christian understanding of justice is, therefore, connected to the *imago Dei*: we are called to be just as God is just. How the weakest or most marginalized member of our community is treated indicates how the community is living out its call to reflect God's likeness. Theologians such as Fletcher, therefore, are wrong to assume that persons with Down syndrome are lacking something important in their humanity and thus deserve to be "put down." Christ declares that mistreatment of the least among us is mistreatment of him (Matt. 25:45). What is more, God expects us to love one another, because love is essential to who God is. Our failure to love and treat one another with dignity and respect does not damage the image of God within us, but it does damage our ability to live as God has commanded and reflect God's character. The image of God, therefore, unites humans in a shared destiny; all persons are given room to flourish when they are cared for and loved. The real work of Christians is not to determine who counts as a person but to discern how to live in just and loving relationships that promote mutual flourishing.

Grace and Flourishing

At its best, Christianity has attempted to uphold the notion that all human beings are persons created by God and deserving of care. Such a notion is grounded in the *imago Dei*, but our flourishing also depends on God's grace. Whereas Fletcher and Singer's notion of personhood excludes certain humans and justifies limiting their care, the Christian emphasis on the care of the needy demands that Christians give special care and attention to society's most vulnerable persons. Simply because a person cannot reason or relate is no reason to treat him or her as less than a person.

In opposition to those who judge the value of a life on the basis of quality-of-life standards or a collection of actualized traits, Christians must recognize the potential in every human being to be transformed by God through grace. Aquinas writes, "Now the gift of grace surpasses every capability of created nature, since it is nothing short of a partaking of the Divine Nature, which exceeds every other nature. And thus it is impossible that any creature should cause grace. For it is as necessary that God alone should deify, bestowing a partaking of the Divine Nature by a participated likeness, as it is impossible that anything save fire should enkindle."[17] Through grace human beings are able to participate in God. The Christian community, therefore, ought not to predetermine what or who any individual will become or is capable of becoming, because God's grace surpasses what we can imagine. Using Aquinas's language, all humans share a capacity to respond to God in love. Christian communities that wish to create welcoming spaces for all people, including those with disabilities, must develop open imaginations and learn to recognize human potential and capacity.

Given human beings' status as bearers of God's image and the potential for grace in the lives of all individuals, Christian theology must reject the assertion that some individuals with diseases or disabilities are less than persons. As discussed in the previous chapter, the doctrine of creation teaches that human existence is not irrational; rather, it is ordered by God's providence. We know from the Genesis creation narrative that God created humankind in God's image, blessed them, and saw them as very good (Gen. 1:27–31). Human worth and goodness are not achieved through humans' mental or physical capacities, rather, they are granted simply by our being made in God's image. In other words, the "is" of the human is synthetic, which means "goodness" is not added as an additional quality to its "esse." Aquinas explains, "Every being, as being, is good. For all being, as being, has actuality and is in some way perfect; since every act implies some sort of perfection; and perfection implies desirability and goodness. . . . Hence every being as such is good."[18] Brought into being by God and finding their end in union with God, human beings are not only persons deserving dignity and respect, they are also essentially good.

After the Fall, the goodness of the world is much more difficult to discern, and many are tempted to deny humans' continued connection to God and God's goodness. Yet the gift of life given from God's love is not begun and ended with God's initial act of *creatio ex nihilo*. It is sustained by God's blessing every day. God did not create only in the Genesis narrative but actively continues to preserve and sustain creation with the same love and care that initiated creation in time. Augustine reminds us, "God is working even now, so that if His action should be withdrawn from his creatures, they would perish. . . . God moves His whole creation by a hidden power, and all creatures are subject to this movement."[19] If God's wisdom and good will did not reach out and cause creatures to continue to move toward God, then all things would cease to participate in God and thus cease to exist. Called into existence by God's purposive will, each finite life (in both body and soul) participates in God's creation and belongs to the intelligible order created by God. Being bound to God through the gift of creation, human beings — along with all of creation — are invested with spiritual depth.

As created beings we are gifted because we are fundamentally dependent on God and one another. Giftedness, then, becomes a quality of our ontology, the logic of being human, which opens us to others in community. The only thing that is deemed "not good" in the Genesis creation story is that Adam is alone. From the start humans are created as social beings; therefore, we know that the goodness of personhood requires other persons to share in that goodness. In opposition to those who think human beings function best when they act independently, theologians throughout the Christian tradition, from Augustine to Aquinas to Calvin, agree that all human life, everything from soteriology to ecclesiology, depends on our receptivity to the Other.[20] In the sacraments, for instance, Calvin explains that faith and the Spirit's power transform participants by restoring them to original communion with God and neighbor.[21] Through our participation in God's otherness, we learn to allow others to be, without trying to make them more like ourselves. Human beings are bound to God, to each other, and to the whole of the universe in indivisible and irreducible unity. Our essential human nature is thus donative, social, and interconnected.

Although many are quick to read dominion and cocreatorship into the Genesis narrative, our first reaction to God's creating life ought to be one of reverence and awe. We must learn to see the beauty, integrity, and freedom in all of creation. With the Psalmist, we should marvel that God would choose to create and love us.

> O Lord, our Sovereign, how majestic is your name in all the earth!
> . . . .
> When I look at your heavens, the work of your fingers,
> The moon and stars that you have established;
> What are human beings that you are mindful of them,
> mortals that you care for them?
> Yet you have made them a little lower than the angels
> And crowned them with glory and honor.
>
> (Ps. 8:1, 3–5 NRSV)

The gift of life can be experienced every day through our mere physical existence. We may experience this gift through the birth of a child, relationships of care, the daily activities of other animals around us, and the seasonal cycles of the earth. Such gifts of life are so gratuitous that they do not fall upon good and righteous people alone; rather, God "makes his sun rise on the evil and on the good, and sends rain on the righteous and on the unrighteous" (Matt. 5:45 NRSV). The proper orientation to this gift of life is gratitude and humility. Reflecting on the Apostles' Creed, Martin Luther contends, "The first article teaches that God is the father, the creator of heaven and earth. . . . This article teaches that you do not have your life of yourself, not even a hair. . . . Do not let us think that we have created ourselves, as the proud princes do."[22] Calvin also cautions Christians not to act as cosmic ingrates.[23] Instead, with all creatures, we should sing a universal hymn of praise to our Creator (Ps. 148). Before we turn to what is corrupt and evil in this world, we ought first to turn to what is good and meditate humbly on all we have been given.

Our response of gratitude is intimately connected to humankind's telos, which is to be with God forever. As previously mentioned, we become who we are meant to be in our encounter with God's grace. The Westminster Shorter Catechism begins, "Q1: What is the chief end of man? A. Man's chief end is to glorify God and to enjoy him forever." Calvin's Geneva Catechism opens similarly: "What is the chief end of human life? To know God."[24] Such answers suggest humans are created for relationship with God. In other words, friendship with God is humanity's telos. All humans are created and lovingly sustained by God and are thus capable of glorifying, enjoying, and being with God. Our capacity to be with God, however, cannot lie with our own human efforts, since we know through the biblical narrative, particularly in Paul's letters, that we are unable to achieve this end without God's aid (John 14:16–17; Eph. 2:8–9; Rom. 9:16). Luther writes, "God looks down from heaven and does not see even one who seeks or attempts to seek him; hence it follows that there is nowhere any power which might attempt or wish to seek him, but instead they all turn aside. . . . For [Paul's] whole concern here is to make grace necessary for all men. But if they were able to initiate anything of themselves, there would be no need of grace."[25] If all human beings, with God's help, are capable of communion with God (and even sea monsters are capable of praising God [Ps. 148]), then the potential for this communion must be open to all persons whom God has promised to be with. Communion with God should perhaps be understood, not primarily as a human achievement, but as a gift from God who chooses to be with humankind. Receiving this gift from the Spirit, even in our frailties, we participate in the life of God and move toward our telos.

THE FALL AND ONTOLOGICAL ESTRANGEMENT

Although Christians affirm that their ultimate destiny is to commune with God forever, they recognize that their ability to do this has been marred by sin. As described in the previous chapter, the Christian understanding of fallenness and sinfulness may initially appear to be in tension with the declaration of creation's goodness. The freedom that structures human life can be used in evil ways. The story of the Fall indicates that our current reality is separated from our true source as a result of the misuse of our freedom. Paul Tillich contends that our lives are marked by a tragic estrangement from our true being, from one another, and from God. In other words, our existence is no longer united with its essence. In this life "Man has left the ground [of divine life] in order to 'stand upon' himself, to actualize what he essentially is."[26] Here we can see how the doctrine of creation and the doctrine of the Fall join and where essence and existence fall away from one another. The Christian narrative does not attempt to fully explain the mystery of human existence as it is experienced, nor does it rationalize the evil of the world; rather, it attempts to express the mysterious possibilities of human freedom. Fallen nature is now a part of human historical existence, an existence that is estranged from its life-giving source.

Outside of the divine life, there is a fracturing of essential and existential being that causes human beings to become separated from each other and the world. Thus the ontological structures of life are experienced in polarities, which are difficult to harmonize. According to Tillich, there are three ontological elements that characterize human existence: individualization and participation, dynamics and form, and freedom and destiny. Tillich believes we know something of God in these ontological polarities because they constitute the rational structure of reality. Human sin distorts the ontological structure of life, so that we frequently act against our good. We tend to value our individual selves over participation with others and God; we direct our creative dynamism away from our essential natures (our energy for life away from its true purpose); and we use our freedom to resist our destiny.[27] There is no capacity of the person that is not skewed by sin and its consequences, and there is no person, community, or institution that is exempt from sin's effects. When Christians say creation is good, they also recognize reality is not what it should be. Many, although perhaps not all, of the problems or hardships in life are thus attributed to the effects of the Fall. The question remains, however: if the medical community deems a person's genes "defective," is this deviation the result of the Fall or a product of God's good and diverse creation?

The question of how the Fall and sin are related to genetic disability is no mere theoretical question. Our answers will bear on the lives of people with disabilities and may have profound effects on how the church community treats and welcomes persons whose bodies and minds differ from our socio-medical norms. In her book *The Disabled God*, Nancy Eiesland discusses the ways in which persons with disabilities have been harmed by particular discussions of sin. The first is by conflating sin and disability. Too often, disability is seen as a punishment for wrongdoing, which mars the divine image in humans.[28] As previously discussed, the divine image in humans cannot be damaged, but the connection between disability and sin remains. Unfortunately, the Bible is full of passages that, on their face, appear to link (both metaphorically and literally) disability with sin.[29] Many theologians presume that prelapsarian bodies were perfect and incorruptible and therefore consider any marker of finitude or limitation to be a direct result of human sinfulness.[30] Still others consider such bodily defects to be potential blessings given for virtuous suffering. Eiesland warns that viewing disability as virtuous suffering does not escape the sin-disability conflation and can lead to passivity and resignation toward those who suffer. The biblical theme of "salvation as healing" also risks identifying bodily disease and disability with individual or communal sin. Disability theology requires an account of salvation in which the un-healable, or "abnormal," body is not an obstacle for human participation or communion with God. How,

then, should we understand the relationship between fallenness, sinfulness, and disease and disability so that it is not injurious to people
who wish to know and love God better? Rather than look to the
prelapsarian bodies of Adam and Eve (of which we know little bibli-
cally) to understand human nature, we ought to look first to Christ,
who took on human nature to be God with us.

Christ's Nature

Reconciling the goodness of creation with the corruption of nature
in the Fall has been a difficult task in Christian theology, and one
that appears to bear directly upon the status of disability in any
Christian conception of ontology, or what it means to be a human
being created by God. If humanity is sinful and all creation groans
and suffers with us (Rom. 8:22), then how can creation still be
counted as good? As noted in chapter 2, thinkers such as Francis
Bacon have gone so far as to assert that all of nature is corrupted as
a result of humankind's fall and so humans must exert mastery over
nature in the service of our neighbors whose bodies bear the brunt of
our fallenness. On this view, disability is a univocal indicator of
original sin, so the fragility of the body is a result of humanity's sinfulness. The causal connection between sin and disability has been
difficult for many people to reconcile with their belief in created
goodness and mercy. Either people have been given disabilities because they in particular have sinned or their bodies bear the universal
marks of original sin. As long as sin and disability are easily correlated, those who appear unwell in the eyes of society either will
provoke moral revulsion and become excluded from our moral
projects or (via their disease) will become the focus of intensive efforts aimed at spiritual or medical cure.

   To understand our fallen situation, we ought to look to Christ's
incarnation for guidance. Although direct knowledge of God's will
remains hidden for Christians, in Christ, God's intentions are most
transparent. In Christ's assumption of human nature we find further
clues about human nature. Christ took on human form to unite
human beings with God once again, but he was able to do so without

sinning. Understanding how Christ could be both God and human in the Incarnation, therefore, may provide a framework for understanding how fallenness and sin are related to human nature. Looking to Christ as an exemplar of human nature might seem strange, considering that Christ, as God, bears a fundamentally different relationship to God than the rest of fallen humanity. As was made clear through the Chalcedonian Creed (451), however, Christ was both fully divine and fully human. The church fathers affirmed that Christ had to take on human nature in order to save it. Against those who denied that Christ had a human mind, Gregory of Nazianzus writes, "For that which he has not assumed he has not healed; but that which is united to his Godhead is also saved."[31] Unable to reach God on their own, humans needed God to come to them, to suffer as they suffered and be tested as they were tested (Heb. 2:17–18). If Christ had not assumed human nature, he could not have saved humankind, but if he had not been God, he could not have completed his task of salvation without sin.

But if Christ took up the fallen nature of humankind, how was he was able to live a sinless life? After all, humans are estranged from God as a result of original sin. The Chalcedonian understanding of "hypostasis" (or "person") helps to clarify Christ's relationship to human nature, fallenness, and sin. The distinction between a hypostasis and a nature allowed early Christians to understand how Christ could have both a divine and a human nature without compromising his divinity. Traditionally, one's hypostasis has been distinguished from one's nature and serves as the ontological basis for distinguishing a "who" (the person as agent) from a "what" (the person as historically conditioned, fallen, and so on). The will allows us to believe the human is not fully described as a some*thing*, but rather as a some*one*.[32] Environmental and genetic factors may play a role in shaping our will's desires, but they can never fully explain human behavior as long as persons experience their self as an "I." The obvious difference between Christ's hypostasis and our own is his will. Unlike the rest of humanity, Christ was able to direct his will to God's will perfectly, even while being tempted to sin as humans are tempted. Christ's ability to take on humanity's fallen nature without sinning reveals that sinfulness is properly attributed to our hypostasis rather than to our nature.

Christ's exceptional hypostasis points us toward the fundamental difference between fallenness (a property of nature) and sin (a property of hypostasis, or person). A nature can be damaged and fallen, but a nature cannot sin, because sin is ascribed to agents. In all humans besides Christ, however, the will's fallenness is experienced hypostatically as one's own sin rather than as damage that exists apart from one's own agency. Ian McFarland explains that Christ shares in our nature without sharing our sin: "He reveals sin as a function of the will that is nevertheless prior to any act of the will . . . and thus allows it to be understood as an ontological rather than an axiological category."[33] This does not mean human beings are ontologically evil but that they are bound to sin. Human sinfulness itself is a mystery, but it is a function of who the human is, even while it resists explanation with respect to cause.[34] Thus the will is not the cause of our sinfulness but the place where our sinfulness is experienced. We therefore cannot talk of sinful natures. Even a fallen nature is good and not evil. Unlike our sinfulness, our nature cannot separate us from God because it only exists in God. In other words, our human nature as created by God is good because all of creation is good. McFarland asserts, "The assumption by Christ of a fallen human nature simply reinforces this basic point: if the nature God assumes is itself damaged and yet is taken on by God as God's own humanity, then the damage our natures suffer is clearly not an occasion for divine revulsion."[35] Taking on human nature, Christ shared in human fragility and vulnerability and was subject to disease, disability, and death, but these frailties did not separate Christ from God. In other words, Christ's own mortality did not follow from his sinfulness. Thus human nature does not stand in the way of God's love.

The Nature of Disability

If disease, disability, and finitude are constitutive parts of our fallen human nature (our whatness) but theoretically distinguishable from our sinful wills (our whoness), then our bodily limitations are loved rather than despised by God. The fragility of our bodies is part of our natural state of existence; therefore, physical vulnerability, illness, and disability are natural components of God's good creation, albeit in its fallen state (the only state of existence we know). Understanding bodily disease and disability within the category of natural human finitude rather than estrangement or alienation from God, the Christian community may be encouraged to alter its conceptions of naturalness in light of a diverse group of bodies. Rather than viewing people with disabilities primarily as a sign of humanity's sinfulness, Christians should be encouraged to see them as part of the natural human condition—lives and natures that are gifted and continually loved by God.

Some may object that disability is part of human finitude, which itself is a consequence of sin or the Fall. The equation of death and finitude, however, is contested in theological circles. Wolfhart Pannenberg, explains, "The finitude that is part of creaturely life will not be set aside by participation in the divine life. It follows, however, that finitude does not always have to include mortality. The eschatological hope of Christians knows a finitude of creaturely existence without death. Hence death cannot be necessarily a part of the finitude of creaturely existence."[36] Paul Tillich goes even further to suggest that finitude and death are not intrinsically evil; rather, they are problematic only when we are separated from God. "Participation in the eternal makes man eternal; separation from the eternal leaves man in his natural finitude. . . . In estrangement man is left to his finite nature of having to die. Sin does not produce death but gives to death the power which is conquered only in participation in the eternal. . . . Sin is the sting of death, not its physical cause."[37] Friedrich Schleiermacher writes similarly when discussing the original perfection of the world. Schleiermacher finds that mortality motivates human development and our care of the world.[38] Death becomes sinful only when it causes humans not to trust in God and God's plan for the world. Moreover, if Christ, as a sinless human, had been naturally immortal before his resurrection, then his suffering to the point of death would have been a mere empty gesture to those who suffer. Whether or not one wants to go as far as Tillich and Schleiermacher in maintaining that death

itself is not caused by sin, there seems room for distinguishing finitude from sin. In either case, our sin separates us from God, not our
finitude. Even in the eschaton, our finitude does not cease to be finitude; rather, it is "taken into" the infinite, the eternal life of God. God
will clothe our mortality with immortality (1 Cor. 15:53).

Understanding genetic disability as part of God's creation, however, does not mean a person will necessarily understand or experience disabilities as gifts, particularly when they are accompanied by
physical pain or existential suffering. Under the conditions of sin,
bodily suffering and limitation take on added dimensions of our
estrangement from God. Tillich elaborates,

> In estrangement man is left to his finite nature of having to die.
> Sin does not produce death but gives to death the power which is
> conquered only in participation in the eternal. . . . The loss of
> one's potential eternity is experienced as something for which one
> is responsible in spite of its universal tragic actuality. Sin is the
> sting of death, not its physical cause. . . . Suffering, like death, is
> an element of finitude. . . . Under the conditions of existence, man
> is cut off from his blessedness, and suffering lays hold of him in
> a destructive way.[39]

That disabilities are "natural" or universal to human existence is not
in itself grounds for minimizing the real and intense suffering that
many persons experience. In a fallen world, suffering affects more
than just our bodies. Genetic disability can cause suffering that
affects our spiritual and relational selves. The bodily pain and suffering that at times accompany genetic disability can cause persons
to feel disconnected from themselves, from other persons, and even
from God, which increases their suffering. The sting of such suffering is amplified in a sinful world.

Moreover, sin gets easily entangled with bodily fragility when
perverted human desire and hubris cause disability. Many of the disabilities experienced by the global population are a result of our mistreatment of the earth and each other. Although bodily frailty may
be a part of human nature, our modern industrial age has produced

many disabilities that are human-made. Furthermore, as many disability scholars have noted, the suffering experienced by many people with impairments is often aggravated and sometimes fully derived from the social, economic, and political structures that impinge upon people's lives.[40] The suffering often associated with bodily limitation can be intimately tied to the hubris of humans who refuse to believe that limitation and finitude are a natural part of the human condition.

The doctrines of creation and the Fall produce a Christian ontology that has repercussions for persons living with genetic disabilities. If life is a gift given by a loving God, no life can be considered worthless. Similarly, if the telos of human life is to be with God, then this potential must be open to all existing creatures through God's grace. Christ's life and resurrection open up the potentiality for all human beings to be joined to him and thus to participate in divine life. The radical and transformational nature of God's grace should prevent Christians from attempting to circumscribe or limit what any person might become in this life. Disability does not distance any human being from God's grace, nor is it a reflection of the evil present within the world. Christ's own vulnerable and mortal body teaches us that these qualities of the human body are not the result of sin, because Christ did not sin. Likewise, the Eucharist body allows us to experience the grace of God within the bodies we now occupy—the same bodies that will be transformed through resurrection and will participate with God in eternity. Imitating Christ and receiving God's grace now, we move toward God and eternal life. A Christian ontology would thus not be complete without understanding the promised future body.

Disease and Disability in Eschatology

Christians look forward to the time when they will achieve their telos, both individually and with the rest of creation. The biblical promise of a "new heaven and a new earth" (Isa. 65:17; Rev. 21:1) implies the Kingdom of God has a universal character. Human beings and the rest of creation suffer now under the conditions of existence, but one day all will become what it ought to be. The doctrine of salvation in Christianity symbolizes the fulfillment of creaturely existence in the eternal. Within classical Christianity, eschatology, or the end of history, is not merely a future event but one that happens in the eternal "now." The "already-but-not-yet" nature of the Kingdom of God demands that we participate in that future now, revealing the "already" and signaling the "not yet" nature of the Kingdom.

One way that Christians can participate in the eternal now and hence symbolize the Kingdom of God on earth is to work toward the relief of suffering. The fact that human frailties are part of our natural condition does not preclude healing or even curing from being gifts of God. Christ's own ministry is replete with stories of individual bodily and mental healing. Few would argue Christians should not use medicine because frailty is part of the human condition. It is not wrong in principle that we seek to mitigate or even eliminate certain effects of human finitude, as long as we do not presume to overcome the natural conditions of vulnerability and dependency. We should recognize that Christians are called to care for one another in dependent relationships, not to overcome all human limitation.

Christians should work toward the relief of suffering, even if that suffering is a result of finitude and not estrangement from God. Even if fallen human nature is counted as good, Christ promises humankind more than its current predicament. In the Last Judgment, human beings will have a *glorified* nature and a *resurrected* body. One of the tasks of the Christian community, therefore, is to prepare for the Kingdom of God and be the representatives of the Kingdom of God in history. In the Kingdom of God, the cosmic, social, and personal elements of Christian theology come together. A frequent biblical theme, the Kingdom of God is represented as a political sphere in which God rules over a new heaven and new earth, a social sphere where peace and justice reign, a personal sphere where individuals come together to commune with God, and a universal sphere where all of creation finds its completion.[41]

Of course, the church does not have a perfect or unobstructed vision of the future Kingdom. With the rest of humanity, Christians frequently display sinful desires, hubris, and concupiscence, which distort their vision of the Kingdom. As discussed in chapter 1, the fundamental flaw of the Social Gospel movement was that some Christians (in particular white, elite Protestants) believed they could bring the Kingdom of God through their own social programs. Consequently, eugenics was easily accommodated into the church's eschatological vision. We must understand the Kingdom as God's gift rather than creation's achievement. All too often, Christians think of the Kingdom as a perfected version of their particular and historically situated society, rather than a radical transformation of the current world order. Christians are also prone to understand bodies within this Kingdom as normalized, rather than transformed. Historically, many theologians have been preoccupied with questions of how individual bodies will appear in the future Kingdom.[42] Affirming the goodness of embodiment has been an important theme within Christian theology, but our cultural conceptions of the natural are liable to restrict our vision of a resurrected, glorified body. For instance, many continue to presume that resurrected bodies will be "blemish-free" and thus without any mark of illness or disability. Curing disease and disability, then, has been viewed as a way of signaling the coming Kingdom. The Bible, however, is ambiguous about the physical appearance of individual bodies in the Kingdom of God. "See what kind of love the Father has given to us, that we should be called children of God; and so we are. The reason why the world does not know us is that it did not know him. Beloved, we are God's children now, and what we will be has not yet appeared; but we know that when he appears we shall be like him, because we shall see him as he is. And everyone who thus hopes in him purifies himself as he is pure" (1 John 3.1–3 NRSV). Recognizing that resurrected bodies bear some resemblance to Christ's resurrected body, some disability theologians have countered the idea that resurrected bodies are "blemish-free" by noting that Christ's own resurrected body displayed the marks of his crucifixion (John 20:27).[43]

Although the Bible does not give substantial content to how bodies will appear in the Kingdom, it has much to say about the community that exists in the Kingdom. Within Jesus's eschatological parables the poor, the crippled, the lame, and the blind are invited to feast with the king (Luke 14:1–24). Individual bodies are not "fixed"; rather, persons are invited to come as they are. New Testament parables about the Kingdom of God are strongly communal in nature. The Kingdom is frequently portrayed as a banquet (Luke 14:15), a wedding feast (Matt. 22:2), or a city—the New Jerusalem (Rev. 21:2). Eternal life is thus not a projection of an individual human existence but an experience of sharing in the community of a loving God. In his book *A Vulnerable Communion,* Thomas Reynolds describes the Kingdom of God as a communal metaphor for a realm shaped by God's empowering rule and constituted in honorable self-giving.[44] Self-giving, as exemplified in the life and death of Jesus, invites Christians to exist together in vulnerability, dependency, and radical openness to others as a prefiguring of God's Kingdom. Living in community with those whose bodies render them most dependent on others signals the Kingdom of which Christ spoke. Participating in physical curing and healing can bring people into community, but these acts ought to be secondary to inviting others to simply *be* in community. If God loves us for simply being, and not because of our efforts and acts, then we should show this same love to others.

Cautionary Notes on Cocreatorship

Unfortunately, many of our technological innovations in medicine fail to allow others to simply be. Our socially constructed understandings of disability influence our decisions about which technologies ought to be developed, standardized, and routinized. Some Christian bioethicists presume that creative engineering (often in the form of medical therapy and genetic engineering) represents the Kingdom of God or that the fullness of life promised in the Kingdom is akin to the enhancement of our current bodies. As previously noted, Francis Bacon was convinced that increasing control over the created order would help humanity regain bodily immortality, which had been lost in the Fall. Bacon believed humans could return to the prelapsarian state of Adam and Eve through technological control of the body. Today, few theologians express a desire to inhabit prelapsarian bodies, but many still believe our desire to enhance human qualities is part of our created nature and eschatologically oriented. This eschatological vision often goes hand in hand with an understanding of the *imago Dei* as expressed in "cocreatorship"—humans bear the image of God by creating as God creates. The idea of cocreatorship, or "created cocreatorship," is rooted in a theological and biblical ethic, and many theologians have a nuanced view of the obligations as well as the limits of cocreatorship. For those who bypass or fail to understand this more nuanced view, however, persons who are seen as physically or mentally deficient may end up paying the cost for eschatological visions that focus on human technological achievement over God's grace.

Most theologians who champion the idea of human genetic engineering (either for therapy or for enhancement) imagine human beings as "cocreators" who participate with God through creating. Karen Lebacqz, for instance, believes that if it is our destiny to be more than we are in our fallen state, and if we are cocreators with God, then medical improvements to the human body (both therapy and enhancement) participate in God's eschatological vision for humanity. "Our very dignity" she writes, "may well lie in our transcendence of limits and in our orientation toward that eschatological call from God."[45] Undoubtedly, Lebacqz has a more nuanced understanding of human dignity, cocreatorship, and the eschatological body than her one short essay on human enhancement allows, and she clearly states there are necessary limits to human transformation and human striving given our fallen natures. Yet Lebacqz does not entertain the idea that human dignity lies in accepting bodily limitation. Instead, she advocates for pursuing technological enhancement of the human body as an eschatological vocation. My fear is that Lebacqz's intimate connection between eschatological transcendence and technological enhancements may be misunderstood as a demand for technological progress and control over the human body. For persons whose bodies resist cure or enhancement, this eschatological call may sound more despairing than hopeful. Without the help of intelligent scientists to cure their limitation, persons with disabilities may feel their human dignity in question.

We ought to be cautious in ascribing redemptive significance to technology, not least because, as described in chapter 1, this kind of thinking led directly to the alliance between Protestant churches and the American eugenics movement. Christians who joined the Social Gospel movement were later criticized for placing far too much trust in their ability to discern God's eschatological intentions for the world.[46] If we concede sin is the human attempt at self-justification and the refusal to see human dignity and identity as defined in and through God, then the attempt to create eschatological bodies through technological means may be sinful rather than eschatologically oriented. As evidenced in the previous section, it is not our finite bodies that limit our communion with God and others but our sinful wills. Dependent bodies actually demand communion with others, rather than limiting that communion. If dignity itself is tied too closely to exceeding our bodily limits, then it is all too easy to disregard the dignity of diseased and disabled persons and fail to come into communion with them. I doubt Lebacqz or other theologians who champion human enhancement technologies would want to question the dignity or personhood of people with disabilities, but their demand for progress may lead some toward a Pelagian quest for perfection that cannot tolerate the imperfect.

Theologians should also be cautious of "cocreator" language when it appears to link God's work in creation with human creations. During the eugenics movement, Roman Catholics resisted the idea that sterilization was God's intention for humanity because their natural law theory placed limits on human interference with humanity's given nature. Morally appropriate medicine can mimic the prior given of natural processes but ought not to thwart them. Knowing the ontology of the natural, therefore, is important for discerning the moral use of medicine and technology. As discussed in the previous chapter, Protestants may be ambivalent about what counts as the "natural," but it is important to remember that God creates *ex nihilo*, making human creativity contingent upon the already given. Human beings are limited and contingent in ways that God is not. Irenaeus writes, "While man cannot make anything out of nothing, but only out of matter already existing, yet God is in this point pre-eminently superior to men, that He Himself called into being the substance of His creation when previously it had no existence."[47] The divine act of creation is a totally unique act, because God is utterly unique. Any analogy between God and human, therefore, must remain paradoxical and mysterious. God is not an actor in space and time as human beings are, so we cannot describe God's deeds literally, as we describe our own. We do not create out of nothing (*ex nihilo*) as God creates. Our creative acts, therefore, are fundamentally different from God's creating. James Gustafson reminds us, "Whether the focus of attention is on human genetics, psychology or nutrition, the sciences inform us regarding the ordering conditions and laws. While we can, in modern cultures, intervene in these processes to alter them, we still consent to them in a significant measure, cooperating with them as they are given. If a chromosomal defect cannot be corrected, we can consent to it (not merely resign ourselves to it) and participate in the development of a limited natural capacity. . . . The conditions both limit possibilities and make possible our cooperation with them for some developments."[48] The distinction between God's acts of creation and our own should warn us against conflating God's creation with human creation. We are situated and responsive participants in the cosmic ecology of God's world, but we are not God.[49]

Of course, the Christian obligation to care for the ill often demands the imagination and creativity of medicine. Christians are called to care for one another through a multitude of means, including the appropriate use of medical technologies. Diseases that were once considered incurable have been treated through advancements in medicine and technology, which has spared countless people immeasurable pain and suffering. Christians should not fatalistically accept that there are limits to medicine and that some people are fated to suffer. There is a place for medical innovation in Christian bioethics, but medicine should never be seen as a replacement for other kinds of care Christians may offer one another. Christians ought never again to see the goal of medicine as the fulfillment of the Kingdom of God. Insofar as medicine enables a person to be who God calls her to be, then medicine is appropriate and even praiseworthy. We cannot assume medicine or medical technologies will always be appropriate, however. Weighing the benefits and burdens of any medical or technological intervention upon the human person will always be a necessary task. Given the medical community's propensity to overtreat or even force treatment upon persons with disabilities, theological bioethicists should be particularly careful when discussing the necessity of genetic technologies.

Salvation and Healing

We also should not confuse physical healing with salvation. The telos of the human life is communion with God. In the Christian narrative, God is not the securer of our health and well-being; rather, God is the one who relinquishes all power and security to live in solidarity with those who are suffering. God is not a faceless Other who fulfills our greatest desires but Jesus Christ, God incarnate, who suffers crucifixion. Any response to suffering and limitation must first call to mind the suffering God. Jürgen Moltmann warns, "Whether or not Christianity, in an alienated, divided and oppressive society, itself becomes alienated, divided, and an accomplice of oppression, is ultimately decided only by whether the crucified Christ is a stranger to it or the Lord who determines the form of its existence."[50] The crucified Christ calls the church to live differently in the world and to understand suffering in light of God's reconciling work on the cross. By humbling himself on the cross, Christ not only saves us, he also teaches us that our eternal security comes through powerlessness, self-surrender, and even suffering. A scandal to both the ancient and modern mind, in Christ's crucifixion, human perfection takes on new meaning (1 Cor. 1:18–25).

From the Christ narrative we learn that the primary threat of suffering is not the destruction of one's body but the alienation that accompanies and exacerbates suffering. Christ's cry on the cross is "God, my God, why have you forsaken me?" (Matt. 27:46; Ps. 22:1). The suffering of Christ occurs primarily in his alienation from the Father. As Karl Barth writes, "Here [on the cross] the alienation from God becomes an annihilating painful existence in opposition to Him. Here being in death becomes punishment, torment, outer darkness, the worm, the flame—all eternal as God himself."[51] Sin is perhaps more appropriately correlated with separation than suffering is; our sin separates us from God, from one another, and from the world.

Suffering as an element of finitude is experienced as evil and destructive only because we are already separated from God, but just as God takes up our finitude, God takes on our suffering. Rather than continue to alienate those who suffer, Moltmann implores, Christians need to come into solidarity with them. "Christian identification with the crucified necessarily brings [a person] into solidarity with the alienated of this world, with the dehumanized and the inhuman. But this solidarity becomes radical only if it imitates the identification of the crucified Christ with the abandoned, accepts the suffering of creative love, and is not led astray by its own dreams of omnipotence in an illusory future."[52] Solidarity with the suffering and alienated is an absolute demand on the church if it wishes to identify itself with the work of Christ. The Christian God does not promise an absence of suffering in this life but calls the Christian to model her life after Christ, suffering with those who suffer. If the Christian community wishes to bear witness to God's redemptive work, then it will need to model the patience, hospitality, and long-suffering that God revealed in Christ.

Our current Christian communities must become less concerned with individual health and instead recover a Christian conception of communal health. This is not to say individual disabilities should be overlooked; rather, caring for those with disabilities must be understood as a political and inherently eschatological act. Our current understanding of "health," which is a wholly individualized commodity, has obscured Christ's vision of God's Kingdom. In their examination of the intersections between medicine and Christianity, Joel Shuman and Keith Meador explain that "in the world of the acquisitive, self-interested individual, illness is a threat because it hinders the pursuit of individual goods. Sick people cannot work or enjoy the fruits of their work, and their sickness is typically understood as a burden to those who care for them, a burden that keeps the caregivers from working or enjoying the fruits of *their* work."[53] If the Christian community understands "health" as a communal endeavor, it should first question how to bring others, particularly those seen as "unhealthy," into the community to be loved and cared for. Rather than understanding the persistence of disability as a sign of the "not-yet-ness" of the Kingdom of God, the community that gathers around the person with disabilities and cares for her is itself a sign of the Kingdom to come as well as its alreadiness.

SCIENTIFIC CONSTRUCTIONS of the human person tend to focus on human "whatness," but Christian theology demands an accompanying "whoness" that is theocentrically determined. We know who we are as human persons only in light of God's action toward humanity. In opposition to contemporary secular debates about personhood, a Christian ontology of the human person points us toward the value of life beyond its capacity or abilities. From the creation narrative, we know that the lives of all human beings are gifts, which constitutes the donative nature of the human being. Through the Incarnation we can recognize that human nature (in all its fragility and limitation) is good, even though our sinfulness directs our wills away from God. To despise our nature would be to despise what God has given and the very nature to which God has promised ultimate communion through Christ's redeeming action. Finally, Christian eschatology leads us toward communal care as witnesses of God's Kingdom in the here and now. Living as witnesses to the Kingdom means recognizing all human persons as worthy of dignity and kinship. As sinful human beings, we tend to pervert our kinship with others and the earth. In response, the church must work to represent God's Kingdom to the world by first relinquishing power and control over our fate and turning toward being with God and others as its primary task.

By welcoming and including all persons into their communities, Christian churches have the opportunity to declare something vital about the worth of human life in its material and nonmaterial aspects, as well as in its actuality and potentiality. Against those who would situate God and the "supernatural" outside of mechanical human life, Christians know they are ontologically determined by a God who took on human form in order to be with humanity in its very nature. The church must assert that our genes are not the essence or defining feature of *who* we are and that even if genes contribute to *what* we are, we should not reduce all human whatness to genetics. We are finite material beings, but we are also creatures of God, which means we are more than mere material, and our DNA is no more sacred than the whole of human life. Christian churches have an opportunity to declare that humans are more than molecules, more than their particular capacities and deficiencies. Our genes are not the key to who we are: Christ is.

Within our current culture, genetic engineering presents itself as a double-edged sword, promising to relieve the suffering of many while simultaneously obstructing deeper conversations about the complexity surrounding genetic diseases and disabilities within human life. The geneticization of all physical difference may hinder our acceptance of persons with phenotypic variation. By focusing on curing abnormality, Christians often neglect the hospitable and patient care that is required of them. All too often, we deploy our techno-medico projects upon the bodies of those we assume suffer as a result of our cultural configurations and assumptions about personhood. If we allow ourselves to be carried away with the achievements of genetic testing and medicine, our good intentions may become weapons against persons with genetic variation (or their parents) when they consider options within health care institutions. As John Swinton warns, "Genetic technology . . . become[s] a conduit through which oppressive attitudes and values easily become embodied in practices that are eugenic in nature if not in intent."[54] We often have diagnoses in mind rather than people when we imagine the products of genetic engineering, precisely because we see people's whatness through the lens of technology. The church must have a constructive role in debates about genetic engineering, prioritizing compassionate care over diagnosis and technological therapies.

As discussed earlier in this chapter, genetic science may compel Christians to reevaluate some aspects of their theological ethics, but perhaps not in the way some churches originally imagined. The materialism and reductionism inherent in much of genetic science, coupled with medicine's focus on cure and the relief of suffering, have caused some people to question the personhood of humans with certain impairments. Unfortunately, Christians have been complicit in our culture's drive toward normalcy, so they stand under judgment with culture for failing to appreciate the dignity of all. To better serve all persons, Christians must reimagine the place of persons with disabilities within God's creation as well as within their own communities. Taking into account the doctrine of creation outlined in chapters 3 and 4, chapter 6 will reexamine the usefulness of natural law and natural theology within Protestant social ethics. A Christian understanding of natural law that takes history and culture seriously can help Christians discover their essential nature and how they must relate to others in order to fulfill the law of their own being.

CHAPTER SIX

The Limits of Natural Law
in Christian Genetics

In the early days of the Human Genome Project, the hopes and fears of theologians were primarily focused on the possible medical applications of human genetic research, but some also began to consider the potential for social discrimination as a result of genetic information. Envisioning such a prospect did not take great imagination, since the eugenics programs of the early twentieth century have now been largely condemned as discriminatory. The Center for Theology and the Natural Sciences at the Graduate Theological Union in Berkeley, California, which received one of the first grants awarded by the HGP's Ethical, Legal and Social Implications Research Program (ELSI), identified a number of religious and ethical issues likely to raise public concern, including genetic determinations of race (biological determinants of race and behavioral traits associated with race) and sexual orientation.[1] Ted Peters, director of the CTNS, recalls that theologians were concerned with how the HGP might positively or negatively affect discrimination against certain racial minorities and the LGBT community.[2] Many predicted the HGP would deconstruct the notion of biological "race" and its corresponding behavioral traits, which would make the public *less* likely to stereotype racial groups. Studies in the early 2000s, however, showed that the public overwhelmingly believes race is linked to genetics and many people use their understanding of genetics to explain intellectual and behavioral differences between the "races."[3]

Similarly, some theologians were optimistic that a genetic link to homosexuality might make the public more sympathetic to homosexual orientations because they were genetic and, therefore, not based on personal choice.[4] Many (including the Human Rights Commission) once thought detaching homosexuality from "choice" would be an effective antistigma campaign, but this assumption was misguided.[5] Studies show that even when homosexual and heterosexual orientations are framed as biologically caused and therefore immutable, negative attitudes about homosexuality remain.[6] Perhaps unsurprisingly, qualitative studies reveal that genetic explanations legitimize or strengthen people's psychological essentialist biases, even when genetic science ultimately shows that some constructs, like race, are scientifically indefensible.[7] The attempt to find the cause of homosexuality or the links between behavior and race betrays our cultural propensity to see gay and raced bodies as deviant, outside of the "normal" (white, straight) body. There remains a powerful presumption in our culture that our true, most essential self is biologically determined and that abnormal or deviant bodies are fated to be disruptive to social cohesion.

Interestingly, among the many concerns CTNS initially raised, the discrimination against persons with disabilities was not mentioned as a potential result of the HGP. For some, this might appear surprising given that discrimination against the mentally and physically "deficient" was at the heart of the eugenics movement. On the other hand, genetic research often presupposes that genetic "defects" should be prevented. James Watson, for example, describes genetic disabilities as "random tragedies that we should do everything in our power to prevent."[8] Intentional or not, disability discrimination can result when there is a proliferation of medical technologies aimed at curing genetic defects. Genetic indicators for disability, however, are rarely awarded the kind of social acceptance many sought for "gay genes." Whereas Peters imagined some might interpret a gay gene as biologically inherited and, therefore, part of "God's will" and a "gift," similar expectations were not held for disabilities linked to chromosomal anomalies, such as Down syndrome.[9] In fact, Peters also worried that if a gay gene were found, some might begin treating it as they do Down syndrome: namely, through abortion.[10]

The "able body" might be the most pervasive hegemonic fiction that exists within our culture. Chromosomal and genetic disabilities are so obviously bad and in need of remediation that they stand as the paradigm by which we judge the potential reactions to other forms of biological deviation. Peters's neglect of disability rights issues in genethics is indicative of a wider trend in mainline Protestantism, which does not see genetic discrimination against the disabled as akin to other forms of discrimination. Although most Christian bioethicists claim they are conscious of the dangers hidden in eugenics, few are willing to concede that their own genethics comes perilously close to a eugenic mind-set.

This chapter attempts to take the problem of disability discrimination seriously as it explores the nuances of a Christian genethic that is constructed from the ontological and metaphysical inferences garnered from the doctrine of creation presented in the previous two chapters. A Christian ethical approach to genetic technologies should take the classical Christian tradition seriously as the foundation for moral discernment. To show how theologians can incorporate their metaphysics and theologies into genethics, I first highlight what Protestants can learn from Roman Catholic conceptions of the natural law and how Tillich's insights will be especially helpful for constructing a thoroughly Protestant understanding of natural theology. Next, I show what natural law brings to the genetic engineering debates, particularly within Roman Catholic thought. Finally, I explore the limits of natural law for Protestants. There remains a place for natural law thinking within Protestantism, but natural law alone will not resolve the more complex ethical issues that arise in genethics.

ETHICS AND NATURAL LAW

In contemporary secular and theological debates about genetics and biotechnology, a kind of natural law thinking is often adopted. Many argue that certain technologies ought to be morally rejected because they interfere with God's creation, Mother Nature, or evolution. Conversely, others argue that the use of biomedical technologies coheres with God's intentions for humanity or is the extension of natural evolution. Some theologians believe they do not necessarily need to appeal to theology or scripture to make natural law arguments that will support or restrict the use of certain technologies. Instead, arguments that appeal to principles derived from human nature are encouraged because they appeal to unbelievers as well as believers.[11] The Protestant resistance to natural law and its claims to universal rational authority, however, is multifaceted and born out of an appropriate skepticism concerning whether ethics can come directly from nature, or, in Hume's construction, if an "ought" can be derived from an "is." As previously shown, the term *nature* has historically had many inconsistent definitions, so it is hard to know what we mean by *nature*, much less what moral obligations can be derived from nature.

Rather than begin with a vision of what nature or biology demands, Christians might begin with the doctrine of creation to form a coherent vision of the natural world, the human's place within it, and the duties and obligations humans have to themselves, each other, and the rest of creation. Clearly, a theological orientation toward nature will not automatically resist the oppressive power relations seen in the past, but using the narrative of creation as a starting point for moral reflection may help to orient Christians toward a theocentric understanding of the natural world and the moral obligations human persons have in and with creation.

For many Roman Catholics, and some Protestants, the moral evaluation of medical technologies can be informed by a theory of natural law. Within the context of medicine and the care of persons with genetic disabilities, natural law can be helpful insofar as it informs how we understand human nature, the ends of human life, and what constitutes deficiencies in the human body and mind. The appropriate or licit use of medicine will be to fix or ameliorate conditions that cause humans to deviate from their natural or normal state and disallow persons from achieving the goods of human life. If we think that people with certain genetic disabilities cannot achieve a particular good of human life, it will become imperative to develop technologies to correct their genetic disabilities. Our tolerance for certain bodies will be influenced by our understanding of what is proper to human nature.

Roman Catholic Conceptions of Natural Law

There are, of course, many versions of the natural law tradition that Christians may use to inform their understanding of human nature and moral obligations, but Aquinas's approach may be the longest-standing and most influential. Although it is beyond the scope of this chapter to describe Aquinas's understanding of the natural law in full detail, it is worth describing it in brief so that Protestant objections, particularly within the reformed tradition, can be better understood. For Aquinas, laws are rules and measures by which we are induced to act or restrained from acting.[12] The law is connected to reason because this is the way human actions and rules are judged. Aquinas believed there are four kinds of law: eternal, divine, natural, and human. The eternal law is law established by God in creation. Eternal law is identical to the mind of God, because God is the eternal creator and ruler of the world. The divine law is God's eternal law as it appears to humans, particularly through revelation. Divine laws are known through the Bible, particularly the Ten Commandments and the teachings of Jesus.[13] The natural law, on the other hand, is instilled in humans by the Creator so they can come to know God through natural reason.[14] Humans participate in the eternal law through natural law. Humans seek out their ends through their reason, which is why Aquinas believed reason is fundamental to human nature. Finally, human laws are laws devised by human reason (according to the natural law) and directed at particular communities for the promotion of the common good.

When discerning how to use medical technologies, Thomists view the natural law as particularly important because natural law helps humans to know what is good for them, or their "proper acts and ends."[15] For Aquinas, the first precept of the natural law is that good is to be done and evil is to be avoided.[16] Natural law, therefore, can be helpful in assessing whether genetic technologies are good for human beings. God gave little direction about the use of such technologies in the Bible, but God did instill in humans a desire for their own good; therefore, we can instinctively know what is good for us. For example, by way of the natural law humans are inclined to preserve their life, to know God, and to live in society.[17] When it comes to applying the general precepts of natural law to specific situations, however, humans can err. Everything we are inclined to is good in some respect, but not necessarily good *for us*. To apply general precepts of the natural law to specific cases, therefore, we must use our conscience. For Aquinas, our conscience is the application of knowledge to a particular case.[18] Even if we are naturally inclined to do good, our conscience can lead us to err or exert bad judgment because our reasoning is flawed. Moving from natural law to moral discernment, therefore, is no straightforward task, but one that requires that we properly understand the facts of a case, reason appropriately about that case, and form a good conscience through education and reflection on church teachings.[19]

Of course, Roman Catholics disagree on whether natural law is the best route to medical and sexual ethics and whether natural law is discernable through rationality alone. Many post–Vatican II moral theologians tried to move beyond natural law arguments, particularly as they related to the church's sexual ethic and the conclusions of *Humanae vitae* on contraception.[20] For those who remain committed to natural law theory, new natural law theologians have challenged whether natural law needs a theological foundation. Some of the so-called new natural law theorists, including Germain Grisez, John Finnis, and Joseph Boyle, believe that one can determine a list of a priori incommensurable goods by reflecting rationally on human nature, often without direct reference to God, divine commands, or human beings' chief end (*eudaimonia*).[21] Instead, practical reason recognizes a number of goods as self-evidently desirable for human beings. Morality thus consists in deliberating on which goods one ought to pursue when faced with a choice between them. Adherents of the new natural law theory (NNLT) propose that they can resolve moral controversies in, among other things, beginning-of-life ethics (e.g., abortion, embryo research, and contraception) through rational argument without invoking the Roman Catholic moral tradition specifically.

New natural law theory has been critiqued on many fronts. First, classic natural law theorists claim one cannot derive an "ought" from an "is" without first having an understanding of human nature.[22] According to classical natural law, the goods that ought to be pursued are those that are conducive to the flourishing of that being's nature. In human beings' case, that good is *eudaimonia*. New natural law theorists, however, argue that the basic goods of human nature are self-evident using practical reason. In other words, one does not need to infer the truth about human nature to know what is good for human beings. Along those same lines, without a theological anthropology, some believe NNLT fails to appreciate that friendship with God should be the highest good for humans.[23] Instead, NNLT proposes that the goods of human life are incommensurable. Other critics believe NNLT is overly optimistic about what moral norms can be deduced from rationality and what kind of moral consensus can be achieved through rational argument.[24]

A critic of NNLT, Jean Porter develops a theological account of natural law that offers an alternative to the notion that moral norms can be discerned rationally and offered universally. Instead, Porter describes natural law as bound to its cultural, theological, and social context, just as all rational inquiry is reflective of its particular socio-historical context.[25] Porter believes natural law, particularly as it was developed in the twelfth and thirteenth centuries, was inherently theological and not purely rational.[26] Clearly, such debates between natural law theorists are beyond the scope of this book, but as Protestants look to whether natural law might ever be useful within their own bioethics, it is important to note that there are multiple natural law theories to engage, even within the Roman Catholic tradition.

Protestant Conceptions of Natural Law

When discerning our ethical obligations, as well as the content of the virtuous life, many Protestants believe the Bible is an (if not *the*) authoritative document for God's revelation of the moral order to humans. While humans may have been able to discern the moral order in their prelapsarian state, human desire, will, and knowledge are now too damaged to know the good or to carry it out. More optimistic about practical rationality, Thomists generally believe the natural law is knowable apart from the biblical witness, but some believe there is biblical warrant for a theocentric and teleological account of natural law theory and that the Bible is a helpful aid in discerning the natural law. According to Matthew Levering, the Bible helps us to connect "the wisdom inscribed in the created order" to Torah, to the Word.[27] From the biblical story we learn that God created with a teleological ordering in which God's eternal law draws creation to Godself. Divine commands and natural law are, therefore, not in competition. Divine law is God's revelation to humanity, which articulates God's wisdom through God's providential plan. Humans participate in God's plan for creation through the natural law and our use of reason. The problem with many natural law theories today, Levering believes, is that they have become anthropocentric and ordered toward "arbitrary power rather than wisdom."[28] Apart from the biblical witness, natural law becomes the construction of human will (which gives too high a status to autonomy) and not divine will. Other Thomist scholars, such as Eugene Rogers, further elaborate on why the natural law does not stand independently of other sources of knowledge. Taking a more historical and metaphysical approach, Rogers believes Aquinas invites us to supplement natural law with biblical interpretation as well as the virtues, empirical facts about the world, and the faith community.[29]

Rogers's conception of natural law as coextensive with the Bible, understood through wise interpreters, received by the priesthood of all believers, and informed by our experience of the natural world (including our bodies) will likely be more appealing to many Protestants than any independent ethical account built upon practical reason alone. Although there are many different kinds of Protestants and it is impossible to summarize a Protestant position on any particular issue, in general, Protestants have a much more devastating account of the effects of the Fall than Roman Catholics. Many Protestants, particularly those influenced by the early reformers, such as Calvin and Luther, acknowledge that humans were naturally inclined toward harmony with the eternal law in the Garden of Eden but say this inclination has been marred by sin. Both our intellect and our desires have been corrupted as a result of the Fall, and we can no longer trust our natural instincts to lead us toward God. Protestants, therefore, are much less likely than their Roman Catholic counterparts to refer back to the Garden when conceptualizing the goods of human life; instead, they look to the Kingdom of God as the fulfillment of human nature and the telos of human life. Made in the image of God, human beings have a special status that awaits fulfillment in the Kingdom. Humans do not simply have an ideal nature to which they must aspire; they anticipate their fulfillment in the new creation. Special revelation and grace are primary if we wish to make sense of the goals of human life.

Calvin had a place for some forms of natural knowledge of God; however, he did not believe natural knowledge of God was tremendously instructive in matters of morality. Without God's grace, we cannot grasp God's infinite love as displayed in the cross, which is crucial for discernment in ethics. For Calvin, conscience, or "the law written on the heart," is a general grace given to all persons by God. The human conscience "responds to God's judgment" and is a "sign of the immortal spirit."[30] In other words, the conscience primarily refers to the relationship between the individual and God. Our conscience can judge us, but moral judgments are not enhanced by a deeper understanding of nature. Instead, to know what we should do in any given situation, we must form a deeper comprehension of God's intentions for humanity, which we understand in part through the doctrine of creation and through special revelation.[31]

Karl Barth likewise dismisses moral natural law as a dangerous reliance on human reason, which places human philosophy over God's revealed Word. For Barth, God has become hidden from us after original sin. As a result of the Fall, our reason is clouded by sin and we are inclined toward malice. The only access we have to God as Creator is in revelation, mainly biblical revelation. Barth was particularly concerned that the pro-Hitler members of the German Church Movement relied upon a moral natural law theory that Lutherans called the "order of creation."[32] Barth did not reject the idea that there is order within creation, but he did not believe humans could perceive it outside of the grace of God as revealed in the Word.[33] With Calvin, Barth believed we might be able to intuit something about God using our reason, but this would not be the Christian God, who can be known only through faith. The specific content of our morality, particularly as it relates to the moral use of medicine, simply cannot be discerned from nature.

The only way to discern moral precepts from nature is to first agree on what nature is, and in the modern world there is considerable disagreement on this front. Moreover, there is no longer agreement that nature is a realm shaped by final causes, much less final causes oriented toward a higher moral good. Our belief about God the Creator must precede our interpretation of the world. Hume's contention that we cannot derive an "ought" from an "is" appears insurmountable, particularly when we are trying to make publicly defensible arguments about morality. Nature, apart from special revelation, cannot tell us whether it is right or wrong to edit our genome, create embryos outside the womb, or abort disabled fetuses.

Barth's contention that natural law arguments have been used to defend unethical, discriminatory practices is undeniable. There are many facts about the world that our culture takes for granted, such as the objective categories of disease and disability, which some theologians contend are "in reality artifacts of cultural traditions."[34] From the German support of Hitler to the justification of racial hierarchies to the degradation of women as inferior humans, it is hard to deny that natural law arguments (Christian or otherwise) have been used to justify unethical social structures and practices.

Even with the aid of the biblical witness and God's grace, however, there will still be disagreements concerning the moral use of genetic technologies. As discussed previously, Aquinas believed the human conscience could err when attempting to apply general principles to specific questions. Aquinas believed that to discern virtue and vice, we need the aid of wise people who are guided by their interpretation of nature and a community informed by scripture.[35] For this reason, Aquinas himself makes room for debate when interpreters of natural law and the Bible come into conflict. Wise people will continue to dispute how to interpret the book of scripture and the book of nature. When it comes to understanding the nature of disability, there seems to be considerable dispute between biblical commentators as well as those who desire to make sense of disability using a natural law account.[36] One may argue that when we read the biblical stories of Jesus healing the sick, the plain sense of scriptures tells us that certain kinds of "sickness" (e.g., blindness, paraplegia, deafness) hinder one's relationship to God and are naturally evil, or at least deficient. Of course, the literal sense of Scripture that is often used to interpret these texts is a class of readings but not the only valid interpretation.[37] Other biblical commentators have pointed out the ways in which the healing narratives bring persons ostracized from community back into relationship. By attending to the restoration of social bonds, Jesus is doing the work of healing broken communities.[38]

To discern moral virtue, or the moral use of a medical technology, we need wise interpreters to help us understand what counts as justice, what counts as natural, what goods should be sought above the others, and what scripture says. When wise interpreters debate the proper understanding of human nature with regard to disability, the most appropriate interpretation of the healing narratives, and the best model for understanding health, disease, and disability, it becomes less clear how we ought to approach the care of persons with genetic disabilities. If, as some presume, genetic conditions that result in disability are always a privation in nature, then our response to these genetic "defects" will be to prevent or cure them, unless there is some other competing good that clearly must take priority. If, however, genetic disabilities are not inherently against human nature and do not render a human a nonperson, then our moral obligations toward people with these disabilities are not so clear-cut. We might look toward a cure, but a cure is not demanded for the sake of justice. Therefore, the Christian response to genetic disability ultimately depends on upstream debates over interpretations of scripture and conceptions of nature.

Tillich on Natural Law

The task of Protestant theologians is to explain how their own version of moral theology, shaped by the natural law, scripture, the tradition, and the wisdom of experience, can be used to evaluate genetic technologies. Most Protestants will concede that there is harmony between the moral order and the cosmic order by virtue of God's eternal law and goodness, but Protestants are wary of any claims that humans can discern the natural law using their practical reason. This is not to suggest, however, that Protestants must then reject any Christian ethics that relies upon any metaphysical foundation, particularly ones built upon the doctrine of creation.

Paul Tillich's version of natural law might look more palatable to liberal Protestants who wish to reunite ethics and metaphysics in their theology. Tillich affirms the classic natural law position but adds to it an account of historical and cultural context while maintaining his reliance on metaphysics. Although Tillich recognizes the many criticisms of using metaphysics as a resource for ethics, he believes ethics and metaphysics are both oriented to the Unconditional moving within culture. Theologian George Lindbeck argues that Tillich strengthens the classic natural law position because he is able to specify the "good act" more often than natural law's traditional formulations; he appreciates "the basic positive emphases of Catholicism and of Reformation Protestantism," and he is able to avoid what some have termed the "naturalistic fallacy."[39] Lindbeck's list of Tillich's "improvements" to natural law are certainly debatable, but Lindbeck is correct that Tillich both affirms and expands upon traditional natural law thinking in a thoroughly Protestant way.

Tillich avoids the naturalistic fallacy by reversing the order of the "is/ought" distinction—he begins with the obligatory and then moves to the natural. Tillich believes that what we acknowledge as *absolutely normative* belongs to our essential nature. Natural laws, in other words, are those that come from our internal compulsions. Crucially, Tillich derives this thinking from his doctrine of creation. "Natural law, according to classical doctrine, is the law which is implied in man's essential nature. It has been given in creation, it has been lost by 'the fall,' it has been restated by Moses and Jesus (there is no difference between natural and revealed law in Bible and classical theology). The restatement of the natural law was, at the same time, its formalization and its concentration into one all-embracing law, the 'Great commandment,' the commandment of love."[40] Like Aquinas,

Tillich believes natural law coheres with divine law, but after the Fall we can no longer rationally discern the divine law without grace. We have become estranged from our essential nature, and in this state no perfect moral act is possible. After the Fall, we can and should obey the divine commandments, but unless we carry them out with joy, they have not been fulfilled. We find ourselves in a paradoxical situation: the law is imposed on us externally, and yet we are asked to unite ourselves willfully with what it commands. Only through grace can we overcome this paradox to find joy in the divine law. Only through grace can we overcome the split between "what we are and what we ought to be."[41]

Tillich advocates for a dynamic morality that resists absolute authority, but he also believes humans have an essential nature that imposes a sense of morality upon them. Morality, as given by God, is unconditional. The moral imperative is not imposed upon us but is the law of our own being. In other words, God's eternal law is built into the human conscience. Because we are estranged from our true natures as a result of the Fall, however, we struggle to fulfill the law of our own being. Yet unlike God's eternal law, human authorities (e.g., political or religious authorities, traditions, or conventions) are conditioned and relative; they are not morality in its pure form. The ways we operationalize the moral imperative, our concrete ethics, are "moralisms," which are conditional and so do not present us with absolute authority. Tillich describes the difference between the Catholic and Protestant teaching on natural law as follows: "Catholicism believes that the natural law has definite contents, which are unchangeable and are authoritatively stated by the Church (e.g., the fight of the Roman Church against birth control). Protestantism, on the other hand . . . determined the contents of the natural law largely by ethical traditions and conventions; but this is done without a supporting theory, and therefore Protestantism has the possibility of a dynamic concept of natural law."[42] Without an authoritative body that discerns how the natural law applies to specific questions over time, such as the Roman Catholic magisterium, Protestants practice a risky morality. Whereas a morality that subjects itself to an unconditional authority is safe, it is also suspect because the church (just like all other systems or ethical authorities) is not absolute.

This is not to suggest, however, that Protestants have no basis on which to understand the eternal law or the law of being. Protestants have the divine commands within scripture, which have an onto-logical basis. According to Tillich we can begin to understand the law of our nature, the eternal law, through the concepts of love, power, and justice. For Tillich, the demands of love, power, and justice have an ontological character—they characterize what it means *to be* as God created us; they are as old as being itself. Power is the vital strength of being and forms the social life as justice, which unites in love. In turn, "Life is being in actuality and love is the moving power of life."[43] Being cannot be actualized without love, which drives every-thing together. Although we are separated from ourselves, each other, and God as a result of the Fall, love drives us toward reunion. Again, we learn from the doctrine of creation that we are not essentially sepa-rated, because if we were, no reunion would be possible. "Without an ultimate belongingness no union of one thing with another can be conceived."[44] Tillich's emphasis on the drive to overcome separation is different from Aristotle's vision of the striving toward actualizing one's own potentialities. In Tillich's scheme, "All natural laws can be subsumed under the law of love."[45]

On this point, Augustine and Aquinas might agree with Tillich. Aquinas also saw creaturely activity as arising from the desire for union with God.[46] Love for Tillich is not simply an emotion but an ontological concept that provides normative moral guidance. Love allows us to seek and discern justice, "the form adequate to reuniting love."[47] In other words, justice gives form to the encounter of beings. When one inappropriately uses power over and against another, in-justice occurs and love is prevented. Just as we become who we are through the power of being and reunion in love, we become who we ought to be by encountering and accepting the Other. Here Tillich follows Martin Buber, "There is no other way of becoming an 'I' than by meeting a Thou and accepting him as such."[48] The demand to accept the Other is true in our relationship with God, other humans, and even creation. Even trees can place demands on us for justice when we attribute worth to their very existence.[49]

The prioritization of love, power, and justice as ontological real-ties begins to give shape to our moral commitments as well as to what it takes to help one another flourish. These ontological realities, however, do not provide precise normative guidance in complex situations, as we might need in discerning how best to use genetic technologies. For this we need moral wisdom and experience, which come from living within culture and participating in the church—both of which I will explore in the next two chapters. Instead, what Tillich provides is a general principle that unless an action is clearly for the greater good it is "unjust to endanger the unifying functions of a society by violating the positive laws and customs—the established social, political, cultural, and economic arrangements—which are the warp and woof of the unity which it fosters."[50] Although this might sound like a rather conservative standard, Tillich radicalizes this ethic by adding to it the natural law ethic of just love, which goes beyond proportional justice or positive law. Tillich calls this "transforming or creative justice," which has its fulfillment in the Kingdom of God.[51] The form of this justice is most clearly expressed by divine forgiveness. God transforms justice, asking us to approximate God's creative justice in our own interactions. When we act out of love, we internalize the external law, which authenticates and enhances our very being. "Every valid ethical commandment is an expression of man's essential relation to himself, to others and to the universe. This alone makes it obligatory and its denial self-destructive."[52] This kind of divine love and transformative justice cannot be effectively written into the law, but insofar as we are able, we are commanded to represent the Kingdom ethic here on earth, because it creates the possibility for justice and reunites all individuals with their true and essential selves, which is the fulfillment of our primal being or that which God originally intended for us.[53] Kingdom justice, or, as Tillich calls it, "theonomous ethics," in other words, is etched into the structure of the universe. As I will show in subsequent chapters, theonomous ethics places a radical demand for charity and hospitality toward others.

THE USE OF NATURAL LAW IN GENETHICS

In general, Roman Catholic theologians have had an easier time than Protestants applying their own theological method, including natural law, to ethical dilemmas presented in certain genetic technologies. As explored in chapter 1, the magisterium has traditionally maintained that science and medicine offer important goods to society but can also produce technologies that transgress natural law and dominate human beings. In response to advances in genetic science and developments in genetic technologies, the magisterium has reiterated its sexual ethic. As outlined in *Humanae vitae,* the magisterium teaches that each conjugal act must be both unitive and procreative. This means that couples cannot use artificial contraception or sterilization and cannot create embryos outside of the conjugal act (as happens in in vitro fertilization). The Congregation for the Doctrine of the Faith (CDF) reiterates this teaching in *Donum vitae:* "Various procedures now make it possible to intervene not only in order to assist, but also to dominate the processes of procreation. These techniques enable man to 'take in hand his own destiny,' but they also expose him 'to the temptation to go beyond the limits of a reasonable dominion over nature.' They might constitute progress in the service of man, but they also involve serious risks."[54] The CDF affirms that "scientific research and applied research constitute a significant expression of this dominion over creation" but says scientific research and its applications are not "morally neutral."[55] The CDF rejects technologies that override the natural goods of the human being (e.g., procreative functions) and any experimentation that overrides the rights of individuals, which includes embryos.[56] For this reason, the magisterium has maintained nontherapeutic experimentation on early-stage embryos to be morally illicit.[57]

Catholic sexual ethics, however, will not resolve all the ethical dilemmas presented in human genetic engineering. For example, while the magisterium has forbidden embryonic stem cell research, it has not condemned all forms of genetic manipulation for therapeutic reasons. In his "Address on Medical Ethics and Genetic Manipulation," Pope John Paul II stated, "A strictly therapeutic intervention having the objective of healing various maladies—such as those stemming from chromosomal deficiencies—will be considered in principle as desirable, provided that it tends to real promotion of the personal well-being of man, without harming his integrity or worsening his life conditions. Such intervention actually falls within the logic of the Christian moral tradition."[58] John Paul II believes the suffering caused by genetic anomalies should be prevented when the technology to do so is morally licit. In theory, both somatic and germline therapies could help to correct genetic defects without the destruction of embryos. Somatic gene therapy, which involves introducing new genetic material into the somatic cells of a patient, is not illicit in principle. Theologian William E. May notes, "Somatic gene therapy raises problems similar to those proposed by other forms of treatment. Such therapy is morally warranted as long as the risks posed by this new type of therapy are not significant when compared with the reasonable expectation that employment of such therapy will indeed bring great benefit to the patient."[59]

Germ-line therapy, on the other hand, introduces new genetic material into cells that produce reproductive cells, which means that genetic alternations are inherited by future generations. In *Dignitas personae*, the CDF prohibits germ-line therapies because of their potential to harm progeny and because they are often used in conjunction with IVF.[60] Of course, it may one day be possible to perform germ-line therapies without IVF. May argues, "Such therapy is *not* to be regarded in any way as intrinsically evil. It is simply that at present . . . it would be better to leave it alone."[61] If, however, germ-line therapies became more beneficial and less risky (as they likely will become using CRISPR), then they might one day be morally permissible.[62]

The Catholic Church also acknowledges moral permissibility of prenatal testing and counseling as long as they are not done to determine whether to abort a fetus.[63] In *Donum vitae* the CDF writes, "[Genetic] diagnosis is permissible, with the consent of the parents after they have been adequately informed, if the methods employed safeguard the life and integrity of the embryo and the mother, without subjecting them to disproportionate risks . . . [but] this diagnosis is gravely opposed to the moral law when it is done with the thought of possibly inducing an abortion."[64] Similarly, *Ethical and Religious Directives for Catholic Health Care* (ERDs) notes, "Prenatal diagnosis is permitted when the procedure does not threaten the life or physical integrity of the unborn child or the mother and does not subject them to disproportionate risks; when the diagnosis can provide information to guide preventative care for the mother or pre- or postnatal care for the child; and when the parents, or at least the mother, give free and informed consent. Prenatal diagnosis is not permitted when undertaken with the intention of aborting an unborn child with a serious defect."[65]

The US Conference of Catholic Bishops acknowledges that prenatal diagnosis can be useful for parents who may need to prepare to care for a disabled child. Directive 54 of the ERDs goes on to suggest that genetic counseling can promote responsible parenthood. This recalls Pius XII's declaration that some people may use genetic testing to determine they ought not to have children. "Certainly it is right, and in the greater number of cases it is a duty, to point out to those whose heredity is beyond doubt very defective, the burden they are about to impose upon themselves, upon their marriage partner, and upon their offspring. The burden might perhaps become unbearable. To advise against, however, is not to forbid."[66] Genetic testing, particularly when done before marriage, may help persons to discern whether they should procreate.

Clearly, Roman Catholics, like most Protestants, recognize the difficulty of making blanket statements about the moral uses of a number of genetic technologies. With the exception of technologies that involve reproduction outside the conjugal act, many Catholics and Protestants share a concern that genetic technologies be considered in the context of their use and that the potential benefits of the technologies be weighed against their risks. What is largely absent from these considerations, however, is how these technologies come to bear on the lives of persons with disabilities. This is not to say Roman Catholic and Protestant churches have not thought about how to create welcoming spaces for persons with disabilities, but most churches have not consistently related their teachings on biotechnology with their teachings on disability.

As technologies advance, however, such considerations may become more pressing. New advances in fetal surgery, for example, such as those that attempt to correct spina bifida, raise new questions about the acceptable risks a woman may endure to prevent having a child with a disability. In weighing the benefits-to-burdens ratio of a fetal operation that is used to correct a mostly nonfatal disability, theologians will need to be clear about the kinds of burdens a disability like spina bifida places on a person's life more generally and what sorts of risks are acceptable to prevent people from living with disabilities. Should we allow parents to be the sole decision makers in instances where correcting genetic disabilities poses serious risks to a fetus's health? Are such procedures eugenic? Does allowing for a high level of risk in fetal surgery implicitly support a culture of discrimination against those with particular disabilities? Catholic and Protestant bioethicists should begin probing more deeply into whether the technologies they support participate in discriminatory practices.

Beyond Natural Law

Christians' moral evaluations of genetic technologies can begin—but must not end—with natural law. Although natural law can provide a normative structure in ethics, discerning the morality of an action typically requires Christians to go beyond natural law considerations. For Aristotle, the moral life is composed of three parts. The first is the natural tendency or telos on which life is based, which is grounded in the biology of a particular kind of being. As discussed, Christians know from the doctrine of creation that we are tied to the earth, meant to live in community, and destined to be with God forever. Next, humans have moral virtue, which comes from practiced habits. Finally, humans need practical wisdom, which comes through study and experience and involves a more sophisticated application of the virtues to particular quandaries. Richard Sherlock provides a helpful example of the relationship between the threefold structure of the moral life: some members of the human species kill other members of their species. By nature, humans live together in organized groups, so killing members of one's group appears dangerous and unnatural. The human capacity for freedom, however, indicates we must refer to more than biology to define the moral life. We must also be reared and trained not to murder (particularly one's enemies) and to recognize that flourishing is enabled when we do not have to worry about our physical safety.

Natural impulses and habituation, however, do not necessarily tell us how to care for a community member who is disabled. Questions central to bioethics and questions of genetic engineering are best answered with practical wisdom that considers respect to the other, "in the right way, at the right time, to the right person, in the right amount."[67] Practical wisdom in situations where the use of genetic technologies is being considered is certainly needed but is critically lacking in many religious communities. For Aristotle and Aquinas, wisdom is not a calculative science but a deliberative one and requires that we know more than simply the dilemma presented in the abstract. Virtue ethics, as expressed by Aristotle and Aquinas, can include deontological and utilitarian considerations.[68] In Roman Catholic theology, the morality of an act (except intrinsically evil acts) depends on the object of the act, its end, and the circumstances in which the act is performed.[69] Celia Deane-Drummond argues that a recovery of Thomistic virtue ethics and its emphasis on wisdom and prudence might help us to reimagine the debates on genetics from within the Christian tradition.[70]

A recovery of virtue ethics, combined with Tillich's ontological categories of love, power, and justice, might enable us to think differently about how we approach difficult moral dilemmas present in genetic engineering. Virtue, as Aquinas described it, encourages a change in attitude and moral character in one's everyday experience. Love and justice, while essential to the human being, have been obscured as a result of the Fall and may need to be cultivated in the moral life. To the categories of love and justice we might want to add Aquinas's intellectual virtue of wisdom. For Aquinas, the three intellectual virtues were "wisdom," "understanding," and "science."[71] Aquinas understood science as knowledge derived from demonstrated conclusions. Understanding is the habit that perfects the intellect in consideration of the truth.[72] Wisdom, which is given priority, "considers the highest and deepest causes."[73] Wisdom, however, can only be received "from the outpouring of the Holy Spirit,"[74] so it is always shrouded in some mystery. Still, wisdom can and should direct human life.

Wisdom must be paired with the virtue of prudence, or practical wisdom, in moral matters. Prudence helps set the particular way a virtue should be expressed, or the "mean" of a virtue in varying circumstances.[75] Although humans may begin moral deliberation with the use of natural reason, we will still need deliberative prudence in the process of our moral judgments. For Aquinas, prudence is not just about individual moral agents but has a political dimension as well. Tillich and Aquinas acknowledge that justice must serve as a guiding principle in our interactions with others because we are social animals who tend toward union with others.

The desire to know God and the ultimate causes of the universe represents the contemplative side of wisdom, whereas the desire to act rightly in accordance with God's will represents the practical side of wisdom. Both Aquinas and Tillich believed metaphysics and ethics are never completely separate endeavors, because they represent the desire for wisdom. Practical decision-making in the use of technologies, then, is an extension of a Christian account of metaphysics as told through the story of creation. In the next chapter, I show how the cultivation of wisdom is taken up in the practical sphere and how the experience of disability will be necessary for the development of wisdom in the Christian tradition.

A CLOSE EXAMINATION of the nuances of Tillich and Aquinas's moral theology reveals how fundamentally different their understanding of the human person and ethics is from that of secular bioethics. Even when Christian bioethicists and secular bioethicists can agree on certain policies or cases, their underlying rationales are often quite different. Love, justice, and power, for example, have particular meanings for Tillich that do not coincide easily with what most secular philosophers or politicians mean when they use the same words. For both Aquinas and Tillich, there is something fundamental or ontologically true about human persons that demands we treat one another with respect and love. As I will show in the next chapter, this ontological orientation toward love and just communion with others should profoundly change our orientation toward persons with disabilities. Persons are valued, not for what they can contribute to society, but because of who they essentially are. In the following chapters, I radicalize this thinking even further by arguing that Christians ought to *prioritize* the experience of persons with disabilities when deliberating on human nature and the ethical life. Liberal democracies often pride themselves on allowing for voices of the marginalized to be heard before moving toward consensus; however, the Christian Church must go further in care for the marginalized, not merely listening to persons with disabilities but centralizing their concerns, experiences, and wisdom. As the next two chapters will show, the wisdom of persons who live with disabilities can transform, not merely inform, genetic policies and the liturgical life of the church.

CHAPTER SEVEN

Practical, Embodied Wisdom

In 2018, a group of scientists gathered at the Second International Summit on Human Genome Editing "to advance the global dialogue . . . by bringing together a broad range of stakeholders."[1] Over five hundred "researchers, ethicists, policymakers, representatives from scientific and medical academics, patient group representatives, and others from around the world" came together to discuss the benefits, risks, and implications of human genome editing.[2] Notably absent from the group of stakeholders, however, were disability rights activists, despite the fact that the organizers of the previous summit had been criticized for not inviting members of the disability community. After the first summit, sociologist Ruha Benjamin remarked that the summit gave "the illusion of opening up science . . . something that appears public but really is meant to insulate the science."[3] By not inviting members of the disability community, who are often critical of gene editing, Benjamin and others claimed the summit had not truly been inclusive of disparate voices in the debate.

Of pressing concern for both international summits was the advancement of CRISPR-Cas9 (or CRISPR for short), which allows parents to avoid passing on incurable genetic diseases to their offspring through gene editing of their embryos and can be used to alter the genes of adults.[4] Like many gene-editing techniques, CRISPR has implications for persons living with disabilities as well as their care-takers, many of whom believe it represents a modern-day eugenics, which impedes disability equity.[5] Such viewpoints, however, are often dismissed by the scientific and bioethics communities as extreme or biased. Embodied experience is rarely sufficient for moral expertise in modern society, but by refusing to include the voices of persons with disabilities, summit organizers overlooked important moral considerations. At neither the first nor the second summit on human genome editing were issues of ableism or discrimination discussed.

Christian bioethics, as both an academic discipline and a practice, also risks overlooking important critiques of genetic technologies when it fails to consider disability theorists and activists as important conversation partners. Christian churches and theologians have typically not prioritized or even included the voices of people living with genetic disabilities within their moral deliberations on genetic technologies. As churches and theologians consider how best to care for persons with disabilities and parents making reproductive decisions, the insights of the disability community must be taken seriously.

In recent years, most mainline denominations have carefully crafted statements and policies on the treatment and value of persons with disabilities, but few have related those statements to the use of medical technologies.[6] Although it may be too much to ask denominations to reply swiftly to advancements in medical technologies, when denominational commissions meet to discuss issues pertinent to the disability community, people with disabilities ought to be included. A theological bioethics that refuses to engage the embodied experience of disability risks producing superficial or self-serving solutions to the moral challenges posed by genetic technologies. When discussing issues that affect persons with disabilities in particular, Christians have a moral obligation to engage people with disabilities to see what insights might be gleaned from their experience.

In this chapter, I argue that the wisdom necessary to discern how best to use genetic technologies must incorporate insights from persons with various disabilities and their allies. An understanding of the experience of genetic disability will be crucial for Christians who wish to provide guidance on the use of genetic technologies. To show why the experiences of persons with disability ought to be attended to, I first expose the perils of ignoring the experience of disability in medicine and bioethics. Unfortunately, it is all too common to find bioethicists, both secular and religious, ignoring or outright dismissing the needs of persons with disabilities in the name of the "common good." Next, I describe why the cultivation of wisdom in the Christian tradition requires Christians to examine disability experiences when considering the use of genetic technologies. Finally, I explore alternative understandings of the human person offered by disability theorists and theologians and how they might influence our evaluation of certain technologies.

Disability and Genethics within Bioethics

Theologians who engage in genethics will need to understand the debates already occurring in the field of bioethics to find points of commonality and departure. Certain groups of people, such as scholars and community leaders, may help to enrich theologians' understanding of what is at stake in genethics debates. In their early days, both disability activists and bioethicists critiqued the power and paternalism of the medical establishment, but their different reactions to the HGP split their agendas. The bioethical support of genetic interventions and bioethicists' lack of awareness of the causes and social constructions of disability caused a lasting rift between the two communities. When formulating their ethical reflections on genetic technologies, Christian ethicists should not make the mistake of secular bioethics and ignore the important critiques of these technologies arising from within the disability community.

The basic metaphysical orientation of genetic science does not easily align with Christian understandings of the human person or the doctrine of creation. In modern biomedical science, scientific inquiries are expected to lead to technological advances that prevent human suffering, so discovering what it means to be human is often accompanied by the development of technologies that reduce human vulnerability. Thus it is not surprising that one of the promises of the

HGP was that it would lead to cures for numerous diseases that plague the human condition. Within this frame, genetic conditions that cause disability are seen as undesirable and in need of amelioration. Persons whose suffering cannot be "fixed" risk being eliminated from our moral projects altogether.

There are at least two consequences of genetic medicine's approach to the body for persons with genetic disabilities. First, the HGP works to normalize certain human characteristics while rendering others "abnormal." Mapping the genome assumed a healthy human genome that can be measured against genetic "defects." Persons whose bodies or genes do not measure up to the norm are thus further medicalized and scrutinized. Second, the HGP created a biopolitical response in which one's current and future health, as well as the health of one's offspring, must be managed and controlled. Although genetic technologies are promoted as value-neutral tools that are optional in health care, the use of such tools is increasingly seen as standard medical care. Without scrutinizing or even acknowledging the metaphysics of genetic medicine, secular and theological bioethicists alike have supported and at times even demanded the use of genetic technologies in the name of health and justice. Rather than helping to expand the vision of human diversity, the HGP helped to further stigmatize persons whose genes fall short of the imagined norm.

"Normal Genes" and "Normal People"

The purpose of the HGP was twofold: to find out what makes humans special (i.e., how we are genetically different from other animals) and to create a general reference against which we can compare individual DNA.[7] From its very inception, the HGP was forced to make certain judgments about "the" human genome so it could be used as a reference guide for detecting genetic abnormality. "The" human genome is of course a compilation of many individuals' genes, but the project of mapping the genome assumes that a normative genome can be found. The philosopher Christine Hauskeller explains, "[The Human Genome] project necessarily results in an idealized reference from which only questionable conclusions can be drawn about genomic species differences. In order to find genomic sequences that are 'not normal,' presuppositions of what a healthy normal human is and what her genome consists of are required. Any such reference genome, therefore, has to be healthy and biologically 'pure,' which is impossible because 'the' human genome is only the product of contemporary knowledge of what is healthy and normal."[8] Genetic variation within a species was considered abnormal from the outset of the HGP. Scientists now know, however, that polymorphisms (normal genetic variations that do not adversely affect individuals) are common in the general population.[9] Researchers have also become concerned that the genomes being analyzed in the HGP were not necessarily representative of the wider population. The National Institute of Health's All of Us research program began in 2015 as a way to gather genetic data from at least one million people, particularly from communities of color and those in lower income brackets.[10] Scientists hope the data gathered from the All of Us program will enable physicians to tailor medical treatment plans to individuals within subpopulations. Yet this research is unlikely to increase tolerance for genetic diversity as it relates to disabilities. Treatments for genetic disabilities will incorporate other sociodemographic characteristics, but what counts as a "defect" remains unchanged. Discovering what makes us human does not seem to have expanded the scientific vision of what constitutes human normality.

Taking up this genetic logic, many bioethicists also assume that deviations from the "normal" genome are problematic for individuals and for society. Bioethicists tend to see disability (whether genetic, congenital, or caused by injury) as an individual, medical, and undesirable problem to be eradicated. The medico-scientific episteme is so powerful that even the direct testimony of persons with disabilities about their experiences, quality of life, and needs (medical or otherwise) is often disregarded. The philosopher Miranda Fricker has described this phenomenon as "testimonial injustice," in which the members of a specific marginalized group are seen as lacking credibility.[11] For example, even though there is ample evidence that people with disabilities rank their quality of life equal to those without disabilities, these accounts are often ignored or undermined by clinicians and bioethicists.[12]

After acknowledging that people with disabilities often rate their quality of life as high, bioethicist Jonathan Glover notes, "Disadvantage can itself shape people's preferences" and deems "the satisfaction of scaled-down preferences" as a form of false consciousness.[13] Like many bioethicists, Glover assumes that disability is bad and that any evidence to the contrary must be due to the unreliability of the persons providing the account of their lived experience. Assuming that people with disabilities are untrustworthy narrators, Glover goes on to dismiss the links between eugenics and genetic screening, noting that the parental choice to abort because of the presence of a genetic disability is an act of "compassion" and not gene pool strengthening. Similarly, after noting that some studies show persons with disabilities rating their quality of life equal to and sometimes even higher than that of nondisabled people, bioethicist Dan Brock calls this a problem of "adaptive preferences."[14] Brock compares disabled people who report a high quality of life to slaves who may report being happy but in fact have an objectively diminished life.[15] Surely, however, coping with impairment is not equivalent to coping with the kinds of severe oppression and injustice that cause a person to lower her expectations within slavery. Without direct access to the experience of disability and because of their bias against disability, Glover and Brock are quick to dismiss the testimony of persons with disabilities as irrelevant to their moral deliberations about technologies that seek to prevent or eliminate persons with disabilities.

Assuming that disability is always bad and ought to be prevented, some bioethicists go even further to advocate for eliminating disabled children from being born. Bioethicist John Harris, for example, believes it is morally wrong to produce children harmed by their genetic makeup.[16] For Harris, genetic disability is a "harmed condition" that ought to be prevented when possible. In addition to gene therapy, Harris promotes fetal genetic screenings to avoid pregnancies that will produce "genetically weak" children. Although Harris advocates for reproductive liberty, he also believes it is morally wrong to bear children with disabilities, particularly when a woman can have healthy children in the future (implying that the moral course of action is to abort a disabled fetus and try again for a "healthy" one). Harris contends, "In suggesting that it is wrong to bring avoidable suffering into the world and in indicating that suffering is avoidable where an individual who is or will be disabled can be replaced with an individual who is not disabled I have assumed that replaceability is unproblematic. . . . It is important to be clear that where we do choose to bring avoidable suffering or injury into the world this is wrong."[17] Not only does Harris presume that children are replaceable and that disabled children should be aborted to make room for nondisabled ones, he also equates disability with suffering. The testimony of persons with disabilities and their caretakers that not all disability produces suffering and that much of the suffering involved with disability is produced by social inequality rather than genetics is also ignored. Couched in the language of the relief of suffering, Harris's "compassion" for persons with disability requires their eradication rather than their accommodation.

Given the imagined misfortune produced by disability, some bioethicists have advocated that there is a moral duty to use genetic interventions (namely IVF and PGD) to avoid producing children with disabilities. For example, the book *From Chance to Choice: Genetics and Justice*, written by four prominent bioethicists and funded by the National Institutes of Health's Ethical, Legal, and Social Implications (ELSI) Research Program, argues that in certain circumstances based on "quality of life" predictors, parents are morally required to undertake genetic interventions to prevent "harmful conditions to their offspring."[18] The views of Allen Buchanan, Dan Brock, Norman Daniels, and Daniel Wikler might appear extreme, but they resonate with goals of the HGP as articulated by James Watson: "We place most of our hopes for genetics on the use of antenatal diagnostic procedures, which increasingly will let us know whether a fetus is carrying a mutant gene that will seriously proscribe its eventual development into a functional human being. By terminating such pregnancies, the threat of horrific disease genes contributing to blight many family's prospects for future success can be erased."[19] Although Watson does not here describe which "mutant genes" result in "horrific diseases," elsewhere he references such conditions as Down syndrome to describe lives that are best eliminated.[20] For Watson, as well as many other bioethicists, disability is the only relevant characteristic for the child, so alternative futures, where suffering and tragedy do not mark the child's life, cannot be imagined.

It is a common trope that technology itself is neutral whereas only its implementation carries moral weight, but advances in technology are frequently paired with a rhetoric of new moral obligations for those who have access to them. Nobel prizewinner and pioneer of in vitro fertilization Robert G. Edwards has been quoted as saying, "Soon it will be a sin for parents to have a child who carries the heavy burden of genetic disease."[21] Certainly, some genetic conditions cause immense physical suffering and are even fatal, but the hyperbolic rhetoric about disability often obscures the reality, experiences, and testimonies of persons living with disability. Among many bioethicists and genetic scientists, the worth and predicted future happiness of a fetus are reduced to genetic normalcy. For parents, the decision to terminate can be based on a single gene or an extra chromosome. Genetic testing bestows a disability-based identity on a fetus, and parents are asked to contemplate abortion based on their knowledge of what it is like to live with this diagnostic label.

Given the technological imperative, genetic technologies are helping to create a world in which we seemingly have the choice between health and disease, normality or abnormality. Scientists who have helped map the human genome are continually adding to the list of identifiable "genetic diseases" while predetermining what constitutes a "disease" or an "abnormality." Meanwhile, the nature of normality is ever-shifting. As more and more diseases and abnormal (antisocial) behaviors emerge in medicine, the norm becomes ever further away for those who do not have the means or desire to "improve" their health. By targeting genetic traits that are undesirable, genetic scientists and bioethicists implicitly uphold a vision of the ideal human genome that is never quite static. In their quest to eliminate what is perceived to be injurious, Harris, Glover, and others blur the boundaries of normalcy by suggesting genetic technologies not only should target disabling abnormalities but can be used to "create healthier, longer-lived, and altogether 'better' individuals."[22] Although few bio-ethicists go as far as Harris and Glover in their support of genetic "enhancements," it is not difficult to see how the prevention of disability can exist on a moral continuum with the enhancement of "normal" children who may physically and socially benefit from "stronger" genes.[23]

Because of their social and material power, clinicians and bio-ethicists have an epistemic authority that eludes many people with disabilities. As a result, it is easy for them to undermine or ignore the embodied experiences and testimony of persons with disabilities in favor of an understanding of disability that is overwhelmingly negative. Persons with intellectual and developmental disabilities (IDDs) are likewise assumed to have nothing at all to offer to our understanding of personhood, much less our bioethical deliberations. As a result, very few scholars bother to do research with people with IDDs to better understand their experiences. Persons with disabilities are thus denied epistemic authority and equal moral status in bioethics.

The Justice Model and the Biopolitics of Genethics

Genetic medicine often implicitly carries with it the rather unresolved question of whether perfect health would make us happy or would even create the necessary conditions of human fulfillment. The idea that health creates more opportunities for individual autonomy is an unquestioned assumption made by many in bioethics. Norman Daniels suggests that intervention for preventing disease may be mandated by Rawls's principle of justice. Daniels's framework depends upon the assertion that justice demands equality of opportunity, which may be lost when disease or disability limits our normal range of opportunities. Daniels believes he is justified in elevating the status of health care because illness fundamentally limits the functioning of those who would otherwise be "normal, active, and fully cooperating members of society over the course of a complete life."[24] Although Daniels acknowledges that not all impairments diminish one's life, there remains an implicit assumption that freedom from disease and disability is conditional for happiness, so that genetic technologies aiming to prevent disabilities are not merely permissible but may be obligatory. The logic goes something like this: the healthier and more physically normal we are, the more opportunities we are allotted in life, and more opportunities create greater autonomy, which leads to—or at least creates the conditions for—justice, which in turn allows us to carry out our quest for the good life.[25]

There remains, however, a more ominous problem at play in the assumption that health creates the conditions for fulfillment or happiness. When fragility and suffering become antithetical to the idealized conditions for human life, imperfect, disabled bodies are placed in grave danger. When society increasingly fixates on the conception of a happy life free of suffering, it becomes more difficult for disabled people to fulfill their social roles and flourish within their communities. An exclusive focus on genetic remediation is likely to lead to continued discriminatory attitudes and policies against those whose bodies fall outside our genetic ideals.

In promoting the use of genetic technologies, bioethicists even go so far as to argue that accommodating persons with disabilities would negatively affect society. For example, in *From Chance to Choice: Genetics and Justice*, Buchanan, Brock, Daniels, and Wikler attempt to dismantle the disability rights critiques against genetic technologies (particularly the use of selective abortions after genetic screening) as well as the disability rights movement more generally. The authors claim that the disability rights movement is not a legitimate civil rights movement and that including persons with disabilities into our social arrangements would harm our economic system and threaten social stability.[26] The analogy the authors use to prove that disability accommodation will be harmful to the nondisabled is a card game: "Suppose we wish to play a card game in which everyone in a mixed group of individuals ranging in age from 5 to 50 years can successfully participate. . . . If the game chosen is contract bridge, then some individuals in the group—namely, the 5 year olds—will not be able to participate effectively. There is another option, however: A simpler game (a less demanding infrastructure for social interaction) can be chosen so that everyone will be able to participate successfully. We can play 'go fish.'"[27] Not only is comparing persons with disabilities to five-year-old children appalling, the analogy is nonsensical. The disability rights movement has never demanded that employers ensure all jobs can be carried out by all people, nor is this the goal of the Americans with Disabilities Act. The authors of *From Chance to Choice* go on to provide examples of demands disability rights advocates *might* have but in reality do not hold. For example, the authors spend much of their time arguing against the (uncited) slogan, "Change society, not people," but critics have pointed out this slogan has never been used by disability advocates and cannot be found in any disability literature.[28] Without a single reference to any disability scholar or activist, these respected bioethicists consistently deconstruct arguments never made by authors within the disability rights community. The result is a book that is methodologically irresponsible as well as bigoted. Had the authors engaged voices from within the disability rights community, they might have been less likely to mischaracterize and ultimately demean disability advocates.[29] By failing to take persons with disabilities seriously, much less draw from their wisdom, these bioethicists' ethical evaluations of genetic technologies lack critical perspective.

When the driving force behind genetics research is the remediation of all genetic diseases and disabilities, it is not surprising that many bioethicists strongly endorse the idea that the use of genetic technologies is morally praiseworthy if not mandatory. Medical technology is never neutral with regard to its purpose. The ability to detect undesirable features and conditions easily becomes a mandate to eliminate them, which can, in turn, mean eliminating some kinds of "defective" future people from existing. The metaphysics of genetic science grounds the bioethical response to genetic disability.

The Baconian project lives on in our genetic machinations. The science of genetics must offer a technological response to human suffering; and if technology cannot cure the suffering we currently experience, it will eliminate the potential for suffering itself. To relieve the human condition, we must relieve some people from being born. Although new medical technologies are promoted as offering people more options and freedom of choice, the advancement of medical technology diminishes as often as it increases our freedom of choice and opportunity. Ironically, although some in the bioethical and bio-medical community attempt to limit the number of persons born with disabilities, advances in medicine are allowing people to live longer than ever before, creating an ever-increasing number of people living with disabilities. Disregarding the testimony of persons with disabilities and instead viewing genetic disability as inherently tragic and socially and economically disadvantageous, we may find ourselves unable to meet the needs of a growing number of people within our society. Moreover, the desire to escape finitude and suffering can eclipse many other goods, such as community, solidarity, and care, which can and should be sought in human life. Health is a poor substitute for *eudaemonia* and may even fail to provide us with the conditions for a good life. Our quest for genetic perfection and our mandate for all to be genetically healthy might, in the end, leave us all a little sick.

WISDOM AND EXPERIENCE IN CHRISTIAN ETHICS

Refusal to incorporate the perspectives of people living with the conditions researchers and physicians are attempting to eliminate impoverishes the fields of medicine and bioethics. Thankfully, a growing number of disability scholars are helping to reveal the un-reflective ableism present within much of bioethics and our modern notions of personhood. Often building upon (and at times challenging) foundational disability scholarship, disability theologians work to critique both our modern notions of disability and the failures of Christianity to adequately attend to the needs and experiences of persons with disability within its theologies and church structures.

Within the Christian tradition, experience is considered a vital source of moral reflection, but diverse experiences have not always been considered. Critically reflecting on the experiences of persons with disabilities within Christian theology has the potential to both affirm and challenge aspects of the tradition as well as Christian ethical deliberations on biomedical technologies. Embodied experience is not the only source of knowledge in Christianity, but it cannot be ignored as a critical source of knowledge. Christian ethicists, therefore, ought to search out and attend to the lived experiences of persons with disabilities, particularly if they wish to make moral judgments about technologies that aim to cure or eliminate people with disabilities. Christian theology in general, and theological bioethics in particular, must open itself up to being transformed by disability epistemology if it wishes to speak to the moral nature of biomedical technologies.

Relying upon experience as a source of moral reflection is hardly new in Christian ethics. Experience has always been central to the theological method. In her essay "The Role of Experience in Moral Discernment," Margaret Farley highlights the importance of experience for normative guidance. Of the many sources used to fund Christian ethics (scripture, tradition, and various secular disciplines) Farley believes experience is unique:

> All of the sources together can be used dialectically in moral discernment. But whatever decisions are made about the use of sources, it seems fair to say that experience is never just one source among many. It is always an important part of the content of each of the other sources and is always a key factor in the interpretation of the others. Scripture, for example, is the record of some person's experience of God; tradition represents a community's experience through time; humanistic and even scientific studies are shaped by the experience of those who engage them. Past experience, therefore, provides content for all of the sources, and present experience provides a necessary and inescapable vantage point for interpreting them.[30]

Christians recognize that multiple sources ought to inform moral theology, but experience is not simply one category among many. Experience gives shape to the other sources. *Diverse* experiences, however, have not always been incorporated into theological reflection, which has led Christian communities to produce the same kinds of epistemic injustices seen in the biomedical realm. If persons with disabilities experience the world in unique ways, then they might also have unique insights that could be valuable to Christian ethics, particularly when ethical deliberations directly affect their future well-being.

As embodied creatures, our theological reflections will necessarily be done through our embodied selves. Embodiment makes our moral reflections possible, and the particularity of our bodies influences how we experience and perceive the world, which inevitably influences our moral and theological perspectives. Christian theology has traditionally paid particular attention to embodiment because Christianity is the religion of the Word made flesh. God became incarnate in a human body, was resurrected in a body, and continues to be embodied through the Eucharist. As followers of Christ, Christians are called to *be* the body of Christ, and we too are promised a resurrected body. Christians experience God through the body, both in their own bodies and through the corporate body. Christianity, in other words, is a religion of the body. Our theologies, therefore, must critically reflect on embodied experience to make sense of how we experience God.

Critically reflecting on the experience of disability can help to reveal many implicit assumptions we make about normalcy as well as which capacities are necessary to live a good life. Persons with disabilities are likely to perceive the world differently than those without disabilities, both because of the exclusion and oppression they experience and because their phenomenological experience of the world is unique. The modes of knowing acquired through disability are likely to be distinctive and formative for how a person experiences the world and, therefore, are constitutive of ethical reflection. For example, as a blind man, the theologian John Hull provides unique insights on the "sighted" assumptions that exist within the Bible text, which tend to equate blindness with unbelief, ignorance, unworthiness, and despair.[31] Hull offers a nonableist perspective on the blind characters in the Bible as well as the meaningfulness of Jesus's tactile ministry. Hull's perspective on the biblical stories is born of his epistemic insights as a blind person. Hull has distinctive ways of knowing that have enabled him to develop reflections that can expand the ways we understand traditional biblical readings. Given the array of disabilities that exist in the world, the opportunities for renewed and refreshing perspectives on classic Christian texts and doctrines by persons with differing disabilities are vast. Christian communities who wish to make wise choices regarding medical technologies would benefit from retrieving these subjugated epistemologies.

Obviously, there is no way to universalize the "disability experience." Even disabilities that are genetic in origin have varying manifestations that will affect one's experience of the world. Yet there are some unique challenges and perspectives held by various persons with disabilities, in large part because of the way persons with disabilities are perceived and treated by society. The situatedness of living with a disability can lead to fresh ways of perceiving the world and the idolatries that normalcy masks for most nondisabled people.

Incorporating the unique revelatory experiences of persons with disabilities can help to develop communal wisdom for the Christian community. Christians have long believed that the cultivation of wisdom is necessary for moral discernment. We can gain wisdom through at least three paths. In the first, wisdom is a gift given by the Spirit, which is not attained all at once but cultivated through experiences where one uses correct judgments concerning ultimate causes. Alternatively, we can gain wisdom from our habits, which makes rational moral deliberation less necessary, or at least less taxing. Finally, we can gain wisdom through charity, which comes from our will and not our intellect. In all three paths, wisdom does not arrive by sudden divine insight; rather, it must be nurtured through our experiences, judgments, virtuous habits, and love for others.

Because wisdom is a gift of the Spirit, there is reason to believe it is not reserved for those who are capable of self-reflexive thought or critical reasoning. For persons with IDDs and others who do not have access to typical modes of reasoning, one's habits and expressions of love can be shaped by the Spirit. Aquinas does not believe that explicit faith—that is, a reasoned faith that is rationally explainable—is necessary for those who are not capable of having it, because of either lack of education or cognitive limitations. Richard Cross notes that Duns Scotus goes even further, implying that all persons have implicit faith and that those with cognitive limitations are capable of being oriented by God toward the good.[32] Although some persons with disabilities will be unable to share their reflective experience with others, they too have a relationship with God and thus an embodied wisdom to gift to their communities. Insofar as wisdom can be a gift of the Spirit that inclines us toward the good, persons with cognitive limitations or intellectual disabilities are capable of wisdom. Moreover, it is possible for persons to gain wisdom from others with cognitive limitations, particularly after entering into relationship with them, because this enables the individual to better perceive the other's acts of faith and love.

If the unique episteme that comes from experiencing the world through disability shapes one's judgments, habits, and relationships with others, then there is reason to believe there is a particular disability wisdom. When Christians are considering the use of genetic technologies, therefore, it would make sense for them to incorporate disability wisdom into their collective deliberations, particularly because the outcomes of these deliberations often affect persons with disabilities directly. Wisdom, for Aquinas, is both contemplative—the desire to know fundamental truths or ultimate causes of the world—and practical—the desire to use "right reason with respect to action."[33] Wisdom, in other words, brings together metaphysics and ethics. For many persons with physical or sensory disabilities, speculation about the cause and purpose of their bodies will have direct impact on how they understand and appreciate themselves as well as how they interact with others, including others who desire to participate in their healing. For those with intellectual or developmental disabilities who are unable to critically reflect on the purpose and meaning of their bodies, the care they receive from others will be based on how the community understands the ontology and worth of their bodies. Likewise, the gifts persons with disabilities bring to their communities may be received differently on the basis of the community's ability to understand the value of those gifts to the life of the community. Speculation about the causes of disability is never neutral; it directly affects how we care for one another and the justice that we seek for members of the community. Incorporating the experiences, perspectives, and wisdom of persons with disabilities, therefore, will help to ensure that our moral deliberations are informed and responsible to others.

If experience shapes our ethical deliberations, then experiencing the world with and through disability, and experiencing the world in relationship with people with disabilities, might yield new moral insights to be taken up in the process of moral discernment. Such experiences should not be taken in isolation but brought into what Farley calls the "hermeneutical circle" that tests experiences against "general moral norms; intelligibility of accounts of experience in relation to fundamental beliefs; mutual illumination when measured with other sources of insight; harmful or helpful consequences of interpretations of experience; confirmation in a community of discernment and integrity in the testimony of those who present their experience."[34] Given these guiding criteria, the Christian community can and should be the ideal place for incorporating the insights of disability experience into its own processes of moral discernment.

INCORPORATING DISABILITY EXPERIENCE IN HEALTH CARE

People with disabilities are not a monolithic group, nor do they share a single "disability ethic," but there are noteworthy critiques of genetic technologies from disability advocates and scholars that have persisted over the past forty years. Members of the disability community have critiqued the "medical model" of disability taken up within genetic science, the disability stigma reinscribed by genetic technologies, and the false narratives of "choice" that surround genetic interventions. These critiques are rarely offered from a Christian perspective and should not be determinative of Christian theology. Many of the philosophical assumptions made by disability scholars ought to be challenged by theologians, whose metaphysics is grounded in an understanding of God as Creator, Sustainer, and Redeemer of life. At the same time, Christian ethicists should explore the ways in which the experiences of people with disabilities and their allies undermine prevalent cultural assumptions concerning the meaning and value of human life that also permeate the church. Disability experience can draw attention to the ways in which Christians have failed to take the Christ narrative seriously and have failed to fully accept, love, and appreciate their neighbors. Most mainline Protestant denominations will not want to make universal declarations about the moral use of each and every genetic technology for each and every person, but they will want to offer theologically sound advice to prospective parents and persons with disabilities who are considering using genetic technologies. To do so responsibly, they must understand the objections coming from members of the disability community, many of whom believe their dignity and very lives are at stake in these deliberations.

Genetic Technology and the Medical Model

Since nearly the advent of prenatal genetic testing in the mid-1970s, scholars and activists have considered the implications of genetic technologies for persons with disabilities. The parents of children with Down syndrome were some of the first to raise concerns. Many worried that prenatal screenings for Down syndrome would lead to increased instances of selective abortion, which in turn would lead to increased social stigma against persons with Down syndrome and decreased aid and services for individuals and their caretakers.[35] Their fears were not unfounded. Down syndrome remains highly stigmatized, despite the fact that individuals with Down syndrome and their parents highly rate their levels of life satisfaction.[36] James Watson once remarked, "We already accept that most couples don't want a Down child [*sic*]. You would have to be crazy to say you wanted one, because that child has no future."[37] The basic assumption of the man who pioneered the Human Genome Project is that people with Down syndrome have no future and that anyone who would want them is "crazy."

Although Watson is known for his shocking language, his sentiments are hardly singular. Much like the Human Genome Project itself, genetic technologies are grounded in a metaphysics of normalcy that positions disability as a negative departure from "normal" human functioning. Naturalistic accounts of normal functioning, such as those previously described by Norman Daniels, presume that there is a standard way that humans should function and that any departure from that normal functionality ought to be considered defective. Disability scholar Elizabeth Barnes points out, however, that such accounts fail because they overgeneralize. Some departures from normal human functioning are advantageous and clearly not disabilities.[38] If we restrict disabilities to *negative* departures from normal human functioning, then the definition of disability is inherently normative and not value-free as Daniels claims. If we take seriously the accounts of people with disabilities who do not view their disability as a lack, absence, or defect, then naturalistic conceptions of disability appear value-laden.

Naturalistic accounts, however, dominate most thinking about disability, particularly within medicine. The so-called medical model of disability has been critiqued by disability scholars for decades. Disability theorist Tobin Siebers claims the medical model has three defining characteristics: (1) it positions disability as an inherent deficit, (2) disability is understood as a medical problem requiring a medical solution, and (3) disability resides in individuals.[39] The medical model of disability reflects the logic of eliminating finitude and contingency articulated by Francis Bacon centuries ago. Without a concept of final ends, medicine offers a technological solution to anomalies that are presumed to cause suffering. The HGP provided a genetic version of the medical model, in which disability is understood in a linear relationship between DNA sequence, phenotypic characteristic, and (negative) human variation. Geneticized disability positions genes as the "problem" because of the phenotypic variation that results.

Part of the trouble with the medical model when applied to genetic technology is that it assumes that all genetic disabilities are bad and that any action that would remove or ameliorate disability is good. When disability is framed solely in negative terms, the question becomes "How do we prevent disabilities?" When discussing disability, bioethicists tend to focus their interest on preventing disabled people from being born (through prenatal testing, preimplantation genetic diagnosis, or more recently CRISPR) and on the ethics of euthanizing disabled people. For this reason, some have claimed that "the relationship between bioethics and disability has traditionally been focused on killing."[40]

The presumption that disability is inherently bad requires us to overlook the heterogeneity of disability as well as the experiences of people with disabilities. Marfan syndrome and Tay-Sachs may both cause disability, but the physical suffering and limitations that result are often quite disparate. When discussing policy matters for abortion and genetic intervention, many geneticists and bioethicists will refer to "severe" disabilities, but what constitutes "severe" is highly contested and rarely explicated. Moreover, if it is assumed that all disability is bad, any experience of disability that is positive must be denied, which is perhaps why so many scientists, clinicians, and bioethicists are reluctant to believe the testimony of persons with disability about their quality of life.

Disability critics of the medical model have traditionally favored a social understanding of disability, but exactly what this entails is contested. Social models attempt to describe disability in ways that are less value-laden than naturalistic or medical approaches by beginning with human difference as the starting point, rather than a "normal" phenotype from which all deviation is measured. Rather than a negative departure from normality, disability is defined as a product of the social environment, including beliefs, attitudes, structures, and institutions.

A purely social model of disability popularized in the 1970s and '80s, which frames disability as a "phenomenon generated by social organizations that discriminate against some embodiments,"[41] is no longer dominant in disability studies. Strong social models seem to deny any place for the body in their formulation, and they risk ignoring people with disabilities who testify that some of their physical experiences, such as chronic pain, are not social and could not be ameliorated through better social arrangements. Instead, hybrid models that consider biology and social environment are preferred. "Relational" models of disability attempt to take seriously both the positive and negative accounts of disability that exist and to attend both to people who affirm that their disability is a positive aspect of their identity and to those whose pain and suffering cannot be rectified through better social accommodations. Relational models understand disability as constituted through the experience of disability as well as disability's associated meanings. We are embodied creatures, but we are also fundamentally social creatures, whose experiences are shaped by cultural assumptions and the meanings we place on bodies. Strong social models of disability risk denying the first claim, whereas purely naturalistic or medical models risk denying the second. Within relational models, we cannot prejudge whether a particular bodily state, much less a genetic sequence, is inherently good or bad, because context matters. We must take seriously disability activists who positively value their disability experience as well as those who do not. Disability is simply too complex to be defined outside of its context, and experiences are shaped by both the social meanings of disability and material manifestations.

Of course, no model of disability can capture each person's experience of disability. Disability is an inherently heterogenous category, which changes across time and space. Stringent models can become totalizing and exclude particular disability experiences and knowledges. Models can reveal subjugated epistemologies, but they can also constrict our vision of which bodies or experiences "count." Still, it would be a mistake to give up on models altogether, because they allow for persons with disabilities to identify themselves as belonging to a marginalized group, which is the first step toward finding community and advocating for shared interests. In a perfect world, this sort of need for a shared minority status would not be necessary, but in our fallen, imperfect world, fighting for the rights of particular groups is often necessary and life-saving. A relational conception of disability, which includes both physical and intellectual disabilities, helps to focus attention on the real harms of disability, which are predominantly the social environments in which disabilities are constructed and not the bodies that are predetermined to be "bad" or "defective." We ought to view disability, not as a natural kind, but as a contingent classification that is constantly shifting.

More recently, critical disability scholars have illuminated the ways in which modern society tends to couple disability with cure.

Alison Kafer refers to this impulse the "curative imaginary."[42] Kafer does not discourage people with disabilities from using medicine; rather, she resists the idea that approaches to disability ought to be limited to cure. For many people with disabilities, flourishing does not require medical interventions. Although critical disability theorists are sometimes criticized for not being attentive enough to the material conditions of persons with disabilities, the decoupling of disability from medical intervention is a crucial insight from the field that will be important for Christian bioethics.[43] When coupled with a relational model of disability, attention to our society's "curative imaginary" can be helpful for a reimagined Christian bioethics that is attentive to disability.

A Christian Response

What can Christians learn from these debates surrounding models of disability? First, they can discover exactly why taken-for-granted medical models of disability are so harshly critiqued within the disability community. A purely medical model of disability that frames all things we call "disability" as inherently bad and in need of a cure must be rejected by Christian theologians. A reductionistic view that locates the badness or harm of disability in a genetic sequence hardly seems Christian. After all, modern scientific understandings of life do not allow for purpose in the universe. In Christian theology, the goodness of life rests upon our ability to receive life as a good gift from God, regardless of our circumstances, and not upon the quality of one's life as defined by medicine. A purely naturalistic model of disability, therefore, will be inadequate because Christians understand their nature as created and fulfilled in God. When we listen to the voices of persons with disabilities, another reason to be wary of medical and naturalistic models becomes obvious: they fail to capture the wide range of disability experience, much of which is about social and not biological oppression. Negative attitudes toward disability and the neglect of disability experience have direct ethical consequences for people who experience disability.

Yet if Christians wish to hold onto a teleological view of human life, then they must believe there is a way that humans ought to be.

For this reason, Christians must also reject a purely social model that does not posit a norm for human life. The demand for an ontological norm justifies why many Thomists argue that disabilities are in fact defects, because they are departures from how God intends bodies to function according to our essential human nature. Yet few Thomists articulate a precise definition of "disability," making for slippery ground when one is trying to articulate why disabilities deviate from an ontological norm. More importantly, however, there appears to be a disconnect between the bodily norms espoused (rationality, sense perception, sociability, etc.) and the capacities necessary to achieve the ultimate human goal, which is friendship with God. Even if a coherent definition of disability could be found, essentialism alone may be inadequate to determine which disabilities are inherently bad for human beings. After all, why should we think that cognitive limitations make a person less capable of friendship with God? Surely, God's grace and capacity for self-revelation far surpass our ability to comprehend them.

Christians should not be too quick to judge the spiritual lives of persons with disabilities. Jill Harshaw provides a compelling account of the spirituality of persons with intellectual disabilities, even those who do not have the capacity for language or self-reflection. Harshaw develops a "theology of accommodation," which challenges the notion that God is inaccessible to persons with intellectual disabilities. According to Harshaw, divine revelation is "attuned to the capacities of its particular recipients to apprehend it."[44] John Calvin has a similar notion when discussing how God communicates with those who cannot comprehend language. God accommodates knowledge of Godself to all human abilities.[45] God must do this for all human beings, but if God can do it for those with the highest IQs, why would we believe God could not be made known to persons who are profoundly intellectually disabled? God meets us where we are, wherever that might be. The ontological difference between us and God is inexhaustible and can be bridged only by God's grace and not by any human capacity.

If there is a norm for human life, it is embodied in Jesus Christ, who became human to be with us. Jesus came to create a body through a body. Jesus's own body, as well as the body he created (the church), are marked by dependency and vulnerability. These are not qualities that should be shunned; rather, they are markers of the body of Christ. Deborah Creamer reminds us that our limits are part of creation, part of what it means to be human and not a negative or evil character-istic.[46] The understanding that we are all vulnerable binds humanity together, disabled and nondisabled alike. Those vulnerabilities are expressed through our individual bodies (made in the image of God's own body in Christ) as well as in our corporate body, which we call the body of Christ. Within the body of Christ, our lives are best expressed not through their radical independence but through our dependent mutuality. Through the Incarnation, Christ became vul-nerable to save. We are incorporated into that body when we carry out Christ's work of caring for the vulnerable and entering into de-pendent relationships.

The dependency expressed by persons with disabilities, therefore, does not make them exceptional, it makes them typical; they reveal the normal expression of ontological personhood. According to Stan-ley Hauerwas, persons with disabilities remind the community who we all are: persons who are wholly dependent. We depend on God for all we are and have. Everything we have is gift and promise.[47] Within this frame, we have nothing to offer God: not our rationality, not our physical capacities, not anything. All we receive is through grace. If we believe that all persons share the same vulnerable, dependent state, then it becomes more difficult to locate what exactly is bad or defec-tive about disability. Finding kinship in our dependency, however, should not mute the differences between us. Some persons are par-ticularly vulnerable because of the ways we have constructed our so-cieties, and it is our Christian duty to recognize patterns of inequality and work toward the equality and inclusion of all. Here the relational model of disability helps to direct Christians toward the social struc-tures that systematically disadvantage certain bodies in our society.

As critical disability theorists note, the disadvantages experienced by persons with disabilities do not always need to be ameliorated through cure. This is not to say the effects of disability should never be mitigated but that our standards for determining whether it is right to prevent or fix disability need to shift. From a Christian perspective, it is only when our disabilities prevent us from enjoying and glorifying God that they ought to be cured or ameliorated. For example, when a disability is accompanied by pain that separates the person from herself, her community, and God, then there is reason to turn to medical interventions. For many, the body in pain will be injurious to the individual's spiritual life as well as the spiritual life of the individual's community. According to Elaine Scarry, pain can cause an "absolute split between one's sense of one's own reality and the reality of other persons."[48] Pain can be isolating because it can cut a person off from community and her own sense of self. For individuals in pain, the use of or hope for a technological cure seems appropriate. Of course, not all disabilities are accompanied by pain, and curing one's pain does not mean that disability itself is cured.

By assuming that all persons with disabilities are in pain or suffering, Christians risk offering healing that is not needed or wanted by persons with disabilities. The inability to accept and appreciate the lives of persons with disabilities can also cut people off from one another and from God. By idealizing or idolizing certain bodily states, Christians may fail to see God at work in the world. In the rush to "fix" or "prevent," we might deny our communities the gifts and wisdom of persons with disabilities. Disabilities can separate us from God, but how they do so is complex and often has as much to do with practices of exclusion as with bodily difference.

Admittedly, using spirituality or communion with God as a standard for appropriate medical intervention is far from a definitive way to determine which disabilities require amelioration or should be prevented, but it begins to shift our attention away from what we presume to be defective bodies and toward bodily states that limit an individual's flourishing. Such a standard is not limited to persons who are capable of understanding and articulating their differences and needs. There is a way bodies ought to be, and that being is both embodied and social. Persons are made to be in community with one another and with God. Thus Christians must be more attentive to the relational and environmental aspects of disability as well as our cultural imaginary, rather than predetermining what differences diminish a person's quality of life or deviate from some sort of idealized biological or genetic norm. Even while positing an ontological norm for human life, Christians should resist definitions of disability that are merely negative and should instead focus on ameliorating conditions that prevent us from being in relationships of mutuality and dependency. Determining when it is appropriate to rely on technologies to prevent or ameliorate conditions requires a moral community of deliberation because, as relational beings, our spiritual lives are intertwined. I will discuss this process of deliberation in chapter 8.

Genetic Technology, Stigma, and Choice

There is room for the development and use of genetic technologies within a Christian bioethic, but genetic technologies should not be viewed as inherently good or morally obligatory. Many disability theorists and theologians raise concern that the attention and investment paid to genetic technologies, including screenings and gene editing, distract us from the real problems within disability: built environments and social attitudes. Hans Reinders notes that preventing disabled lives through reproductive technologies is at odds with the full inclusion of persons with disabilities.[49] There is a duplicity at the heart of liberal societies that claim to value persons with disabilities while at the same time desiring a world without them. By prizing self-determination, liberal morality has excluded persons with disabilities, particularly those with intellectual disabilities, from full personhood and thus positions them as less worthy of protection. Nearly two decades after Reinders's writing on genetic technologies, there is little evidence that societies that invest considerable public funds into genetic science and technologies are less willing or able to improve disability access. Yet the tension Reinders points out remains. Bioethicists continue to push the idea that parents who refuse prenatal intervention are irresponsible, and prejudices against disability continue to abound.

For many disability advocates, genetic technologies that lead to selective abortion send the message that it is better to be dead than disabled. According to the pioneering disability bioethicist Adrienne Asch, "For people with disabilities to work each day against societally imposed hardships can be exhausting; learning that the world one lives in considers it better to 'solve' problems of disability by parental detection and abortion, rather than by expending those resources in improving society so that everyone—including those people who have disabilities—could participate more easily, is demoralizing. It invalidates the effort to lead a life in an inhospitable world."[50] Asch was one of the first disability scholars to raise concerns that prenatal genetic testing and selective abortion sent the message that a disabled life is not worth living. This argument, dubbed the "expressivist argument," has been contentious, even among disability scholars, but it remains a powerful critique of the assumption that selective abortion of a disabled but otherwise wanted child is a reasonable if not moral choice.

Of course, proponents of prenatal genetic testing and gene editing claim they are merely enhancing opportunities for choice, not trying to send a "message" about the value of disability. Genetic counselors are trained to be nondirective; they are merely providing prospective parents with options. Yet embedded within the development and implementation of prenatal screenings is the implicit idea that preventing the births of children with disabilities is good, or at least desirable. If no woman chose to abort a child because of prenatal screening, the large investment in screenings by basic scientists or counseling in health care systems would hardly seem worth the cost.[51] Genetic counselors may strain to be neutral or nondirective, but they mediate a technology undergirded by a metaphysics that positions disability as an undesirable defect of human life.

Modern societies falsely view technology as neutral. Genetic test results are neither moral nor immoral, but access to the "facts" produced by these technologies is instrumental in decision-making and comes to shape our "genetic imaginary."[52] Genetic technologies allow for choice but also constrain choice by defining the situation as one that calls for a choice. Women who undergo prenatal genetic screening are now presented with a choice of what to do with those results. In the future, many more might be presented with the choice of using CRISPR or other technologies to edit embryos or eliminate their own genetic disabilities. Such technologies do not force any particular choice on individuals, but they do require a response. We must either choose to use the technologies or not, and then we must choose what to do with the results of our choice. It is becoming increasingly likely that the choice not to use technology will be viewed as an immoral one.

Disability theorists question whether the choices offered in genetic testing and prenatal screenings are truly informed given the strong biases against disability that exist within medicine and popular culture. It is questionable whether most parents are given adequate information about individuals' quality of life or what it is like to live with a disability by their genetic counselors or physicians.[53] Additionally, parents are rarely provided the perspectives of persons living with the genetic condition their child is expected to have. Without such information, informed consent is severely constrained. Anita Ho notes, "The societal treatment and professional viewpoints of disability continue to shape the meaning of pregnancy and the role of screening programs, pre-determining people's decision-making framework and feasible options while giving the illusion of autonomy."[54] Many disability advocates do not believe reproductive "choice" will be sufficiently free until health care providers and prospective parents are better educated on disability experience and people with disabilities are included in all aspects of health care.[55]

Countless narratives from parents and persons with disabilities testify to the limitations of "choice" in medicine. Some patients with disabilities report being pressured or chastised for their reproductive choices. Teresa Blankmeyer Burke, for example, shares how, as a woman who is hard of hearing, she has been chastised as selfish, cruel, and abusive by medical professionals for having biological children.[56] Brian and Stephanie Brock claim that medical professionals pushed genetic testing on them numerous times before and after the birth of their son Adam. The Brocks were repeatedly bombarded with questions about why they had not agreed to genetic testing and were accused of refusing helpful knowledge that could benefit their son. In their desire to be helpful and humane to the Brocks, medical professions forced their views of responsible parenthood on them. The Brocks write, "[The medical professionals'] belief in the neutrality of genetic information masked a sharply normative claim that no *good* parent would resist genetic testing."[57] As genetic screenings become more routine, the "choices" involved are likely to become increasingly constricted. A focus on individual autonomy in the informed consent process means that the nuances of social pressure and the power of medicine are often ignored.

A Christian Response

Disability theorists are right to point out that prenatal testing and selective abortion reveal the implicit values of our society and that genuine choice in medicine is constrained because of a systematic bias against disability. At the same time, the insistence on the goodness or necessity of free, informed choice is prejudicial against persons who do not have the capacity for autonomous choosing. By over-valuing free choice, bioethicists, and even some disability theorists and theologians, risk implicitly endorsing other values such as self-sufficiency, rationality, and individualism, which can work to de-value the lives of persons who are determined to lack such traits. Moreover, it is highly unlikely that fully informed consent to pre-natal genetic testing would eradicate prejudicial attitudes toward disability. A much deeper social reform concerning disability would be required before this could happen.

Undoubtedly, informed consent is essential for the practice of medicine. Without it, physicians could run roughshod over pa-tients, determining what was best for them without their input. Yet choice ought not to be valued in such a way that it becomes an ulti-mate good. Overvaluing choice risks excluding people who do not have the capacity for choice from our moral frameworks. When per-sonhood is tied to notions of rationality, individual autonomy, and self-determination, persons with intellectual disabilities are likely to suffer. In opposition to modern constructions of personhood, however, theologians offer accounts that are more inclusive of who "counts" as a person and what we owe to one another based on the recognition of personhood. Combined with a conception of life as a "gift," a new understanding of the value of persons with disabilities in the body of Christ emerges.

The German Catholic theologian Robert Spaemann believes modern constructions of personhood (such as the one proposed by Peter Singer) that separate those who are "persons" (with rights) from those who are merely "human beings" risks misunderstanding the moral meaning of personhood. All human beings are persons, not because they have a certain set of capacities, or because they belong to a particular species or genus, but because they exist in a community of reciprocal recognition. We discover we are persons in recognition of the other as a person. Against Singer, Spaemann insists that human animality is not mere animality but a "medium of personal realization."[58] Humans are not merely a natural kind, they are kin who stand in relationship to one another. We belong to a human family that is not predicated upon empirically demonstrated properties; humans are not the sum of their predicates.[59] Severely disabled infants, therefore, belong to the human race and "participate in the community of persons" even if they do not recognize themselves as such.[60] In fact, in lacking particular properties that we attribute to humanity, persons with disabilities become the "paradigm for a human community of recognizing *selves,* rather than simply valuing useful or attractive *properties.*"[61] Like Hauerwas, Spaemann believes persons with severe intellectual disabilities are not an exceptional case of being human but the very paradigm of personhood.

Recognizing the other as a person is not merely an ontological recognition but an ethical one as well. Persons have an inherent claim on us because we belong together; we are gifts to one another. Perhaps no theologian has done more to explicate the theology of the "gift" than John Milbank. Building on the anthropology of "gift giving" in the work of Marcel Mauss and the pneumatology of Augustine (for whom "gift" is the name of the Holy Spirit), Milbank articulates a Trinitarian metaphysics of gift exchange that invites reciprocity (in the form of "gratitude and charitable giving-in-turn") between the Godhead and human beings and between human beings.[62] Our mutual recognition of one another as persons is rooted in the gift exchange of God's own Trinitarian life. God is always giving and receiving within Godself. God also gives us the gift of our own being in our creation. *Creatio ex nihilo* marks creation as a gratuitous gift such that our very lives are gifts to ourselves.[63] Unlike gifts as we typically consider them, the divine gift cannot be refused; God's gift "established creatures *as* themselves gifts."[64] That does not mean, however, that God's gift is forced upon us unilaterally. We receive God's gift as an "active reception," in which we give and receive God's love. The divine gift, therefore, is inherently a reciprocal one, which we extend to our neighbors.[65] Although Milbank is highly critical of reformed theologies of grace because they appear to render the human passive to God's activity, Todd Billings makes a powerful case for why Calvin's theology of grace is similar to Milbank's theology of the gift and may even provide a clearer picture of how grace relates human and divine agency.[66] Whether one agrees with Billings's critique of Milbank or not, both Milbank and Calvin ground their notion of what we owe to one another in God's gratuity in the creation and redemption of the world.

The notion that life is a gift is good news for people who are viewed as "unproductive" nonpersons in our market-based economy as well as those who feel the pressure to constantly "produce" to prove their worth to society. There is nothing that we must *do* to be accepted. All persons bring gifts to the community because we are gifts. Our worth is not based on our productions or our capacities but on God, who created all persons. Insofar as we exclude, reject, or fail to recognize the personhood of people with disabilities, we reject God's gift and diminish the body of Christ.

Against the bioethicists, philosophers, and politicians who believe accommodating persons with disabilities harms our economic and social systems, a theology of gift offers an opposing understanding of what enables communities to flourish. There is no room in Christian ethics for a world where the maximization of economic efficiency comes at the expense of social inclusion of persons with disabilities. Of course, accepting all persons as gifts does not mean persons with disabilities should not be challenged to grow into their relationship with God or attain virtue through their habits. Simply because all persons are good creations does not mean they are already who they are meant to be when creation is completed in the Resurrection. All persons should be encouraged and enabled to flourish, but this does not mean that those who do not live up to our culturally determined standards for normalcy are any less worthy of care or encouragement. As genetic tests and interventions proliferate, informed consent should be sought from all who are capable of giving it, but the exercise of free choice does not establish our personhood or confer our dignity.

The theological assertions that all humans are persons and that life is a gift have implications for the use of genetic technologies. Rather than viewing technological intervention as a moral obligation, a theology of gifted personhood implies that we cannot view life as a right or a possession that we can manipulate as we wish. Accepting life as a gift is in direct opposition to the notion that it is best to control all aspects of our life to improve ourselves and our communities. Our lives are not good because we chose them. Our lives are good because they are given by a good God. Eugenics and genetic engineering tempt us to value choice over giftedness. The acceptance of disability can help to defeat rampant hubris that prevents us from valuing vulnerability in the human condition.

AT THEIR BEST, modern liberal democracies listen to the hopes and concerns of persons with disabilities before making policies that will radically affect their lives and the lives of future people living with disabilities. The Americans with Disabilities Act (ADA) represented a milestone achievement in the protection of persons with disabilities against discrimination. Although the ADA demands that a certain amount of reasonable accommodations be made to persons with disabilities, America (along with many other countries) has a long way to go before persons with disabilities are fully incorporated into the dominant structures of society. Many Christian churches have also attempted to make their physical and social structures more accommodating to persons with disabilities, but for the most part disability continues to be seen as a difference to be accommodated, rather than as a natural part of the human life cycle and an inevitable product of human finitude. Our contemporary culture is in danger of making an idol of able-bodiedness, a sinful illusion that denies the inherent vulnerability and dependency that mark all our lives. Until persons with disabilities are understood as gifts that belong in the community, their dignity and their lives will be at risk, and technology will become a necessary mode of their salvation.

If, however, the wisdom of persons with disabilities is truly valued, it should inform our understanding and evaluations of genetic technologies. The critiques leveled by disability activists cannot be ignored when we are discerning the ethical use of genetic technologies. Denominational statements on genetic technologies should be attentive to disability concerns and actively seek out persons with disabilities to serve on commissions tasked with writing such statements. Churches should connect parents considering the use of genetic screenings or selective abortion with persons with disabilities in the community who can offer them perspective on what it is like to live with a disability. Of course, for either to happen, churches must first create spaces of belonging for persons with disabilities.

As the next chapter will show, the wisdom that comes from living with disabilities may also challenge how the Christian community sees itself, its values, and its obligations toward others. Such a challenge is necessary because church ought to be the place where persons with disabilities belong. When placed within the Christian narrative, disability narratives can serve as a reminder to the body of Christ of who they are and who they are called to be. Living as the body of Christ requires not only that Christians care for one another but also that they begin to cultivate virtues that help them to see the gifts present in one another. Only by first seeing the other for who she is and who she is meant to be within a Christian ontology can the church practice its theonomous ethic. By centralizing rather than marginalizing the experience of disability, Christians can reimagine the role of the virtues in the church's communal life and help communities re-envision their role in the process of moral discernment.

CHAPTER EIGHT

Disability Inclusion and
Virtue within the Church

A Christian bioethic built upon the notion of gifted personhood offers a counternarrative to that of late modern liberalism. Whereas
people in late modernity tend to view their bodies as possessions to
be used as they desire, in the Christian tradition bodies are understood as gifts. If all persons are gifts, then we can never view ourselves or others as objects of our control or mere tragedies to be fixed.
A Christian ontology of personhood places notions of autonomy and
self-determination as secondary to the goods of mutuality and dependency. Acknowledging our shared status as dependent, gifted
creatures, Christians must first accept one another before determining what needs to be changed in the other. The notion that we seek
first to accept people as they are is radical in a society that tends to
view difference as deviant and medical technologies as salvific.

Acceptance is not merely a concept, however. More fundamentally, it is a practice. By practicing radical acceptance, Christians offer
a counterpraxis to modern liberalism, which treats bodies as infinitely
malleable and upgradeable. Of course, this is not to suggest that
"natural bodies" are somehow fundamentally unalterable. Instead, the
alteration of the individual body must have a justifiable reason. What

counts as a "good" reason will be debatable, which is why Christian bioethics must embrace an ontology that can inform their understanding of the goods of the human body. For Christians, interventions upon the body will be judged on whether they promote or hinder human flourishing, or, in ontological terms, whether or not they enable humans to achieve their final end.

Questions concerning the ethical nature of genetic interventions are not merely individual, however. Christians must also consider the effects of interventions on the ecclesia, because in God all things are essentially connected. The body that is primary in Christianity is not the individual body but the body of Christ. Robert Song argues that in modern societies we tend to regard the individual, physical body as primary, but "in Christian theology, it is the body of Christ, the ecclesia, which forms the basic context for interpreting the psychophysical body of the individual, the corpus."[1] The Pauline texts, particularly 1 Corinthians, turn on the idea that individual bodies participate in a greater reality, which is Christ.[2] Within the body of Christ all members have a role to play because each member brings his or her own gifts to the beloved community.

The connection between individual bodies and the ecclesia has two direct implications for Christians attempting to better understand genetic disabilities. First, Christians cannot view their bodies (or the bodies of others) as objects or possessions to manipulate as they see fit. We do not create our identities from scratch, nor can we perfect ourselves by altering our bodies to fit our desires. Our bodies are not something other than ourselves, nor are they wholly separate from other bodies. Our bodies are gifts that we share with one another. The health of the individual is bound up with the health of the community. Our interdependence, therefore, has direct implications for the ethics of altering bodies through genetic manipulation or genetic selection.

Second, how Christians treat the least among them is a direct reflection on the unity of the body.

> The eye cannot say to the hand, "I have no need of you," nor again the head to the feet, "I have no need of you." On the con-

trary, the members of the body that seem to be weaker are indispensable, and those members of the body that we think less honorable we clothe with greater honor. . . . God has so arranged the body, giving the greater honor to the inferior member, that there may be no dissension within the body, but the members may have the same care for one another. If one member suffers, all suffer together with it; if one member is honored, all rejoice together with it. (1 Cor. 12:21–26 NRSV)

How Christians welcome those with genetic disabilities into the ecclesia reflects the strength of that community. Song argues that just as Paul appeals to those in the Corinthian church with higher status to change their behavior to favor those with lower status, so too should nondisabled Christians honor the experiences, insights, and needs of disabled Christians.[3] Disabled and nondisabled Christians need one another; the health of the Christian community depends upon their mutual recognition and care.

In this chapter, I highlight how Christian communal practices reflect the community's underlying theological, metaphysical, and ethical commitments to persons with disabilities as well as ways in which churches might improve their ecclesial practices to make them more inclusive. To show how inclusive practices can aid Christians in discerning the proper role of genetic technologies, I first describe how members of the body of Christ can create welcoming spaces for persons with genetic disabilities and future parents to reconceive the possibilities for communal life together. Only once persons with disabilities feel the church is a place where they belong will the choices concerning genetic technologies be free from the social demands of mandated normativity. Second, I consider how the liturgy informs and forms ethical practices. Liturgies of radical acceptance can reorient congregations to the value of all persons within the body of Christ. Finally, churches can help make explicit how they engage in the work of moral discernment. Church should be the space where Christians' most pressing moral dilemmas, including medical care, are deliberated. Although not every congregant will want to share the intimate details of his or her health care decisions with the whole community, churches can still support members when they struggle with difficult moral decisions. As an embodied community, Christians must learn to care for one another's physical, mental, and spiritual needs.

CREATING HOSPITABLE CHURCHES

As noted in the previous chapter, social structures and attitudes make it difficult to imagine how persons with disabilities can flourish in our society. Our culture's tendency to ostracize and demean persons with disabilities means the choices about using genetic technologies will be constrained. In an inhospitable world, "treatments" for genetic disabilities—such as experimental gene therapy, genetic screenings, PGD, or abortion—appear necessary. The body of Christ, on the other hand, ought to foster a different imagination regarding the meaning and purpose of the body. Before Christians can begin to help others in their decisions regarding the use of genetic technologies, they must first create churches that are hospitable to all bodies. Creating a hospitable community where all members feel they belong will not prevent all forms of suffering or make all medical considerations simple, but it may help to alleviate many of the social and attitudinal obstacles people with disabilities face. The church must be open to all people in all of their uniqueness.

In his book *Vulnerable Communion: A Theology of Disability and Hospitality*, Thomas Reynolds lays out three principles the church should use to make itself available or hospitable to persons with disabilities. Reynolds describes "availability" as "a sympathetic attunement in which I am brought into relation with the other's own way of being, experiencing the other's invocation as of moral substance by disposing myself to it in three interrelated postures: respect, fidelity, and compassion."[4] Being available to the other is a willingness to accept the other's difference and participate in the other's life. The first way we make ourselves available is by respecting one another enough to let the other be, in the same way God grants us all freedom to be. We seek first, not to change the other, but to accept her as she is, including her dependency upon others. Accepting the other's dependency requires we make ourselves dependable. Parents and caretakers should never feel alone in their caretaking responsibilities; they ought to be able to rely upon members of their church to share in their practices of care as each is able. Offering care to persons with disabilities and their families may require special training and education, but congregations should invest in practices that allow all members to flourish. Relationships of dependency and caretaking should be extended to all members of the community, who will inevitably need to rely on others to ensure their well-being and flourishing.

At the same time, the acceptance of everyone's dependency must be balanced against each person's individuality. As with all people, respecting the lives of persons with disabilities means allowing them space to develop their own individuality. Philosopher Eva Feder Kittay acknowledges this need when she discusses her daughter Sesha, who is developmentally disabled. Kittay describes how many people refuse to see Sesha as her own individual or to allow her personality to develop in its own time.[5] Many people assume Sesha has no capacity for individuality because of her obvious dependencies. The problem with this thinking is that it fails to appreciate how Sesha is unique and why she is deserving of friendship. Many nondisabled persons in our society overvalue individuality and fail to recognize the dependency we all share. At the same time, persons with disabilities are often seen as *only* dependent and not as unique gifts to the community on their own terms.

Because all persons are dependent individuals, the well-being and flourishing of the body of Christ requires that all persons grow in their relationship with God and with one another. Some in the Christian tradition have described persons with intellectual disabilities as "holy innocents" who do not have the ability to sin and, therefore, do not need to grow in their faith. Holy innocents are otherworldly creatures who exist only to remind Christians of who they are, but they are not unique persons. The notion of holy innocence denies people with disabilities their individuality, but it also denies them their spirituality. We ought to relate to persons with disabilities not as angels but as our friends. In his work *Receiving the Gift of Friendship*, Hans

Reinders claims Christians must consider people with disabilities, even profound intellectual disabilities, to be just like other people and thus deserving of friendship.[6] Unfortunately, many people with disabilities, particularly intellectual disabilities, are not befriended by the nondisabled. This is problematic, not only because it reveals a failure on the part of nondisabled Christians to fulfill their duty to love their neighbors, but also because the only way to discern and foster one another's spirituality is through friendship. We cannot befriend those we discount as unique individuals. It is only in the practice of friendship that persons with disabilities are valued for what they bring to the community.

Second, availability means fidelity or faithfulness to the other over time. "Fidelity requires giving time to others on their own terms, patiently and persistently, and without treating them as a means to some other end that I may have in mind, like being helpful."[7] To practice fidelity, we must not view others as objects or moral lessons given for our benefit. Being in relationship with persons with disabilities will likely benefit nondisabled persons, but persons with disabilities are not created solely for the enlightenment of others or to make the nondisabled feel useful. Fidelity requires the practices of friendship and mutuality.

Fidelity to the other may require that we enter relationships that are nonreciprocal, however. When discussing friendship with persons with profound intellectual disabilities, Jason Greig writes, "Friendships based on mutuality are marked by an openness and orientation toward the other that invites and draws out a response without demanding an equal exchange."[8] Christians offer friendship (*philia*) to one another for the sake of relationship. We do not extend love in order for it to be returned. Just as God offers us friendship despite the asymmetry between creatures and God (and despite our continual infidelity to God), so too are all Christians expected to offer friendship to others regardless of their ability or willingness to reciprocate that friendship. "In God's gift of friendship, Christians receive their personhood and ultimate value and learn how to recognize the same beauty in others that God sees in them."[9] Without expecting anything in return, Christians extend love to others and delight in one another's gifts. In so doing, we may be surprised by the gifts we are able to receive from others. Such mutuality is necessary for Christian flourishing, which is accomplished only in community.

Finally, availability as compassion allows us to "undergo, feel, or suffer with the other."[10] Compassion desires the other's well-being but does not try to eradicate suffering to make oneself feel better. Following Bacon, the eradication of suffering is a moral mandate in contemporary medical practice. In modern liberal society, compassion is understood through a techno-scientific lens as requiring the elimination of suffering through technological means. Selective abortion, assisted suicide, and euthanasia are merely the latest instantiations of our abhorrence of suffering and dependency. When suffering is understood as irredeemably bad, it is better to be dead than to suffer. Christians should not delight in suffering, but they do not understand the relief of suffering as a requirement of the good life, particularly if the relief of suffering requires the eradication of a person. Compassion requires a suffering with, rather than the elimination of all suffering.

Suffering is often read onto the bodies of persons with disabilities. Without a doubt, many persons with disabilities (much like those without) experience suffering as a result of their embodiment. To truly understand the suffering of another, however, requires that we know the other. Compassion, therefore, is a virtue practiced in relationship with others. Compassion requires imagining ourselves as the other, because we cannot truly feel their pain. As previously described, however, most nondisabled people are not very good at imagining what it is like to have a disability. To truly have compassion, we must experience life with the other, and we must identify our own vulnerabilities in these encounters. The more we practice compassion, the more likely we are to extend it to others, even those whose lives and experiences initially appear foreign to us. Practices of compassion resist eliminating or medically manipulating the vulnerable.

To Reynolds's categories I add two more: charity and mercy. Unfortunately, the meaning of Christian "charity" has become distorted over time. Charity for the ill or persons with disabilities has become a way for people to practice benevolence by donating money. The primary aim of many charity organizations is to "cure" illness or eradicate disability. Rather than explore relationships of mutuality, "nice" people donate to the needy without having to admit any need for them in return. In the Christian tradition, however, charity is a form of love rather than a form of pity. "Charity" or *caritas* was the predominant Latin translation of the Greek word *agape*, which has traditionally been understood as the highest form of Christian love because its original source and ultimate end is God. Aquinas understood charity to be a theological virtue that draws us toward the good. Charity is what enables human beings to be God's friends and directs us toward our ultimate goal of enjoying God.[11] Thus charity is not about being nice or giving away money; it is primarily about our relationship with God, which we extend to others and to our own bodies.[12]

Mercy, or *misericordia*, for the suffering is an effect of charity. Aquinas writes, "For just as charity makes us rejoice with those who rejoice, it makes us weep with those who weep."[13] Sadness over another's perceived misfortune is not mercy; rather, mercy is the ability to see another's misfortune as one's own.[14] Ultimately, we are all connected to the body of Christ; therefore, the misfortune of one is the misfortune of all. Again, the referent body in Christianity is the body of Christ. As Christians consider how best to relieve one another's suffering, they look first to communal practices of recognition and care. Describing practices of anointing in the Roman Catholic tradition, Therese Lysaught notes how the sacrament establishes a formative practice that reinscribes meaning onto the suffering body.[15] Suffering within the medical context is an isolated and isolating experience. Anointment, on the other hand, validates the individual's pain while also giving it a place within the body of Christ.

The practices of charity and mercy require persons with and without disabilities to become connected in acts of giving and receiving mercy. Aquinas believed the virtues did not exist in their fullest sense apart from one another. To imagine oneself in the place of another who suffers also requires that we imagine allowing others to give us that same mercy. Nancy Mairs in her book *Ordinary Time* describes how her own physical deterioration due to multiple sclerosis forces her to receive charity as well as to willingly give it to others. True charity demands conversion from simply giving from one's abundance to receiving as one who also needs. Mairs believes all persons have abundances and all have lacks. She writes, "True, your abundance may complement someone else's lack, which you are moved to fill, but since your lacks are being similarly filled, perhaps by the same person, perhaps by another, reciprocity rather than domination frames the interchanges."[16] For Mairs, "abundance" may take any form, and it often takes the form of suffering. Mairs believes living in real community means recognizing that one's own lack (for example, one's lack of another to give to) can be met only by the other's abundance of need (one's need for the mercy of the other). Each one of us is in need, and each of us lacks something only another can fill. Refusing to give care or refusing to be cared for, as if you were a "burden" on the community, affects the health of the community.

To practice radical acceptance, the ecclesia must encourage the virtues of respect, fidelity, compassion, charity, and mercy. These virtues are not merely extended to persons with disabilities but are reciprocally cultivated between all members of the body of Christ. Radical acceptance is not merely about the receptivity of the members of a congregation, however; it also requires the church to develop practices of mutuality and care. The liturgy offers space for such practices to occur.

LITURGICAL REORIENTATION

The church's liturgical life can help reflect, rehearse, and form the ethics of the church. Liturgies that maximize the participation of all members of the congregation are in the best position to reflect the value of the body within the Christian narrative. According to Lysaught, "The body is both necessary for and central to the entire enterprise of the Christian life. . . . The liturgy is the workout or training ground by which our very bodies are transformed from their current state of being to something radically different—bodies that we might call 'christo-form.'"[17] In other words, liturgy produces Christian bodies that faithfully follow Christ.

The Methodist liturgical scholar L. Edward Phillips notes that there are at least four ways liturgy is connected to ethics: (1) the liturgy can be informative for ethical reflection, (2) the liturgy can be morally formative, (3) the liturgy can offer an ethical critique of society, and (4) worship of God within the liturgy can be an ethical practice.[18] For churches that seek to welcome persons with disabilities and their caretakers, the liturgy can witness to all four of these connections to ethics.

Liturgy as Ethical Reflection

Liturgical texts and rites can help to inform Christians how the church understands the corporate and individual body. Services of healing offer a unique space for Christians to reflect upon the meaning of the body, as well their shared need for healing and reconciliation. Although most mainline churches have liturgies for healing services, their use is relatively rare and can sometimes reflect ableist sentiments that disability advocates seek to eradicate. Perhaps unsurprisingly, healing rituals have been used to single out persons with disabilities as pitiable and in special need of healing and wholeness. Yet there is the potential within such rituals for Christians to respond to the suffering that people with disabilities experience with God's good news. Healing services can allow the community to make their love visible to one another and to strive toward more equitable and just relationships.

There are at least four things the ecclesia can do to create liturgies of healing and wholeness that are disability-friendly. First, allow people to name their needs. Christians should not assume that persons with non-normative or disabled bodies desire physical cure. Rather than assume that disabled bodies are broken and in need of healing, we should first assume they are sufficient. Many persons with disabilities see their bodies not as obstacles but as vehicles for their spirituality.[19] Moreover, persons with disabilities may require healing, but healing will mean different things to different people. Individuals may desire physical health, spiritual renewal, or reconciliation with their neighbors. Services of healing should reflect the diverse ways people understand and seek out healing.

Second, services of healing should be careful not to conflate disease and disability with moral failing. In her book *Illness as Metaphor*, Susan Sontag writes, "Illness is not a metaphor, and . . . the most truthful way of regarding illness—and the healthiest way of being ill— is the one more purified of, most resistant to, metaphoric thinking. Yet it is hardly possible to take up one's residence in the kingdom of the ill unprejudiced by the lurid metaphors with which it has been handicapped."[20] Metaphors for illness and disability abound. Persons who are stubborn are called "deaf," the foolish are "blind," the fearful are "paralyzed," and so on. With such a rich metaphoric tapestry, it is not surprising that disability and disease are often conflated with tragedy and sin. Rather than rely on tropes such as blindness or paralysis to speak to our spiritual condition, pastors and congregants should use precise language that avoids conflating disease and disability with our communal failures and iniquities.

Third, liturgies should universalize the need for healing. Decoupling sin from disability does not require us to forgo the understanding of Jesus as a Healer and Savior. The most productive way to do this might be to position Christ's power to heal as signaling a new reality. The power of Christ as the cosmic healer is best understood as reconciling all of human existence to Godself, not correcting individual bodies that are perceived to be lacking. All people suffer, not simply those with disabilities. It may be that people with disabilities are suffering as a result of the discrimination and isolation they experience. As the great liberator, Christ urges us toward reconciliation with one another and justice in our communities. Healing services must acknowledge our universal need for healing as well as how we have collectively failed to extend grace to all of God's people.

Finally, liturgies of healing and wholeness should allow space for lament. Public lament is difficult for many people with disabilities, because they fear that others will associate their pain with their disability alone. The lack of such a space in our churches is tragic. Christians must work to create spaces where people with disabilities feel safe to lament without fear that they are confirming the worst stereotypes about people with disabilities. Of course, there are many reasons why people with disabilities may wish to lament their circumstances. They may wish to lament the loss they feel as a result of their disability. Alternatively, they may wish to lament what Andrew Sung Park refers to as "Han," or their feelings of sadness and resentment at being marginalized or victimized.[21] Until people with disabilities feel they belong in the church, they will be reluctant to lament corporately. Churches that struggle to faithfully include people with disabilities into their liturgical practice ought to consider allowing a person with a disability to lead the healing service.

Liturgy as Morally Formative

The embodied practices of worship can also help habituate Christians in the virtues and reorient them toward God. Liturgy provides Christians with another set of experiences to incorporate into the hermeneutical circle of moral discernment through the church's liturgical life. Traditionally, the priest and congregation faced the same direction—east—during mass following the Jewish practice of facing toward Eden in the east (Gen. 2:8).[22] Although few churches maintain the practice of both the minister and congregation facing in the same direction, the idea of a liturgical reorientation remains.[23] Liturgy requires congregants to orient themselves differently to experience the divine. Many aspects of the liturgy demand congregants comport their bodies, minds, and spirits differently during worship. Protestants have abandoned many formal bodily comportments (e.g., kneeling, prostrating), but these have been replaced by informal practices (e.g., raising of the hands, shouts of praise, spontaneous call and response)—all of which are based in the tradition but rarely instructed. Many of these bodily comportments are physically difficult for certain parishioners, while others require auditory, visual, or mental processing skills that leave others out. Rather than abandon embodied movement in liturgy, however, churches should seek out creative alternatives for persons who wish to participate in their own unique ways.

In her book *Accessible Gospel, Inclusive Worship*, Barbara Newman discusses several practices churches can adopt to include persons with intellectual and developmental disabilities into their liturgies. Newman encourages congregations to get to know each of their members, both their strengths and their struggles. Many people with disabilities will be perceived through their limitations. Most of our communal definitions of disability focus on what persons cannot do, which qualifies them for disability benefits. Instead, Newman suggests the right question for the church is, What *can* the person do? When getting to know persons with disabilities in our congregations, we ought to consider how they take information in (e.g., orally, visually, kinetically), how they get information out (e.g., speech, writing, gestures, picture identification), and what movement they can do (eg., run, walk, move wheelchair, move eyes, hold utensils). By understanding what a person can do and what he or she enjoys doing, the church can begin to think creatively about how each individual can participate in the liturgy.

Newman gives the example of her friend Yolanda, who is nonverbal and enjoys waving a streamer during worship. This is the way Yolanda says, "I love you" to God without using words.[24] Ideally the whole congregation should know Yolanda and how she expresses her love so that her participation in worship is seen not as a distraction but as a gift to her community. By allowing persons with disabilities to praise God as they desire, the entire congregation benefits from the gift of their presence and their expression of *philia*. Newman believes congregations should make similar efforts to help persons with intellectual and developmental disabilities form virtuous habits through other aspects of the liturgy, including confession, lament, illumination, petition, gratitude, service, and blessing.[25] By teaching and practicing these habits as each is able, congregations form themselves as the body of Christ.

Liturgy as Ethical Critique

The embodied practices of liturgy are capable of undermining the discrimination practiced against many persons with disabilities as well as undermining our common cultural understandings of "normalcy." Unfortunately, the liturgy can sometimes be malformative. The church's perpetuation of exclusion and marginalization represents a failure to embody its theonomous ethic. Margaret Farley observes,

Those who continue to be marginalized in the church (whether because of sex or race or class or whatever) are acutely aware that we have never adequately asked what it means to worship together as equals. We have not yet worked out patterns of authority that fully satisfy the gospel norms. We have not yet found creative answers to the questions of roles, degrees, and forms of participation in liturgy. We violate in our symbols and structures of worship both our teaching regarding the church as *koinonia* and our teaching regarding social justice in the world.[26]

By first modeling justice and inclusion in its sacramental and liturgical life, the church can begin to embody its teaching of justice. This requires the church to examine whom it marginalizes and how best to include those persons into the life of the church with true equality. Standing under the judgment of the gospel, the liturgical life of the church ought to be examined and possibly reconstituted to include the gifts of all its members.

Liturgical practices can serve as a direct challenge to the metaphysics of modern medicine. Whereas modern medicine tends to view the body a meaningless machine, Christians understand the body as a sacred gift, made in the image of God's own body in Christ. Jason Greig argues that the result of this Christian ontology is a "spirit of nonviolent care."[27] Christians accept bodies as they are without demanding that they first change to match our conceptions of normalcy or acceptability. Reflecting on his time spent in L'Arche, Greig believes the ecclesia offers an alternative imagination to that of Baconian medicine.[28] L'Arche communities are made up of people with and without intellectual disabilities who share life together in friendship. L'Arche presents an alternative form of community where persons with intellectual disabilities are not socially excluded but integrated and valued. When we enter into friendship and community with people who are devalued, we may come to understand their pain and vulnerability as markers of humanity to be "nonviolently accompanied," rather than as evils to be eliminated.[29]

Greig sees the practice of footwashing as symbolizing the alternative logic of power and justice embodied in the Christian community. Footwashing is a nonviolent practice that attends to the body of the other without trying to eliminate or alter it. "In washing one another's feet, Christians follow Jesus in recognizing the other as another self, as a fellow friend, no matter the embodiment or (dis) ability."[30] Whereas modern medicine seeks to overcome the finitude of the body for the sake of human flourishing, the Christian practice of footwashing embodies an alternative vision of flourishing, one born of humility, patience, and attentiveness rather than efficiency and domination. Through footwashing, nondisabled persons can come to a new understanding of the body as a gift and sign of God.

As a nonviolent, embodied practice, footwashing also helps to signal a future vision of the Kingdom of God in which "the weakest and most humble are given the most prominent place."[31] In this new moral order, people with disabilities are given an exalted place as friends of God and exemplars of human creatureliness. Footwashing inaugurates a new political order, in which persons with disabilities are treated as precious rather than disposable. Just as Jesus affirmed his friendship with his disciples when he washed their feet, so too do people with and without disabilities confirm their friendship by washing one another's feet. All persons in the body of Christ must learn to be givers and receivers of embodied practices. This mutuality establishes all persons as united in the same body. It also helps all persons learn how to endure practices that are often uncomfortable. In a society that values self-determination and self-sufficiency, allowing others to care for us can be difficult. The liturgical rite of footwashing shapes the eschatological imagination of Christians and subverts the logic of modern hierarchies.

Liturgy as Ethical Practice

Finally, the liturgy allows Christians to enact its theonomous ethic by practicing or living out the Kingdom ethic in the here and now. To do this well, the church must acknowledge the holiness of being along with the holiness of what ought to be.[32] According to Paul Tillich, Protestants tend to focus on the prophetic nature of the body, whereas Roman Catholics tend to focus on the sacramentality of bodies. Both notions of the body, however, are essential for Christian communal life. Protestants need to be reminded of the sacred foundation of all bodies "without which the prophetic-eschatological attitude has no basis, substance or creative power."[33] The Catholic emphasis on sacramental substance reminds Christians that all persons are gifts who must be celebrated. The church allows people to come before God as they are, relying not on their own abilities but on God's gracious presence among them. The Protestant emphasis on prophecy complements this thinking by driving the church to look beyond the present moment and toward fulfillment, proleptically signaling God's future Kingdom by working for it now.

Fully including persons with disabilities into the body of Christ requires properly attending to both the sacred and eschatological nature of the body. We must celebrate bodies as they are and anticipate the ways we will be transformed as the resurrected body. Biblical scholar Louise Gosbell notes how Jesus's parable of the banquet in Luke 14 imagines a new way of communal living that subverts the ancient practices of vying for high-ranking positions at banquets.[34] In the Kingdom of God, banquets include everyone, even the marginalized members of the community. Earthly banquets should reflect this Kingdom ethic. Whereas people with various disabilities were often servants or were even displayed for entertainment during ancient banquets, Jesus asks us to invite them as honored guests.[35] In the future Kingdom, equality will be shared among diverse bodies. Within the eschatological body of Christ, equality and diversity are the norm. To live out our ethical life together, Christians must honor one another as gifts from God and embrace our diversity through equality of participation within the body of Christ. The practice of inclusion within the liturgy, therefore, is an ethical practice.

Christian communities that fully integrate persons with disabilities into the life of the church (where they belong) practice what Rev. Dr. Bethany McKinney Fox calls "the way of Jesus." As the founder of Beloved Everybody Church, Fox leads a congregation where the gifts of people of all abilities are intentionally shared within the liturgy. Fox believes the church is not whole until all people are able to fully participate, so she encourages the active participation of persons with and without intellectual disabilities.[36]

For Fox, an ability-inclusive church requires that persons with intellectual disabilities be included at all levels of the congregation, including in leadership. The intentional inclusion of persons with intellectual disabilities in leadership roles has meant that those roles cannot be narrowly prescribed; rather, she has helped to develop positions of leadership for persons who feel called to lead.[37] Welcoming the voices and leadership of people with intellectual disabilities requires both creativity and constant adjustment. Fox quickly realized that the things she had come to value in church leadership, such as "high verbal capacity, intellect, skill for strategizing, and a strong presence," are rarely the gifts of persons with intellectual disabilities.[38] Surely, many Protestants have been led to believe the same. By overvaluing certain kinds of verbal communication and rational assent to belief, Protestants have neglected many other practices within the liturgy that might help persons to grow in their faith. Attending to the gifts of persons with disabilities reveals that many of the traits and practices we value in Christian worship exclude persons with disabilities as well as others whose spiritual experiences and practices are not rooted primarily in rational, verbal acceptance of doxological pronouncements.

When the liturgy attends to the unique presence and gifts of persons with disabilities, some liturgical practices might be revealed to be less relevant and efficacious than we once presumed. Instead, a spirit of openness takes their place. As Fox describes, during the liturgy of the Beloved Everybody Church, members act out biblical passages, bring in objects that remind them of God, play instruments during times of music, draw the biblical narratives as they are read, and call out their needs to God during times of prayer.[39] Openness to the movement of the Spirit allows the congregation to find creative ways of participating in the Christian narrative within the liturgy. Such a liturgy might sound chaotic, but inclusive churches that encourage active participation of all members are likely to be ordered to the wildness of the Spirit. Liturgies that include persons with intellectual disabilities remind the entire congregation that the liturgy must be open to disruption, both by members of the body and by the uncontainable Spirit.[40] Wildness might frighten us, but we are called to be open to the unpredictability of love. Just as God cannot be domesticated, so too should we not seek first to contain the worship of persons in the body of Christ.

By attending to and including people with disabilities in Christian liturgy, we can see how the liturgy offers space for ethical reflection, formation, critique, and practice. Creating spaces of radical acceptance creates an alternative imagination with regard to the place of disability in our society. Inclusive liturgies offer a necessary corrective to an ableist society that adds suffering to disability by excluding persons with disabilities from our shared social life. Within radically accepting spaces, persons with disabilities and their caretakers are free to consider the moral use of biotechnology outside of the pressure to normalize or fix the body. Of course, members of the body of Christ will be truly equal only in the Kingdom of God, but Christians can proleptically signal this Kingdom in their liturgical life here and now.

CREATING COMMUNITIES OF MORAL DELIBERATION

Church communities that actively care for one another through loving and just relationships and enact liturgies that incorporate persons with disabilities are in a better position to come together in the processes of moral deliberation surrounding the use of genetic technologies. Such deliberation continues to be necessary because few Christian denominations have rejected all genetic interventions in principle. Rather than a simple yes or no to genetic technologies, Christians ought to acknowledge the complexity involved in using these technologies and accompany one another when deliberating on their use.

Unfortunately, many Protestant churches have not offered space for members to share their medical concerns with one another or even with their pastors. Even though most Americans claim their faith is important to them when making medical decisions, they are not always sure how to apply church teaching to their medical choices, and many are unable or unwilling to discuss their medical choices with members of their faith tradition.[41] Most Christians want to discuss their faith with their physicians, but few physicians feel comfortable addressing patients' religious questions.[42] In my experience as a hospital chaplain and clinical ethicist, many pastors also feel uncomfortable visiting their parishioners in the hospital because they do not feel equipped to help them make medical decisions. As a result, medical decisions become highly individualized and do not involve a wider community. If we are all members of the body of Christ, however, then churches must make it clear that bodies are never merely individual. Not only does this mean that congregants share in the practice of visiting the sick, it also means churches should encourage parishioners to relate their individual medical concerns to the (church) body as a whole.

So how should congregations help one another in discerning the moral use of medical technologies? Many Christian communities have institutional hierarchies that bear most of the responsibility for deliberation about moral issues. In general, the Roman Catholic magisterium has been more directive than mainline Protestant denominations in its evaluation of medical technologies, including genetic interventions. As described in previous chapters, there are various official Roman Catholic Church teachings on the moral use of medical technologies, many of which are highly proscriptive. The *Ethical and Religious Directives for Catholic Health Care Services* further explicates the "ethical standards of behavior in health care that flow from the Church's teaching about the dignity of the human person" and provides "authoritative guidance on certain moral issues that face Catholic health care today."[43] Using the Catholic natural law tradition, Catholic bioethicists claim some acts done to patients are intrinsically evil, or evil regardless of context or rationale, while other actions support the basic goods of life. Of course, the magisterium does not provide a simple "yes" or "no" directive to all medical interventions, nor do Catholic laity always agree with the church's moral evaluations. Roman Catholics continue to debate the moral use of many technologies and medical procedures, but in general they have clearer and more prohibitive moral evaluations than mainline Protestants when it comes to issues in health care.

As described in chapter 1, mainline Protestants are less likely to describe medical technologies as morally illicit. Unlike their Catholic counterparts, most Protestant denominations do not run large health care systems, nor do they adhere to a natural law tradition. Much like Roman Catholics, however, mainline Protestants tend to work out their denomination's moral stances through special committees that use a process of moral discernment to decide where the denomination stands on important ethical issues. And while many have been reluctant to use the term *metaphysics*, their understanding of the meaning of human life, suffering, and death is informed by their beliefs of how God interacts with creation. As I have argued previously, Protestant denominations would benefit from being more thoughtful and explicit about their metaphysics and how it informs their understanding of the good life, the body, and the limits of medicine.

Even once their theological anthropology and metaphysics are properly worked out, however, denominations will still need to relay their bioethical evaluations to the laity. Even the clearest moral position statements will need to be interpreted and contextualized for each individual case. To draw upon the church's wisdom when making important medical decisions, the laity must be trained in the denomination's processes of moral discernment.

In many instances, mainline Protestant denominations have written eloquently on how they resolve moral debates as a denomination. For example, the Evangelical Lutheran Church of America (ELCA) has a document outlining the denomination's use of moral discernment. It advocates that church members come together in the study of scripture, the creeds, the tradition, and each person's ability to will, reason, and feel when deliberating on matters of moral discernment. The ELCA encourages a group of diverse people come together to share their experiences, knowledge, and imagination "in order to have the best possible information and understanding of today's world. To act justly and effectively, this church needs to analyze social and environmental issues critically and to probe the reasons why the situation is as it is."[44] In particular, the ELCA advocates that persons who "feel and suffer with the issue," and "those whose interests or security are at stake," be included in the processes of moral deliberation along with theologians and social experts.[45]

The United Methodist Church's *Social Principles* also outlines a variety of principles and ethical considerations for assessing one's social and moral life. The document acknowledges that conflicting moral commitments and ethical principles create real moral dilemmas and tragedies, such as the conflicts between the sacred life of an unborn child and the well-being of the child's mother.[46] The UMC provides guidelines for navigating difficult moral disputes, but, crucially for Protestants, it refuses to be dogmatic in the face of complex realities.[47]

Few parishioners will have the opportunity to be involved in the commissions formed to deliberate on ethical issues, so many are likely unaware of their denomination's specific stances on many issues or how the denomination deliberates on important issues. Relaying these stances and processes of discernment is important, however, not only because many parishioners will seek guidance when making moral decisions, but also because the denomination's method of moral discernment may be replicated on the local and individual level. When individuals are struggling with moral choices, they could benefit from understanding the resources and processes the denomination uses to come to its position statements. Understanding how leaders of the denomination employ scripture, creeds, prayer, rational discernment, and conscience can shape how parishioners approach moral dilemmas. For this reason, moral deliberation should be taught and modeled to local congregations by congregational leaders.

In addition to communal processes of moral deliberation, denominations should prepare pastors to counsel parishioners through difficult medical decisions. Health care is one of the most common areas of life in which people go to their ministers for moral guidance, so local pastors should be attuned to the health care decisions their congregants are likely to face.[48] Not all parishioners will want to discuss difficult moral dilemmas with the whole congregation, which is why the pastor is crucial for guiding moral decision-making. Church statements on genetic technologies and guidelines for moral deliberation may guide discussions between the pastor and parishioner. Pastors should not be expected to know everything about every medical technology, but when asked they should at least know the ethical and theological debates surrounding the issue (or how to access them) and how to apply these debates to their own pastoral care. Knowing how to apply genethical debates in theology to the question at hand will require the expertise of a well-trained and sensitive pastor. In the case of genetic technologies, pastors must listen to the real concerns of parishioners and use their theological knowledge to guide them through the process of moral discernment.

When deliberating with parishioners, pastors can help them develop a Christian understanding of conscience, which will ask the individual to consider more than simply her own concerns. Since the Enlightenment, "conscience" has come to be understood as free from external authority and bound only to one's personal authenticity and integrity.[49] As mentioned in chapter 6, however, in the Christian tradition the conscience is believed to be given by God and developed through education and reflection so that we can apply general knowledge to particular cases. Our conscience, therefore, exists within a social matrix—it is socially formed and must respond to relationships that exist outside itself, including one's relationship with God and others.[50] The communal nature of conscience demands that pastors help parishioners raise larger questions about their "personal" decisions, such as whose interests are truly being served. In other words, pastors should probe deeply into the individual's concerns, but they should also raise larger questions about how the individual's decisions will affect the community, particularly the vulnerable within the community. Pastors may consider asking the parishioner, "What do you believe the body is for?" "What do you think is the purpose of having children?" "What are our obligations to our bodies/our children's bodies?" and "What do you fear about disability?" Pastors should have their own answers to these questions, but they should help parishioners consider how their individual understandings and narratives fit within the larger Christian narrative about the body.

Exploring whose interests are being served within any medical decision is particularly important to discuss when parishioners consider using genetic technologies. Ted Peters notes there is a fine line between compassion and convenience when parents consider having children with genetic disabilities. "We should distinguish between eugenic purposes and compassion purposes . . . [but] the line between eugenics and compassion . . . is not clear. We should distinguish between preventing suffering and enhancing genetic potential. [The] risk of commodifying children and evaluating them according to standards of quality control increases, especially when they are sold to paying parents."[51] Peters's concerns should be cautiously discussed with parishioners seeking guidance. As Ellen Painter Dollar and others have noted, one can consider using genetic technologies such as PGD without viewing children as commodities.[52] Only through careful discussion can pastors help to bring forth the parishioners' true concerns and motives. Once they do so, pastors must help to test those concerns and motives against the teachings of the church. Sensitive and informed pastors are essential for discussing the debates that arise within Christian bioethics and applying them in individual cases.

Pastors are not the only persons capable of leading conversations about the use of biotechnology. The worshipping community should be a place where Christians feel free to share their concerns and their decisions. The whole community should be encouraged to pray for one another, accompany one another to the hospital, encourage one another, suffer with one another, and engage one another in deliberation. What makes Christian bioethics Christian is both the resources we use to make medical choices (e.g., scripture, ritual, liturgy) and the gathered community who make up the body of Christ. Moral discernment in Christianity, in other words, is always communal discernment.

SEVERAL FACTORS CAUSE individuals and parents to consider using genetic technologies. Genetic disabilities can have devastating effects on children and adults, some of which can be lethal. At the same time, the effects can be less extreme, causing disabilities that can make life difficult but not impossible. The medical model permeates contemporary thinking on the meaning of disability, causing many to believe disability is always a "bad thing" or a tragedy to be avoided at all costs. Since at least the beginning of the disability rights movement, however, countless activists have tried to recast disability as something other than tragic. Christians have not always been allies in this movement. Historically, many American Protestants have supported sterilizing, euthanizing, ostracizing, and pitying persons with disabilities. It is no wonder then, that so many see biotechnology as salvific; they share medicine's metaphysics.

If Christians wish to affirm that persons with disabilities can flourish with or without genetic interventions, however, they must be willing to create spaces where this can happen. Church ought to be the place where people are accepted as they are, participate in communal life, and worship as they are able. In church, persons with disabilities should feel they belong. Most of our communities have a long way to go before this is a reality. It may require a liturgical reorientation, one that is open to the wildness of the Spirit. If we can create communities of radical acceptance, then the question of genetic intervention will never be an individual one. The choice concerning whether to use a genetic intervention may still be difficult, but it will be less constrained by the forces of social oppression that make life for persons with disabilities isolating and difficult. Only when we first accept persons with disabilities as they are can we hope to make wise decisions about genetic interventions.

Conclusion

The moral considerations surrounding the use of genetic technologies, including genetic screenings, therapy, and enhancement as well as prenatal diagnosis and selective abortions, are complex and require careful moral deliberation. As I have attempted to show, simple valuations of humanity's ability to cocreate fall flat in debates about genetic technologies. Many major themes of Christian theology (sin, salvation, evil, suffering, incarnation, natural law, ecclesiology, sacraments) can be reframed to address the multiple concerns raised in the use of genetic technologies and their impact on our communities. To evaluate the use of genetic technologies, we must know something about the Resurrection, bodies in the Kingdom of God, the effects of sin on the body, and God's action in nature. Throughout these final chapters, I have attempted to reframe these classic Christian doctrines in light of the questions of genetics. I have not sought to provide a definitive Christian response to particular uses of genetic technologies; rather, I have attempted to provide a theological account that should be considered in the processes of moral deliberation. Ultimately, each case of moral deliberation on these topics will be unique, and generalized principles may be more or less useful as technologies evolve. Theologians, ministers, and churches must act as guides in moral discernment both for parishioners and for the wider public, without demanding absolute adherence to their logic and teachings. The church's instruction should be followed joyfully, as an authentication of one's true and essential being.

THEOLOGIANS HAVE BEEN DEBATING genetic engineering for decades, but what has been missing from many of our theological debates is a concern for the lives of persons with disabilities, particularly disabilities that are genetic in origin. Not only does this represent a failure within theological bioethics, but the church cannot be what it is called to be until it takes the wisdom of disability seriously. Without the transformative wisdom that the experience of disability brings, the church cannot properly discern the moral complexities present in genetic engineering. Christians have long proclaimed they find Christ in "the least of these," but they are often complicit in excluding, degrading, and marginalizing certain groups of people. Before the church can begin to make declarations about the medical advances that promise to cure disability, they must acknowledge their participation in excluding and harming those with disabilities. Along with the wider culture, the church stands under God's judgment for mistreating vulnerable persons. Helping to connect people making difficult decisions about genetic technologies to others in the disability community will give flesh to the processes of moral discernment. In fact, disability theology is likely to disrupt many aspects of church life that unconsciously participate in the cult of normalcy. By prioritizing disability, the church may be reminded of its moral obligations as the body of Christ.

IN HIS BOOK *Remaking Eden: Cloning and Beyond in a Brave New World*, geneticist Lee Silver asks us to imagine a world where we have the capacity to genetically alter our children to make them more desirable in our industrialized world. In this future, the rich will have control over the genetic makeup of their children through the insertion of synthetic genes and the poor will have to live with natural genetic inheritances. Our nation will be split between the *Naturals* and the *Gene-enriched* or *GenRich*.[1] The *GenRich* are smarter, more athletic, and more resistant to disease, and after a couple hundred years of genetic modification, there will be little chance of moving from one class to the other. The *GenRich* rule nearly all aspects of society, including the economy, the media, the scientific fields, and the entertainment industry, whereas the *Naturals* are low-paid service providers or laborers who lack the financial and genetic means to give their children a shot at bettering their predicament.[2] Eventually, the *GenRich* and the *Naturals* will become so genetically dissimilar that they will be considered separate species.

Silver's work sounds like the stuff of science fiction, but he maintains this is the inevitable outcome of technologies that already exist or are currently being investigated. Most geneticists and bioethicists argue that genetic and reproductive technologies today are not eugenic because the government is not forcing their use; instead, parents are allowed to make autonomous decisions about which technologies they will use. In Silver's account, however, the ability of the wealthy to seize control of largely unregulated reproductive and genetic technologies creates the conditions for his dystopian eugenic vision. Silver argues that it is hard to see how we could prevent a future where the wealthy will have more access to genetic technologies than the poor given the state of the global marketplace combined with our society's emphasis on parental rights and individual freedom. Couples who wish to make their children in their own image, but with more genetic advantages, create a world that is perhaps even more nightmarish than the one imagined by twentieth-century eugenicists.

Current government regulations and bioethical debates do not pose a serious threat to Silver's vision. Although Silver's book is nearly thirty years old at this point, all the scenarios he imagines are based on technologies that already existed in the 1990s. (Silver updated and rereleased the book in 2007, evaluating new developments in reproduction, but his overall thesis remains the same.) Silver believes bioethics debates about genetic enhancement are superfluous because parents will demand these technologies and the government will be powerless to intervene. For Silver, the line between genetic therapy and enhancement cannot be adequately drawn because they share a similar logic. In the end, Silver wants to resist the future he imagines, but he cannot see how to do so from either a practical or an ethical standpoint. Surveying the ethical and religious literature, Silver comes up empty-handed. Religious communities in particular ought to feel indicted by Silver's claims that their ethical teachings are too flimsy and contradictory to stand up against the arguments for reproductive liberty.

Only a theology with a strong and consistent metaphysical account of the world can resist the future Silver imagines. At the same time, only an apologetic theology that can speak to the current situation can remain relevant to those both inside and outside the church. What Christians need is a theological bioethics that is both metaphysically grounded and culturally compelling. This is no easy task, but Christians might find some resources for this type of theology in the work of theologians like Tillich who remain faithful to the Christian tradition while seriously engaging the deep questions posed by culture. Tillich's belief that metaphysics and ethics are inherently interconnected urges Protestants to reconsider the usefulness of metaphysical thinking within their theological ethics as well as in their engagement with the natural and medical sciences.

Against Silver's fatalism, Christians must resist a future in which the poor are fated to become a separate species from the rich. In such a world everyone suffers because ultimately our fates are intertwined. I want to imagine an alternative future where the lives and experiences of the vulnerable are given ethical priority. In this world, disabilities are sometimes mitigated or cured through medical techniques and sometimes they are not, but either way persons with disabilities are always invited into and equally included in our communities. Here, the disabled body is embraced rather than annihilated. In this world, persons with genetic disabilities are looked upon, not as mistakes or aberrations to be avoided, but as human beings with inherent dignity and a wealth of embodied knowledge and gifts to share. In this world, we do not demand that all people conform to a prescribed normalcy; rather, we embrace difference and diversity. Communities in this imagined future create space for others without demanding that they conform to predetermined standards for physical or mental normalcy. Persons with disabilities both belong in the community and are frequently leaders within the community. Here, all are welcomed as gifts from God who have abundances and lacks that must be shared and filled by others. In this world, we see the potential in all people, and we strive to help all people flourish. In this future, we meet each other face to face at the Eucharist table, where we see the holiness of the body as it is and for what it will be in the Kingdom. The Eucharist table comes to symbolize the final banquet where the poor, the crippled, the lame, and the blind are invited.

Only an alternative ontological view of the human person can inspire us to see the body and the value of human life differently. Far too many of us have bought into a powerful myth that our lives are reducible to our genes and that the ideal body is young, physically and mentally "fit," and able-bodied. This is the body persons strive for and want for their children, but this is not the body of Christ. Christ's resurrected body is not the powerful and beautiful body of Adonis, it is the damaged body of a crucified man who gave up ultimate power and security to be with the vulnerable. The body of Christ is wounded and yet whole. Christ's body is the one we should strive to conform to as individuals and as a corporate body. Taking Christ's body as the norm challenges our modern conceptions of normalcy as well as our social ethic. By taking the disabled body as our new normal, we can learn to appreciate others as the good creations of a loving God.

NOTES

PREFACE

1. PCUSA (Presbyterian Church USA), "The Covenant of Life and the Caring Community and Creation: Theological Reflections on Contraception and Abortion," 195th General Assembly (1983), www.pcusa.org/site _media/media/uploads/_resolutions/covenant-of-life-and-covenant -and-creation.pdf.

2. Ibid., 14–15.

3. PCUSA, "On Providing Just Access to Reproductive Health Care," 220th General Assembly (2012), #2, www.presbyterianmission.org/resource /presbyterian-church-us-general-assembly-resolution/.

4. PCUSA, "Covenant of Life," 11, 16, 20, 27.

5. Ibid., 24.

6. Ibid., 28.

7. Ibid., 27.

8. Philip Clayton, "Theology and the Physical Sciences," in *The Modern Theologians: An Introduction to Christian Theology since 1918*, ed. David F. Ford and Rachel Muers (Malden, MA: Blackwell, 2005), 342–56.

CHAPTER ONE. Science, Religion, and the Ideal Eugenic Man

1. Jonathan Peter Spiro, *Defending the Master Race: Conservation, Eugenics, and the Legacy of Madison Grant* (Burlington: University of Vermont Press, 2009), 47.

2. Quoted in Mitch Keller, "The Scandal at the Zoo," *New York Times*, August 6, 2006, www.nytimes.com/2006/08/06/nyregion/thecity/06zoo.html.

3. Spiro, *Defending the Master Race*, 47.

4. Ibid., 48.

5. Quoted in ibid., 48.

6. Peter Harrison, *The Bible, Protestantism and the Rise of Natural Science* (Cambridge: University of Cambridge Press, 1998).

7. Peter Harrison, *The Territories of Science and Religion* (Chicago: University of Chicago Press, 2015), 77–78.

8. Peter Harrison, *The Fall of Man and the Foundations of Science* (Cambridge: Cambridge University Press, 2007), 3.

9. John Calvin, *Institutes of the Christian Religion*, vol. 1, trans. Ford Lewis Battles, ed. John T. McNeill (Louisville, KY: Westminster John Knox Press, 1960), 64–65.

10. Ibid., 68.

11. Harrison, *Territories of Science*, 139.

12. Francis Bacon, "New Organon," in *The Works of Francis Bacon*, ed. James Spedding, Robert Ellis, and Douglas Heath (London: Longman, 1857–74), 299.

13. Philip Melanchthon, *Orations of Philosophy and Education*, trans. S. Kusukawa (Cambridge: Cambridge University Press, 1999).

14. Harrison, *Fall of Man*, 167–68.

15. Amos Funkenstein, *Theology and the Scientific Imagination from the Middle Ages to the Seventeenth Century* (Princeton, NJ: Princeton University Press, 1986), 6.

16. Harrison, *Fall of Man*, 243.

17. David Hume, *An Enquiry into the Principles of Morals*, ed. L. A. Selby-Bigge, 3rd ed., rev. P. H. Nidditch (Oxford: Oxford University Press, 1975).

18. Immanuel Kant, *Groundwork for the Metaphysics of Morals*, trans. Thomas E. Hill and Arnulf Zweig, Oxford Philosophical Texts (Oxford: Oxford University Press, 2002).

19. Friedrich Schleiermacher, *On the Christian Faith*, ed. H. R. Mackintosh and James Stuart Stewart (London: T. & T. Clark, 1999), 126.

20. Harrison, *Territories of Science*, 170.

21. Ibid., 144.

22. George M. Marsden, *Fundamentalism and American Culture*, 2nd ed. (Oxford: Oxford University Press, 2006), 124.

23. Leslie A. Muray, *Liberal Protestantism and Science*, ed. Richard Olson (Westport, CT: Greenwood Press, 2008), 51.

24. Ibid., 31.

25. Henry Emerson Fosdick, *Christianity and Progress* (New York: Fleming H. Revell, 1922), 87.

26. Ibid., 94.

27. Edwin W. Bishop, "Eugenics and the Church," *Eugenics: A Journal of Race Betterment* 2 (1929): 8, www.eugenicsarchive.org/eugenics/topic_images .pl?theme=32&search=&matches=&dpage=1. This sermon was preached May 13, 1928, to the congregation of the Plymouth Congregational Church in Lansing, Michigan.

28. Christine Rosen, *Preaching Eugenics: Religious Leaders and the American Eugenics Movement* (Oxford: Oxford University Press, 2004), 15.

29. Amy Laura Hall, "To Form a More Perfect Union: Mainline Protestantism and the Popularization of Eugenics," in *Theology, Disability and the New Genetics: Why Science Needs the Church*, ed. John Swinton and Brian Brock (London: T. & T. Clark, 2007), 80–81.

30. Rosen, *Preaching Eugenics*.

31. Marsden, *Fundamentalism and American Culture*, 2.

32. Ibid., 27–28.

33. William Jennings Bryan, "Testimony," in *Orthodox Christianity versus Modernism* (New York: Fleming Revell, 1923).

34. For example, most historians do not believe Aimee Semple McPherson is properly called a fundamentalist, even though she crusaded with William Jennings Bryan against teaching Darwinism in schools. See Margaret English de Alminana, "Aimee Semple McPherson's Pentecostalism, Darwinism, Eugenics, the Disenfranchised, and the Scopes Monkey Trial," *Pneuma* 41 (2019): 255–78.

35. Stephen Gaukroger, *The Emergence of a Scientific Culture: Science and the Shaping of Modernity, 1210–1685* (Oxford: Oxford University Press, 2009), 212–14.

36. Reinhold Niebuhr, "Ten Years That Shook My World," *Christian Century*, April 26, 1939, 542–46, 543.

37. Devan Stahl, "Moral Evaluations of Genetic Technologies: The Need for Catholic Social Doctrine" *National Catholic Bioethics Quarterly* 15, no. 3 (2015): 155–59.

38. Wilfred McClay, "Chesterton's Warning," *American Interest* 6, no. 1 (2010), www.the-american-interest.com/2010/09/01/chestertons-warning/.

39. G. K. Chesterton, *Eugenics and Other Evils* (London: Cassell, 1922).

40. Charles P. Bruehl, *Birth Control and Eugenics in the Light of Fundamental Ethical Principles* (New York: Joseph F. Wagner, 1928).

41. Pope Pius XI, *Casti connubii*, December 31, 1930, no. 71.

42. Herman J. Muller, *Out of the Night: A Biologist's View of the Future* (New York: Vanguard Press, 1935).

43. Ibid.

44. Ibid.

45. John Hyde Evans, *Playing God? Human Genetic Engineering and the Rationalization of Public Bioethical Debate* (Chicago: University of Chicago Press, 2002), 54.

46. David J. Kevles, "Out of Eugenics: The Historical Politics of the Human Genome," in *The Code of Codes: Scientific and Social Issues in the Human Genome Project*, ed. Daniel J. Kevles and Leroy Hood (Cambridge, MA: Harvard University Press, 1992), 16.

47. Ibid., 17–18.

48. John Hyde Evans, *Playing God?*, 57.

49. S. E. Luria, "Directed Genetic Change: Perspectives from Molecular Geneticists," in *The Control of Human Heredity and Evolution*, ed. Tracy M. Sonneborn (New York: Macmillan, 1965), 17.

50. H. Bentley Glass, *Science and Ethical Values* (Chapel Hill: University of North Carolina Press, 1965), 90.

51. See Lee Silver, *Remaking Eden: How Genetic Engineering and Cloning Will Transform the American Family* (New York: HarperCollins, 1998).

52. Pope Pius XII, "Moral Aspects of Genetics," address to those attending the Primum Symposium Geneticae Medicae, September 7, 1953, in *The Human Body: Papal Teachings*, ed. Monks of Solesmes (Boston: Daughters of Saint Paul, 1960), 257–58.

53. Vatican Council II, *Gaudium et spes*, December 7, 1965, n59.

54. Vatican Council II, *Gaudium et spes*, n36.

55. Pope Paul VI, *Humanae vitae*, July 25, 1968, trans. US Conference of Catholic Bishops (Washington, DC: USCCB, 1968), n2.

56. Ibid., n17.

57. Marsden, *Fundamentalism and American Culture*, 240.

58. Langdon Gilkey, "Religion and Science in an Advanced Scientific Culture," *Zygon* 22, no. 2 (1987): 171–75.

59. Frank Newport, "In U.S., 46% Hold Creationist View of Human Origins," Gallup Politics, June 1, 2012, www.gallup.com/poll/155003/Hold-Creationist-View-Human-Origins.aspx. More people also believe that humans evolved but that God had no part in the process (9 percent in 1982 vs. 15 percent in 2012).

60. The Creation Museum in Petersburg, Kentucky (http://creation museum.org/), is a testament to the continued determination of some evangelical Christians to provide an alternative scientific account of the universe.

61. Joseph Fletcher, *Medicine and Morals: The Moral Problems of the Patient's Right to Know the Truth, Contraception, Artificial Insemination,*

Sterilization, and Euthanasia (Princeton, NJ: Princeton University Press, 1954), 168.

62. Joseph F. Fletcher, *The Ethics of Genetic Control: Ending Reproductive Roulette* (Garden City, NY: Anchor Press, 1974), 52.

63. United Methodist Church, Resolution 3185, "Repentance for Support of Eugenics," 2008, in *Book of Resolutions of the United Methodist Church 1992* (Nashville, TN: The United Methodist Publishing House, 1992), www.umc.org/en/content/book-of-resolutions-repentance-for-support-of-eugenics; United Church of Christ, "A Call for the Study of Our Church's Involvement in the Eugenics Movement (A Prudential Resolution)," approved in 2009 at the 27th General Synod of the UCC, https://uccfiles.com/pdf/gs27minutes.pdf. Of course, the UCC was founded in 1957, so it was not a denomination during the eugenics movement, but they recognize that their "predecessor denominations" were involved in eugenics.

64. United Methodist Church, "New Developments in Genetic Science," in *The Book of Resolutions of the United Methodist Church 1992* (Nashville, TN: United Methodist Publishing House, 1992).

65. Episcopal Church, *Journal of the General Convention of the Protestant Episcopal Church in the United States of America: Otherwise Known as the Episcopal Church. Held in Anaheim, California, from September Seventh to Fourteenth, Inclusive, in the Year of Our Lord 1985* (New York: General Convention, 1986), 179, www.episcopalarchives.org/sites/default/files/publications/1985_GC_Journal.pdf; Episcopal Church, *Journal of the General Convention of the Protestant Episcopal Church in the United States of America: Otherwise Known as the Episcopal Church. Held in Minneapolis, Minnesota, from July Thirtieth to August Eighth, Inclusive, in the Year of Our Lord 2003* (New York: General Convention, 2004), 209, www.episcopalarchives.org/sites/default/files/publications/2003_GC_Journal.pdf.

66. See United Church of Christ, "Resolution on Concern about Moral and Ethical Implications of Genetic Engineering," 14th General Synod, Resolution 19, 1983, and "The Church and Genetic Engineering: A Pronouncement and Proposal for Action," 17th General Synod, Resolution 15, 1989, both available on request from Common Services Ministry, Mr. Edward C. Cade, Archivist and Records Manager, United Church of Christ, 700 Prospect Ave., Cleveland, OH 44115; and United Methodist Church, "New Developments."

67. Episcopal Church, *Journal of the General Convention of the Episcopal Church in the United States of America: Otherwise Known as the Episcopal Church. Held in Phoenix, Arizona, from July Eleventh to Twentieth, Inclusive, in the Year of Our Lord 1991* (New York: General Convention, 1992), 251; United Methodist Church, "New Developments"; United Church of Christ, "Church and Genetic Engineering."

68. Episcopal Church, *Journal [Anaheim 1985]*, 179.

69. In Bernard Häring, *Manipulation: Ethical Boundaries of Medical, Behavioral, and Genetic Manipulation* (Slough, UK: St. Paul Publications, 1975), 64.

70. United Church of Christ, "Resolution on Concern."

71. See Section II of United Methodist Church, "New Developments."

72. Ibid.

73. James Gustafson, "Theology Confronts Technology and the Life Sciences," in *On Moral Medicine: Theological Perspectives on Medical Ethics*, ed. M. Therese Lysaught et al. (Cambridge: Eerdmans, 2012), 59.

74. Clayton, "Theology."

75. David Masci, "Public Opinion on Religion and Science in the United States," Pew Research Religion and Public Life Project, November 5, 2009, www.pewforum.org/2009/11/05/public-opinion-on-religion-and -science-in-the-united-states/.

76. Adana Botoseneanu, Jeffrey A. Alexander, and Jane Banaszak-Holl, "To Test or Not to Test? The Role of Attitudes, Knowledge, and Religious Involvement among U.S. Adults on Intent-to-Obtain Adult Genetic Testing," *Health Education Behavior* 38, no. 6 (2011): 617–28.

77. Nigel M. de S. Cameron, "Bioethics: The Twilight of Christian Hippocratism," in *God and Culture: Essays in Honor of Carl F. H. Henry*, ed. D. A. Carson and John D. Woodbridge (Grand Rapids, MI: Eerdmans, 1993), 88.

CHAPTER TWO.   Theological Influences on the Scientific Revolution

1. "What They Said: The Genome in Quotes," BBC News, June 26, 2000, http://news.bbc.co.uk/2/hi/science/nature/807126.stm.

2. Daniel J. Kevles and Leroy Hood, preface to *The Code of Codes: Scientific and Social Issues in the Human Genome Project*, ed. Daniel J. Kevles and Leroy Hood (Cambridge, MA: Harvard University Press, 1992), vii–x.

3. Quoted in Sanger Centre, "The First Draft of the Book of Humankind Has Been Read, the Wellcome Trust and the Sanger Centre in Cambridge, Together with International Partners, Are Announcing Today," press release, June 26, 2000, www.sanger.ac.uk/news_item/first-draft-book -humankind-has-been-read/.

4. Quoted in Leon Jaroff, "The Gene Hunt," *Time*, March 20, 1989, http://content.time.com/time/magazine/article/0,9171,957263,00.html.

5. Walter Gilbert, "A Vision of the Grail," in *The Code of Codes: Scientific and Social Issues in the Human Genome Project*, ed. Daniel J. Kevles and Leroy E. Hood (Cambridge, MA: Harvard University Press, 1992), 83.

6. Richard Dawkins, *The Blind Watchmaker* (New York: Norton, 1986), 272.

7. Gaukroger, *Emergence*, 50.

8. Cf. Thomas Aquinas, *Summa theologica* II-II, q. 9, art. 2, and I, q. 1, art. 6, trans. Fathers of the English Dominican Province (Oxford: New Advent, 1947) (hereafter *ST*), https://dhspriory.org/thomas/summa/.

9. Gaukroger, *Emergence*, 58.

10. Augustine, *Enchiridion on Faith, Hope, and Charity* 3.9, trans. and ed. Albert C. Outler, www.tertullian.org/fathers/augustine_enchiridion_02_trans.htm.

11. Augustine, *On Christian Doctrine*, trans. D. W. Robertson Jr. (Indianapolis: Bobbs-Merrill, 1958), 65–66.

12. Harrison, *Bible, Protestantism*, 15.

13. Funkenstein, *Theology*, 49.

14. Harrison, *Territories of Science*, 68.

15. Gaukroger, *Emergence*, 136–37.

16. Aristotle, *Physics* 7.1.241b24–36, in *Aristotle: Complete Works*, ed. Jonathan Barnes (Princeton, NJ: Princeton University Press, 1984), 2:1–267.

17. Simon Oliver, *Philosophy, God, and Motion* (London: Routledge, 2005), 25.

18. *ST* II-II, q. 167, art. 1.

19. *ST* II-II, q. 167, art. 2.

20. Gaukroger, *Emergence*, 48.

21. Many of these scholastics actually misread Thomas, trying to replicate Thomas by doing philosophy before theology. For more, see Timothy L. Smith, *Thomas Aquinas' Trinitarian Theology: A Study in Theological Method* (Washington, DC: Catholic University of America Press, 2003).

22. Larry S. Chapp, *The God of Covenant and Creation: Scientific Naturalism and Its Challenge to the Christian Faith* (London: T. & T. Clark, 2011), 37.

23. Ibid., 41.

24. Ibid., 42.

25. Ibid., 89.

26. Francis Oakley, "The Absolute and Ordained Power of God and King in the Sixteenth and Seventeenth Centuries: Philosophy, Science, Politics, and Law," *Journal of the History of Ideas* 59, no. 4 (1998): 669.

27. Bronislaw Szerszynski, *Nature, Technology and the Sacred* (Malden, MA: Blackwell, 2005), 43.

28. Ibid., 43.

29. Ibid., xiii.

30. Harrison, *Territories of Science*, 76.

31. Harrison, *Fall of Man*, 91.

32. Harrison, *Territories of Science*, 141.

33. Funkenstein, *Theology*, 3.

34. Ibid.

35. Gaukroger, *Emergence*, 249.

36. Ibid., 5.

37. Szerszynski, *Nature, Technology*, 46.

38. Funkenstein, *Theology*, 6.

39. Gaukroger, *Emergence*, 246–47.

40. Gaukroger, *The Collapse of Mechanism and the Rise of Sensibility: Science and the Shaping of Modernity: 1680–1760* (Oxford: Oxford University Press, 2010), 5.

41. Ibid.

42. Funkenstein, *Theology*, 292.

43. Ibid.

44. Oakley, "Absolute and Ordained Power," 674.

45. Funkenstein, *Theology*, 323. This new ideal for knowledge is why Francis Bacon could see science as power; why Descartes believed, against the teachings of Aristotle not to mix scientific methods (which had begun to erode by the fourteenth century), that physics could use geometry to reconstruct the creation of the universe; and why Thomas Hobbes believed the science of politics, which was constructed, was superior to the science of nature. Knowledge created by doing displaced the contemplative knowledge (knowledge found) held up in the ancient and medieval periods, which reasoned that knowledge ought to be found through introspection, not constructed.

46. René Descartes, *Oeuvres*, ed. Charles Adam and Paul Tannery, 2nd ed., 11 vols. (Paris: Vrin, 1974–86), 251.

47. Bacon, "New Organon," 4:120.

48. Harrison, *Territories of Science*, 79.

49. Ibid., 80.

50. Ibid., 77–78.

51. Descartes, *Oeuvres*, 238–39.

52. Ibid., 153–54.

53. Ibid., 7.

54. Gaukroger, *Emergence*, 456.

55. Thomas Hobbes, "Human Nature," in *The English Works of Thomas Hobbes of Malmesbury*, ed. Sir William Molesworth, 11 vols. (London: John Bohn, 1839–1845), 4:1–76.

56. Thomas Hobbes, "Seven Philosophical Problems," in *English Works*, 7:1–68.

57. Thomas Hobbes, "Leviathan," in *English Works*, 3:1–2.

58. Ibid., 3:80.

59. Ibid., 3:22.

60. Ibid., 3:25.

61. Gaukroger, *Emergence*, 378.

62. Steven Shapin and Simon Schaffer, *Leviathan and the Air-Pump: Hobbes, Boyle, and the Experimental Life* (Princeton, NJ: Princeton University Press, 2018), 65–66.

63. Ibid., 340.

64. Gaukroger, *Emergence*, 373.

65. Robert Boyle, "Letters," in *The Works of the Honourable Robert Boyle*, ed. Thomas Birch, 6 vols. (1772; repr., Hildesheim: George Olms, 1966), 1:cxxx, https://archive.org/details/bub_gb_LqYrAQAAMAAJ/page/n10.

66. Shapin and Schaffer, *Leviathan*, 337.

67. Ibid., 306–7.

68. See Robert Boyle, "The Christian Virtuoso," in *Works*, 5:508–40.

69. Ibid., 5:319–40.

70. Boyle, "Disquisitions about Final Causes," in *Works*, 5:401.

71. Harrison, *Territories of Science*, 108–15.

72. Gaukroger, *Emergence*, 505.

73. For a thorough examination of the Victorian "crisis of faith," see Timothy Larsen, *Crisis of Doubt: Honest Faith in Nineteenth-Century England* (Oxford: Oxford University Press, 2009).

74. Harrison, *Fall of Man*, 243.

75. Gaukroger, *Emergence*, 505.

76. Michael Hanby, *No God, No Science? Theology, Cosmology, Biology* (Oxford: Wiley-Blackwell, 2013), 112.

77. See Benedict Spinoza, *Theological-Political Treatise*, 2nd ed., trans. Samuel Shirley (Indianapolis: Hackett, 2001).

78. Gaukroger, *Emergence*, 505.

79. Ibid., 3.

80. See Stephen Jay Gould, *Rocks of Ages: Science and Religion in the Fullness of Life* (New York: Ballantine, 1999).

81. Szerszynski, *Nature, Technology*, 8.

82. Ibid., 22.

CHAPTER THREE. The Metaphysics and Theology of Genetic Medicine

1. Francis Galton, *English Men of Science: Their Nature and Nurture* (London: Macmillan, 1874), 260.

2. Ibid., 259.

3. Ibid.

4. See Thomas Henry Huxley, *Science and Christian Tradition: Essays* (New York: D. Appleton, 1896), https://archive.org/details/sciencechristian 00huxlrich.

5. Ibid., vii.

6. Thomas Henry Huxley, *Lay Sermons, Addresses, and Reviews* (Cambridge: Cambridge University Press, 2009).

7. Quoted in John Hedley Brooke, *Science and Religion: Some Historical Perspectives* (Cambridge: Cambridge University Press, 1991), 298.

8. Ernst Haeckel, "Ueber die Naturanschauung von Darwin, Göthe und Lamarck," in *Tageblatt der 55. Versamm-lung Deutscher Naturforscher und Aerzte in Eisenach, von 18. bis 22. September 1882* (Eisenach: Hofbuchdruckerei von H. Kahle, 1882), 91, trans. Robert J. Richards in "Ernest Haeckel and the Struggles over Evolution and Religion," *Annals of the History and Philosophy of Biology* 10 (2005): 89–115.

9. Sam Harris, *The End of Faith: Religion, Terror and the Future of Reason* (New York: Norton, 2004).

10. Carole Jahme, "Richard Dawkins Wants Evolutionary Science to Be 'the New Classics,'" *The Guardian*, June 12, 2012, www.theguardian.com /science/blog/2012/jun/12/richard-dawkins-evolution-new-classics.

11. Darwin's evolutionary theory is actually not a single theory but several theories. For more, see Walter J. Bock, "Multiple Explanations in Darwinian Evolutionary Theory," *Acta Biotheoretica* 58 (2010): 65–70.

12. Ibid. According to Bock, variational evolutionary theory is a series of related but independent theories advocated by Darwin including "a) variational evolution; (b) gradualism rather than large leaps; (c) processes of phyletic evolution and of speciation; (d) causes for the formation of varying individuals in populations and for the action of selective agents; and (e) all organisms evolved from a common ancestor" (65).

13. Ernst Mayr, "Darwin's Influence on Modern Thought," *Scientific American*, November 24, 2009, www.scientificamerican.com/article/darwins -influence-on-modern-thought/.

14. Ibid.

15. Ibid.

16. Richard W. Burkhardt Jr., "Lamarck, Evolution and the Inheritance of Acquired Characters," *Genetics* 194 (2013): 793–805.

17. Ibid., 797.

18. Ibid., 801.

19. Charles Darwin, *The Variation of Animals and Plants under Domestication*, vol. 2 (London: John Murray, 1868).

20. Ibid., 17.

21. Hanby, *No God, No Science?*, 254.

22. Ibid., 210.

23. Charles Darwin, *The Origin of Species*, 6th ed. (1872; repr., Amherst, MA: Promethus Books, 1991), 405–6.

24. Mayr, "Darwin's Influence."

25. Ibid.

26. Adam R. Shapiro, "William Paley's Lost 'Intelligent Design,'" *History and Philosophy of the Life Sciences* 31, no. 1 (2009): 57.

27. William Paley, *Natural Theology* (Boston: Lincoln and Edmans, 1829), 25.

28. Shapiro, "William Paley's Lost 'Intelligent Design,'" 56.

29. Connor Cunningham, *Darwin's Pious Idea: Why Ultra-Darwinists and Creationists Both Get It Wrong* (Grand Rapids, MI: Eerdmans, 2010).

30. Brooke, *Science and Religion*, 276.

31. See Cunningham, *Darwin's Pious Idea*.

32. Ernst Haeckel, *Monism as Connecting Religion and Science: A Man of Science*, trans. J. Gilchrist (Project Gutenberg Ebook, 2003), www.gutenberg.org/files/9199/9199-h/9199-h.htm.

33. Wilhem Boelsche, *The Evolution of Man*, trans. Ernest Untermann (Chicago: Charles H. Kerr, 1905).

34. Brooke, *Science and Religion*, 278.

35. Ibid., 311.

36. William James, *Is Life Worth Living?* (Philadelphia: S. Burns Weston, 1896).

37. Augustine, *Confessions*, trans. R. S. Pine-Coffin (London: Penguin Books, 1961), 262.

38. Ernst Haeckel, *Evolution of Man: A Popular Scientific Study* (New York: G. P. Putnam's Sons, 1905).

39. Cunningham, *Darwin's Pious Idea*, 266.

40. Ibid.

41. Karl Raimund Popper, *Objective Knowledge: An Evolutionary Approach* (Oxford: Clarendon Press, 1972), 44.

42. L. Jones, "Social Darwinism Revisited," *History Today* 48 (1998): 7.

43. Bock, "Multiple Explanations," 69.

44. Jean Gayon, "From Mendel to Epigenetics: History of Genetics," *Comptes Rendus Biologies* 339 (2016): 226.

45. Yongsheng Lui, "A New Perspective on Darwin's Pangenesis," *Biological Reviews* 83, no. 2 (2008): 141–49.

46. Gayon, "From Mendel to Epigenetics," 27.

47. Maclyn McCarty, "Discovering Genes Are Made of DNA," *Nature* 42, no. 406 (2003), www.nature.com/articles/nature01398.

48. James D. Watson, *The Double Helix: A Personal Account of the Discovery of the Structure of DNA* (New York: Touchstone, 2001).

49. National Institutes of Health, "An Overview of the Human Genome Project," accessed July 31, 2021, www.genome.gov/12011239/a-brief -history-of-the-human-genome-project/.

50. National Human Genome Research Institute, "What Is the Human Genome Project?" National Institutes of Health, updated October 28, 2018, www.genome.gov/human-genome-project/What.

51. National Human Genome Research Institute, "The Ethical, Legal and Social Implications Research Program," accessed July 31, 2021, www .genome.gov/10002329/elsi-research-program-fact-sheet/.

52. Heidi Chial, "DNA Sequencing Technologies Key to the Human Genome Project," *Nature Education* 1, no. 1 (2008): 219, www.nature.com /scitable/topicpage/dna-sequencing-technologies-key-to-the-human-828.

53. Quoted in Nicolas Wade, "A Decade Later, Genetic Map Yields Few New Cures," *New York Times*, June 12, 2010, www.nytimes.com/2010 /06/13/health/research/13genome.html?pagewanted=print.

54. Ibid.

55. Nina P. Paynter et al., "Association between a Literature-Based Genetic Risk Score and Cardiovascular Events in Women," *JAMA* 303, no. 7 (2010): 631–37.

56. Wade, "Decade Later."

57. Many scientists initially assumed that human complexity necessarily meant more genes, perhaps close to one hundred thousand, but it turns out that humans only have around twenty-one thousand protein-coding genes, just one thousand more than a roundworm.

58. Ann Robinson, "Genomics: The Future of Healthcare and Medicine," *Prescriber*, April 2016, http://onlinelibrary.wiley.com/doi/10.1002/psb .1454/pdf.

59. Ann K. Daly and Ingolf Cascorbi, "Opportunities and Limitations: The Value of Pharmacogenetics in Clinical Practice," *British Journal of Clinical Pharmacology* 77, no. 4 (2014): 583–86.

60. US National Library of Medicine, "What Is Precision Medicine?" *Genetics Home Reference,* August 28, 2018, https://ghr.nlm.nih.gov/primer /precisionmedicine/definition.

61. US National Library of Medicine, "What Are Some of the Challenges Facing Precision Medicine and the Precision Medicine Initiative?," *Genetics Home Reference*, August 28, 2018, https://ghr.nlm.nih.gov/primer /precisionmedicine/challenges.

62. Kamil A. Lipinski et al., "Cancer Evolution and the Limits of Predictability in Precision Cancer Medicine," *Trends in Cancer* 2, no. 1 (2016): 49–63, www.sciencedirect.com/science/article/pii/S2405803315000692.

63. William J. Clinton, "Remarks at Robert Morris College in Cora-polis, Pennsylvania, September 25, 1996," in *Public Papers of the Presidents of the United States: William J. Clinton* (1996, Book II) (Washington, DC: US Government Printing Office, 1997), 1660.

64. Gareth J. Hollands et al., "The Impact of Communicating Genetic Risks of Disease on Risk-Reducing Health Behavior: Systematic Review with Meta-analysis," *British Medical Journal* 352, no. 1102 (2016): 1–11.

65. Companies such as 23 and Me, which as of 2017 has FDA approval for advertising and releasing these risk profiles, asks consumers to opt in to receive results for such diseases. See 23andMe, "Learn More about 23and-Me's New Genetic Health Risk Reports," *23andMeBlog*, May 19, 2017, https://blog.23andme.com/health-traits/learn-23andmes-new-genetic -health-risk-reports/.

66. Katherine Harmon, "How Useful Is Whole Genome Sequencing to Predict Disease?," *Scientific American*, April 2, 2012, www.scientific american.com/article/whole-genome-sequencing-predict-disease/.

67. P. J. Beurton, "A Unified View of the Gene, or How to Overcome Reductionism," in *The Concept of the Gene in Development and Evolution: Historical and Epistemological Perspectives.* ed. Peter Beurton, Raphael Falk, and Hans-Joerg Rheinberger (Cambridge: Cambridge University Press, 2000), 305.

68. Bock, "Multiple Explanations," 69.

69. Richard Dawkins, *The Selfish Gene* (Oxford: Oxford University Press, 1989), 21.

70. Dawkins, *Blind Watchmaker*, 111.

71. Evelyn Fox Keller, "Nature, Nurture, and the Human Genome Project," in Kevles and Hood, *Code of Codes*, 285.

72. On intelligence as heritable and tied to race, see Richard J. Herrn-stein and Charles A. Murray, *The Bell Curve: Intelligence and Class Struc-ture in American Life* (New York: Simon and Schuster, 1996). On the welfare state as unnatural, see Richard Dawkins, *The Selfish Gene*, 30th anniversary ed. (Oxford: Oxford University Press, 2006), 126. On genetic sources of male over female success, see E. O. Wilson, "Human Decency Is Animal," *New York Times Magazine*, October 12, 1975, 38–50. Wilson believes that we may achieve gender equality in society but that it will be difficult given genetic differences. On genetic origins for territoriality, tribalism, xeno-phobia, genocide, violence, and rape, see Richard C. Lewontin, Steven P. R. Rose, and Leon J. Kamin, *Not in Our Genes: Biology, Ideology, and Human Nature* (New York: Pantheon Books, 1984), 29. Wilson does not endorse xenophobia, although he does demand a "genetically accurate and hence completely fair code of ethics." It is also worth noting that Wilson's claims have been taken up by organizations such as the National Front seeking to keep Britain a "white nation."

73. Quoted in Nick Jackson, "Against the Grain: There Are Questions That Science Cannot Answer," *The Independent*, September 20, 2007, www .independent.co.uk/news/science/against-the-grain-there-are-questions -that-science-cannot-answer-402864.html.

74. E. Keller, "Nature, Nurture," 285.

75. Lewontin, Rose, and Kamin, *Not in Our Genes*, 264.

76. Linda L. McCabe and Edward R. B. McCabe, *DNA: Promise and Peril* (Berkeley: University of California Press, 2008), 1.

77. E. Keller, "Nature, Nurture," 282.

78. See, for example, Nessa Carey, *The Epigenetics Revolution: How Modern Biology Is Rewriting Our Understanding of Genetics, Disease, and Inheritance* (New York: Columbia University Press, 2012).

79. Steve Talbott, "Getting over the Code Delusion," *New Atlantis* 28 (2010): 145.

80. Ibid., 15.

81. John Cloud, "Why Genes Aren't Destiny," *Time*, January 18, 2010, 48–53.

82. Ibid.

83. See ibid.; Evan Jones and Blaine Smith, "Epigenetics and Pastoral Counseling the Science Behind What We Preach," *European Journal of Science and Theology* 8, no. 2 (2012): 47–52; Stephen M. Roth, *Genetics Primer for Exercise and Health* (Champaign, IL: Human Kinetics, 2007); Dawson Church, *The Genie in Your Genes: Epigenetic Medicine and the New Biology of Intention* (Santa Rosa, CA: Energy Psychology Press, 2009).

84. James D. Watson and Andrew Berry, *DNA: The Secret of Life* (New York: Alfred A. Knopf, 2004), xii.

85. Cunningham, *Darwin's Pious Idea*, 267.

86. Francis Bacon, "Magnalia Naturae," in *The Advancement of Learning and New Atlantis*, ed. Arthur Johnston (Oxford: Clarendon Press, 1974), 249.

87. Gerald P. McKenny, *To Relieve the Human Condition: Bioethics, Technology, and the Body* (Albany: State University of New York Press, 1997), 18.

88. René Descartes, *Meditation from First Philosophy* (1641), in *The Philosophical Writings of Descartes,* trans. John Cottingham, Robert Stoothoff, and Dugald Murdoch, vol. 2 (Cambridge: Cambridge University Press, 1984), 10.

89. McKenny, *To Relieve the Human Condition*, 21.

90. Ibid., 19.

91. Jeffrey P. Bishop, *The Anticipatory Corpse: Medicine, Power, and the Care of the Dying* (Notre Dame, IN: University of Notre Dame Press, 2011), 20.

92. Gilbert, "Vision of the Grail," 96.

93. Ibid., 83. Emphasis mine.

94. Ibid., 96.

95. Evans and Hudson, "Religion and Reproductive Genetics." It is worth noting that this relationship is correlational and not necessarily causal. As Evans and Hudson have shown, there are other factors, such as religious groups' understanding of suffering that factor into their approval or disapproval of reproductive genetic technologies.

96. In Bryan's closing statement (which he was never able to give), he attacks Darwin's view of the natural elimination of the weak from the population as leading to "Social Darwinism." In the speech Bryan also praises science and technology as a Christian endeavor, nothing that "Christianity welcomes truth from whatever source is comes." For the full text of the speech, see William Jennings Bryan, "Text of the Closing Statement of William Jennings Bryan at the Trial of John Scopes, Dayton, Tennessee, 1925," California State University, Dominguez Hills, website, www2.csudh.edu /oliver/smt310-handouts/wjb-last/wjb-last.htm.

97. Richard C. Lewontin, *It Ain't Necessarily So: The Dream of the Human Genome and Other Illusions* (New York: New York Review of Books, 2000), 161.

CHAPTER FOUR.   Natural Theology and Genetic Ontology

1. Paul Tillich, *Systematic Theology*, 3 vols. (Chicago: University of Chicago, 1957–63), 2:7.

2. Augustine, *City of God*, ed. G. R. Evans, trans. Henry Bettenson (London: Penguin, 1987). Augustine points out that if a baby with two heads is marvelous then the baby with one head is equally, and possibly even more legitimately, a source of wonderment.

3. See Gould, *Rock of Ages*.

4. Steven Weinberg, *The First Three Minutes: A Modern View of the Origin of the Universe*, updated ed. (New York: Basic Books, 1993), 154.

5. Mary Midgley, "Criticizing the Cosmos," in Drees, *Is Nature Ever Evil?*, 11–26.

6. Ibid., 26.

7. See Luciano Onori and Guido Visconti, "The GAIA Theory: From Lovelock to Margulis. From a Homeostatic to a Cognitive Autopoietic Worldview," *Rendiconti Lincei* 23, no. 4 (2012): 375–86.

8. See Weinberg, *First Three Minutes*, 154.

9. According to Christopher Boorse, all organisms have goals they pursue, but we need not give value to these pursuits. For humans, our goals

are survival and reproduction, so the activities that allow us to pursue these goals, such as eating and sex, are natural. Environmental conditions that prohibit us from pursing these goals are rightly called diseases. In Boorse's understanding, disease remains value-free because it derives from empirically given goals, which enable us to conform to "a generally excellent species design." Christopher Boorse, "On the Distinction between Disease and Illness," *Philosophy and Public Affairs* 5, no. 1 (1975): 26.

10. Clayton, "Theology," 353.

11. Wolfhart Pannenberg, *Metaphysics and the Idea of God* (Grand Rapids, MI: William B. Eerdmans, 1990), 3.

12. Ibid., 3. Notably, Pannenberg's reading of Harnack is disputed.

13. Ibid., 6.

14. Tillich, *Systematic Theology*, 1:24.

15. Ibid.

16. Ibid.

17. Ibid., 1:38.

18. Ibid., 1:237.

19. Paul Tillich, *The System of the Sciences According to Objects and Methods*, trans. Paul Wiebe (Lewisburg, PA: Bucknell University Press, 1981), 201.

20. A. James Reimer, *Paul Tillich: Theologian of Nature, Culture and Politics* (New Brunswick, NJ: Transaction, 2004), 186.

21. Tillich, *System of the Sciences*, 201.

22. Thomas Aquinas, *Summa theologica* I, q. 104, art. 1, trans. Fathers of the English Dominican Province (hereafter *ST*).

23. Rudi te Velde, *Aquinas on God: The Divine Science of the Summa Theologiae* (Burlington, VT: Ashgate, 2006), 125–26.

24. Michael J. Dodds, *Unlocking Divine Action: Contemporary Science and Thomas Aquinas* (Washington, DC: Catholic University of America Press, 2012), 220.

25. Petr Dvořák, "The Concurrentism of Thomas Aquinas: Divine Causation and Human Freedom," *Philosophia* 41, nos. 617–34 (2013): 623.

26. Ignacio Silva, "Thomas Aquinas Holds Fast: Objections to Aquinas within Today's Debate on Divine Action," *Heythrop Journal* 54, no. 4 (2011): 664.

27. Thomas Aquinas, *Summa contra Gentiles*, bk. III, chap. 70, trans. Vernon J. Bourke, ed. Joseph Kenny (New York: Hanover House, 1955–57), online ed., http://dhspriory.org/thomas/ContraGentiles.htm.

28. Ibid., bk. III, chap. 70.

29. Ibid., bk. III, chap. 140.

30. Ibid., bk. III, chap. 139.

31. Ibid., bk. III, chap. 140.

32. David Bentley Hart, "Providence and Causality: On Divine Innocence," in *The Providence of God: Deus Habet Consilium*, ed. Francesa Aran Murphy and Philip G. Ziegler (London: T. & T. Clark, 2009), 47.

33. Ibid., 41.

34. Ibid., 43.

35. Ibid., 36.

36. David Bentley Hart, *The Doors of the Sea: Where Was God in the Tsunami* (Grand Rapids, MI: Eerdmans, 2005), 82.

37. Ibid., 49.

38. Ibid., 57–58.

39. Alister E. McGrath, *A Scientific Theology*, vol. 1, *Nature* (Grand Rapids, MI: W. B. Eerdmans, 2003), 87.

40. Aristotle, *Physics* II.1.192b13–19, in *Physics: Books 1–4*, Loeb Classical Library, trans. Cary J. Nederman in "The Puzzle of the Political Animal: Nature and Artifice in Aristotle's Political Theory," *Review of Politics* 56, no. 2 (1994): 288.

41. Aristotle, *On the Soul* 432b16, trans. W. S. Hett, Loeb Classical Library (Cambridge, MA: Harvard University Press, 1957), www.loeb classics.com/view/aristotle-soul/1957/pb_LCL288.9.xml?rskey=sj2Vp3 &result=3.

42. Edwin A. Burtt, *The Metaphysical Foundations of Modern Science* (Garden City, NY: Doubleday, 1954), 98–99.

43. For Aristotle, men are by nature political animals. The distinction between nature and culture thus was not as essential for Aristotle as it is for many modern philosophers. See Nederman, "Puzzle."

44. Bruno Latour, *We Have Never Been Modern*, trans. Catherine Porter (Cambridge, MA: Harvard University Press, 1993), 31.

45. Ibid., 144.

46. Elizabeth Barnes, *The Minority Body: A Theory of Disability* (Oxford: Oxford University Press, 2016), 53.

47. Velde, *Aquinas on God*, 123.

48. Nicholas of Cusa, *On Not-Other (De Li Non Aluid)*, trans. Jasper Hopkins (Minneapolis, MN: Arthur J. Banning Press, 1987).

49. Brian D. Robinette, "The Difference Nothing Makes: *Creatio Ex Nihilo*, Resurrection, and Divine Gratuity," *Theological Studies* 72, no. 3 (2011): 525.

50. Council Fathers, *Fourth Lateran Council*, 1215 AD, Papal Encyclicals Online, www.papalencyclicals.net/councils/ecum12-2.htm.

51. Ian McFarland, *From Nothing: A Theology of Creation* (Louisville, KY: Westminster John Knox Press, 2014), 34–55.

52. Hanby, *No God, No Science?*, 316.

53. Augustine, *The Trinity* II.1.2, trans. Edmund Hill, ed. John E. Rotelle (Hyde Park, NY: New City Press).

54. McFarland, *From Nothing*, 42.

55. Hans Urs von Balthasar, *Cosmic Liturgy: The Universe According to Maximus the Confessor* (San Francisco: Ignatius Press, 2003), 96.

56. McFarland, *From Nothing*, 53. See also John Milbank, "The Second Difference: For a Trinitarianism without Reserve," *Modern Theology* 2 (April 1986): 230.

57. McFarland, *From Nothing*, 53.

58. Ibid., 49.

59. Augustine, *City of God* 9.24, ed. Evans, trans. Bettenson.

60. *ST* I, q. 47, art. 1.

61. McFarland, *From Nothing*, 68.

62. Augustine, *On Genesis* 6.17, trans. Edmund Hill, ed. John Rotelle (Hyde Park, NY: New City Press, 2002), 311.

63. McFarland, *From Nothing*, 71.

64. Hanby, *No God, No Science?*, 351.

65. Augustine, *Confessions*, trans. Pine-Coffin, 340–41.

66. McFarland, *From Nothing*, 74.

67. See, for example, the Christian debates over monogenesis and polygenesis. Kenneth Kemp, "Science, Theology, and Monogenesis," *American Catholic Philosophical Quarterly* 85, no. 2 (2011): 217–36.

68. Hugh Miller, *The Testimony of the Rocks* (Edinburgh: T. Constable, 1857), 229.

69. Ibid., 200.

70. Though certainly not all. In 2018, genetics professor David Reich wrote an op-ed in the *New York Times* declaring there were genetic differences among the "races," including for things like intelligence. He was accused of scientific racism almost immediately, and debates raged anew about the supposed gap between IQ scores between Caucasians and African Americans. See David Reich, "How Genetics Is Changing Our Understanding of 'Race,'" *New York Times*, March 23, 2018, www.nytimes.com/2018/03/23/opinion/sunday/genetics-race.html.

71. Leo P. Ten Kate, "Victims of Nature Cry Out," in Drees, *Is Nature Ever Evil?*, 171.

72. This is known as the Epicurean trilemma.

73. Arthur C. Petersen, "Contingency and Risk: Comment on Smit," in Drees, *Is Nature Ever Evil?*, 99.

74. See Havi Carel, *Illness: The Cry of the Flesh* (Durham, NC: Acumen, 2007).

75. See Richard Swinburne, *Providence and the Problem of Evil* (Oxford: Oxford University Press, 1998).

76. Gilkey, *Maker of Heaven and Earth*, 227.

77. Swinburne, *Providence*.

78. Paul Tillich, "Heal the Sick; Cast Out the Demons," in *The Eternal Now*, ed. Religion Online (New York: Charles Scribner's Sons, 1963), 61.

79. Shane Clifton, "Theodicy, Disability, and Fragility: An Attempt to Find Meaning in the Aftermath of Quadriplegia," *Theological Studies* 76, no. 4 (2015): 773.

80. Ellen Painter Dollar, *No Easy Choice: A Story of Disability, Parenthood, and Faith in an Age of Advanced Reproduction* (Louisville, KY: Westminster John Knox Press, 2012), 24–25.

81. Julian of Norwich, "Revelations of Divine Love," in *Medieval Writings on Female Spirituality*, ed. Elizabeth Spearing (London: Penguin Books, 2002), 189.

82. See Hans Reinders, *Disability, Providence, and Ethics: Bridging Gaps, Transforming Lives* (Waco, TX: Baylor University Press, 2014), 17–21.

83. Sharon V. Betcher, *Spirit and the Politics of Disablement* (Minneapolis, MN: Fortress Press, 2007), 41.

84. See Alasdair MacIntyre, "Is Understanding Religion Compatible with Believing?," in *Rationality*, ed. Bryan R. Wilson (Oxford: Basil Blackwell, 1977), 62–77.

85. Stanley Hauerwas, *Naming the Silences: God, Medicine, and the Problem of Suffering* (Grand Rapids, MI: Eerdmans, 1990), 49.

86. Kenneth Surin, *Theology and the Problem of Evil* (Oxford: Blackwell, 1986), 7.

87. Augustine, *Confessions*, trans. Pine-Coffin, 148–49.

88. Ian McFarland, "The Problem with Evil," *Theology Today* 74, no. 4 (2018): 325.

89. Augustine, *City of God* 11.9.

90. *ST* I, q. 49, art. 1, ad. 4.

91. Thomas Aquinas, *Summa contra Gentiles*, bk. III, chap. 10, trans. Vernon J. Bourke (New York: Hanover House, 1955–57), https://dhspriory.org/thomas/ContraGentiles3a.htm.

92. Thomas Aquinas, *On Evil* 1.1, trans. Richard Regan, ed. Brian Davies (Oxford: Oxford University Press, 2003).

93. Richard Cross, "Aquinas on Physical Impairment: Human Nature and Original Sin," *Harvard Theological Review* 110, no. 3 (2017): 317–38.

94 *ST* I, q. 48, art. 5, ad. 1.

95. Jason T. Eberl, *Thomistic Principles and Bioethics* (New York: Routledge, 2006).

96. In fact, Aquinas believed humans could have at least five different kinds of defects: organic, sense, intellect (both in theoretical reason and practical and moral reason), and spiritual. For more see John Berkman, "Are Persons with Profound Intellectual Disabilities Sacred Icons of Heavenly Life? Aquinas on Impairment," *Studies in Christian Ethics* 26, no. 1 (2013): 83–96.

97. *ST* III, q. 14, art. 1.c.

98. Thomas Aquinas, *Scriptum super sententiis*, III, d. 15, q. 1, a. 2.c, trans. Cross in "Aquinas on Physical Impairment."

99. *ST* I-II, q. 85, art. 5.c.

100. *ST* I, q. 48, art. 5, ad. 1.

101. *ST* I, q. 96, art. 3, ad. 3.

102. *ST* I, q. 92, art. 1, ad. 1. Aquinas sees women as a kind of planned failure intended by God for the good of reproduction. The idea that Aquinas thought women were defective men, however, is contested. See Michael Nola, "Aristotelian Background to Aquinas' Denial That 'Woman Is a Defective Male,'" *The Thomist* 64, no. 1 (2000): 21–69.

103. *ST* I-II, q. 87, art. 7.c.

104. *ST* II-II, q. 123, art. 1, ad. 1.

105. *ST* II-II, q. 47, art. 14, ad. 3.

106. Jason Eberl, "Disability, Enhancement, and Flourishing," paper presented at the annual meeting of the International Academy of Bioethical Inquiry, July 17, 2018.

107. *ST* II-II, q. 32, art. 2, ad. 2.

108. *ST* II-II, q. 75, art. 2.

109. I believe Aquinas does escape some of the critiques laid out by Hans Reinders in his book *Receiving the Gift of Friendship: Profound Disability, Theological Anthropology, and Ethics* (Grand Rapids, MI: Eerdmans, 2008).

110. Aquinas, *The Sermon-Conferences of St. Thomas Aquinas on the Apostles' Creed* XIV.2, trans. and ed. Nichola Ayo (Eugene, OR: Wipf and Stock).

111. The "disability as mere difference" perspective is often refuted by scholars, but the characterization of this view is often a strawman. See, for example, Greg Bognar, "Is Disability Mere Difference?," *Journal of Medical Ethics* 42, no. 1 (2016): 46. Elizabeth Barnes holds a "mere difference" view that sees disability as neutral, while allowing disability (independent of social context) to involve the loss of intrinsic goods. See Barnes, *Minority Body*, 58.

112. John Swinton, *Becoming Friends of Time: Disability, Timefulness, and Gentle Discipleship* (Waco, TX: Baylor University Press, 2016). Swinton

says this is the key point of Nancy Eiesland's *The Disabled God: Toward a Liberatory Theology of Disability* (Nashville, TN: Abingdon Press, 1994).

113. Julia Watts Belser, "God on Wheels: Disability and Jewish Feminist Theology," *Tikkun* 24, no. 4 (2014): 63.

114. Eugene F. Rogers, "Aquinas on Natural Law and the Virtues in Biblical Context: Homosexuality as a Test Case," *Journal of Religious Ethics* 27, no. 1 (1999): 29–56.

115. McFarland, "Problem with Evil," 334.

116. John Calvin, *Commentary on Genesis*, 2 vols., trans. John King (Grand Rapids, MI: Baker, 1996). 62–63, www.ccel.org/ccel/calvin/calcom 01.pdf. Rather than privations, Calvin believed all these things were created by "God as an avenger."

117. John Swinton, *Raging with Compassion: Pastoral Responses to the Problem of Evil* (Grand Rapids, MI: W. B. Eerdmans, 2007).

118. See Clifton, "Theodicy, Disability, and Fragility."

CHAPTER FIVE.   Disability and Personhood

A version of this chapter was previously published as Devan Stahl, "A Christian Ontology of Genetic Disease and Disorder," *Journal of Disability and Religion* 19, no. 2 (2015): 119–45.

1. United Methodist Church, *Book of Resolutions*, 332.

2. Ibid., 329. Italics mine.

3. United Methodist Church, "Joint Appeal against Human and Animal Patenting," press release by General Board of Church and Society, May 17, 1995, quoted in Steven Goldberg, *Seduced by Science: How American Religion Has Lost Its Way* (New York: New York University Press, 1999).

4. Quoted in Edmund L. Andrews, "Religious Leaders Prepare to Fight Patents on Genes," *New York Times*, May 13, 1995, www.nytimes.com /1995/05/13/us/company-news-religious-leaders-prepare-to-fight-patents -on-genes.html; Ted Peters, "Patenting Life: Yes," *First Things: A Journal of Religion, Culture, and Public Life* 63 (May 1996): 18.

5. Joseph F. Fletcher, *Humanhood: Essays in Biomedical Ethics* (Buffalo, NY: Prometheus Books, 1979).

6. Ibid.

7. Peter Singer, *Practical Ethics* (Cambridge: Cambridge University Press, 1979), 122–23.

8. Helga Kuhse and Peter Singer, *Should the Baby Live? The Problem of Handicapped Infants* (Oxford: Oxford University Press, 1985), 235.

9. Peter Singer, *Practical Ethics*, 2nd ed. (Cambridge: Cambridge University Press, 1993), 186.

10. Daniel Dennett, *Brainstorms: Philosophical Essays on Mind and Psychology* (Cambridge, MA: MIT Press, 1978), 285.

11. Hans S. Reinders, "Understanding Humanity and Disability: Probing an Ecological Perspective," *Studies in Christian Ethics* 26, no. 1 (2013): 40.

12. Reinders, *Receiving the Gift*, 154.

13. John F. Kilner, *Dignity and Destiny: Humanity in the Image of God* (Grand Rapids, MI: Eerdmans, 2015).

14. Emil Brunner also believed that protection for people who are "grossly retarded" was not warranted because they do not bear God's image. Emil Brunner, *The Christian Doctrine of Creation and Redemption* (Philadelphia: Westminster, 1952).

15. Bernard Bard and Joseph Fletcher, "The Right to Die," *Atlantic Monthly*, April 1968, 59–64.

16. Devan Stahl and John Kilner, "The Image of God, Bioethics, and Persons with Profound Intellectual Disabilities," *Journal of the Christian Institute on Disability* 6, nos. 1–2 (2017): 19–40.

17. Aquinas, *Summa theologica* I-II, q. 112, art. 1, ad. 3, trans. Fathers of the English Dominican Province (hereafter *ST*).

18. *ST* I, q. 5, art. 3.

19. Augustine, *The Literal Meaning of Genesis* 5.20.40–41, ed. Johannes Quasten, Walter J. Burghardt, and Thomas Comerford Lawler, trans. John Hammond Taylor, 2 vols., vol. 1, *Ancient Christian Writers* (New York: Newman Press, 1982), 171–72.

20. In his book *Calvin, Participation, and the Gift: The Activity of Believers in Union with Christ* (Oxford: Oxford University Press, 2007), J. Todd Billings shows Calvin had a similar understanding of participation. Against the "gift theologians" of radical orthodoxy (John Milbank, Catherine Pickstock, Graham Ward, and Simon Oliver), Billings argues that Calvin does not see humans as mere passive receptacles of God's grace. For Calvin, God's gift of grace is a gift that enlivens, solicits, and includes the recipient's action. Calvin's way of thinking about justification coming from outside us also drives home the falsity of thinking we are our best when we are independent.

21. Calvin, *Institutes*, ed. McNeill, trans. Battles, 2:1284–85.

22. Martin Luther, *Sermons I*, ed. John W. Doberstein and Helmult T. Lehmann, vol. 51 of *Luther's Works* (Minneapolis, MN: Fortress Press, 1959), 162–63.

23. Calvin, *Institutes*, 39–43, 55.

24. PCUSA, *Our Confessional Heritage: Confessions of the Reformed Tradition with a Contemporary Declaration of Faith* (Atlanta, GA: Materials Distribution Service of the PCUSA, 1978), 19.

25. Martin Luther, "On the Bondage of the Will," in *Martin Luther's Basic Theological Writings* 3rd ed. ed. Timothy F. Lull and William R. Russell (Minneapolis, MN: Fortress Press, 2012), 146.

26. Tillich, *Systematic Theology*, 1:255.

27. Ibid., 1:105–9.

28. Eiesland, *Disabled God*, 72.

29. E.g., John 5:3, Acts 13:4–12, Deut. 28:28–29, 1 Kings 13:4, Isa. 42:18–20. For more disability-friendly interpretations of these passages and others, see *The Bible and Disability: A Commentary*, ed. Sarah J. Melcher, Mikeal C. Parsons, and Amos Yong (Waco, TX: Baylor University Press, 2017).

30. In his evangelical response to the genetic revolution, for example, John Jefferson Davis writes, "Creation as man experiences it, however, is not in its original state but fallen and imperfect and subject to 'bondage and decay.' Birth defects, including those of genetic origin, can be understood in relation to this fallenness of creation." John Jefferson Davis, "Christian Reflections on the Genetic Revolution," *Evangelical Review of Theology* 28, no. 1 (2004): 70.

31. Gregory of Nazianzus, "Letter CI ('To Cledonius against Apollinaris')," in *Christology of the Later Fathers*, ed. Edward R. Hardy (Philadelphia: Westminster Press, 1954), 218. The passage continues: "If only half Adam fell, then that which Christ assumes and saves must be half also; but if the whole of his nature fell, it must be united to the whole nature of him that was begotten, and so be saved as a whole."

32. Ian McFarland, "Fallen or Unfallen? Christ's Human Nature and the Ontology of Human Sinfulness," *International Journal of Systematic Theology* 10, no. 4 (2008): 410.

33. Ibid., 415.

34. Ibid.

35. Ibid., 413.

36. Wolfhart Pannenberg, *Systematic Theology* (London: T. & T. Clark International, 2004), 271.

37. Tillich, *Systematic Theology*, 2:67.

38. Friedrich Schleiermacher, *The Christian Faith*, §59, ed. H. R. Mackintosh and James Stuart Stewart (Edinburgh: T. & T. Clark, 1928).

39. Tillich, *Systematic Theology*, 2:67–70. Schleiermacher writes similarly in *The Christian Faith* that suffering is experienced as evil only because of the reality of sin.

40. Kelly Dahlgren Childress, "Genetics, Disability, and Ethics: Could Applied Technologies Lead to a New Eugenics?," *Journal of Women and Religion* 19, no. 20 (2003): 154.

41. Tillich, *Systematic Theology*, 3:358–59.

42. Methodius of Olympus believed human bodies would be melted down and reforged from the same material, so that their defects and damages would be eliminated. Similarly, Peter Lombard claimed in *Four Books of Sentences* that resurrected bodies would be reconstituted with all their defects purged, "shining like the sun." He also claimed that bodies would appear around thirty years old, but with every blemish removed. Augustine concurred that the resurrected body would show the "flower of its youth" but believed the martyrs would continue to bear scars, which would enhance the appeal of the saints' bodies.

43. Eiesland, *Disabled God*, 89–105.

44. Thomas E. Reynolds, *Vulnerable Communion: A Theology of Disability and Hospitality* (Grand Rapids, MI: Brazos Press, 2008), 220.

45. Karen Lebacqz, "Dignity and Enhancement in the Holy City," in *Transhuman and Trascendence: Christian Hope in an Age of Technolgoical Enhancement*, ed. Ron Cole-Turner (Washington, DC: Georgetown University Press, 2011), 59.

46. See Reinhold Niebhur, "Ten Years," 542–46.

47. Irenaeus of Lyons, *Against Heresies* I.10.4, trans. Dominic J. Unger (New York: Newman Press, 1992). Thomas Aquinas reiterates and strengthens this insight, writing, "Now among all effects the most universal is being itself; and hence it must be the proper effect of the first and most universal cause, God. . . . Now to produce being absolutely, and not merely as this or that being, belong to the nature of creation. Hence it is manifest that creation is the proper act of God alone." *ST* I, q. 45, art. 5, and I, q. 42, art. 2.

48. Gustafson, *Ethics*, 241.

49. Douglas Ottati, *Theology for Liberal Protestants: God the Creator* (Grand Rapids, MI: William B. Eerdmans, 2013), 292.

50. Jürgen Moltmann, *The Crucified God: The Cross of Christ as the Foundation and Criticism of Christian Theology* (London: SCM Press, 1974), 3.

51. Karl Barth, *Church Dogmatics*, vol. 3, pt. 2, *The Doctrine of Creation*, ed. G. W. Bromily and T. F. Torrrance (Edinburgh: T. & T. Clark, 1960), 603.

52. Moltmann, *Crucified God*, 25.

53. Joel James Shuman and Keith G. Meador, *Heal Thyself: Spirituality, Medicine, and the Distortion of Christianity* (Oxford: Oxford University Press, 2003), 130.

54. John Swinton, "Introduction: Hauerwas on Disability," in *Critical Reflections on Stanley Hauerwas' Theology of Disability: Disabling Society, Enabling Theology*, ed. John Swinton (New York: Haworth Pastoral Press, 2004), 4.

CHAPTER SIX.   The Limits of Natural Law in Christian Genetics

1. Ted Peters, "Human Genome Project," in *Encyclopedia of Science and Religion* (New York: Macmillan, 2003).

2. Ibid.

3. Morris W. Foster and Richard R. Sharp, "Race, Ethnicity and Genomics: Social Classification as Proxies of Biological Heterogeneity," *Genome Research* 12, no. 6 (2002): 844–50; Toby Epstein Jayaratne et al., "White Americans' Genetic Lay Theories of Race Differences and Sexual Orientation: Their Relationship with Prejudice toward Blacks, and Gay Men and Lesbians," *Group Processes and Intergroup Relations* 9, no. 1 (2006): 77–94.

4. Peter Hegarty, "'It's Not a Choice, It's the Way We're Built': Symbolic Beliefs about Sexual Orienation in the US and Britain," *Journal of Community and Applied Social Psychology* 12, no. 3 (2002): 723–35.

5. Human Rights Campaign, "HRC Welcomes Scientific Study Exploring Genetic Basis of Sexual Orientation and Gender Identity," press release, October 20, 2003, collected on Enviroshop site, https://enviroshop.com /hrc-welcomes-scientific-study-exploring-genetic-basis-of-sexual-orienta tion-and-gender-identity/.

6. Nick Haslam et al., "Psychological Essentialism, Implicit Theories, and Intergroup Relations," *Group Processes and Intergroup Relations* 9, no. 1 (2006): 63–76. Interestingly, a recent Gallup poll shows the percentage of Americans who believe gay/lesbian relations are morally acceptable has risen steadily in the past decade; however, positions on the nature/nurture debate (whether people believe homosexuality is predominantly something a person is born with or due to factors such as upbringing and environment) have fluctuated between 35 percent and 51 percent between 2009 and 2019. Gallup, "Gay and Lesbian Rights," Gallup News, May 2019, https://news .gallup.com/poll/1651/gay-lesbian-rights.aspx.

7. Steven J. Heine et al., "Essentially Biased: Why People Are Fatalistic about Genes," *Advances in Experimental Social Psychology* 55 (2017): 137–92; Toby Epstein Jayaratne et al., "The Perennial Debate: Nature, Nurture, or Choice? Black and White Americans' Explanations for Individual Differences," *Review of General Psychology* 13, no. 1 (2009): 24–33; John Monterosso, Edward B. Royzman, and Barry Schwartz, "Explaining Away Responsibility: Effects of Scientific Explanation on Perceived Culpability," *Ethics and Behavior* 15, no. 2 (2005): 139–58; S. Shostak et al., "The Politics of the Gene: Social Status and Beliefs about Genetics for Individual Outcomes," *Social Psychology Quarterly* 72, no. 1 (2009): 77–93.

8. James Watson, *A Passion for DNA: Genes Genomes, and Society* (Plainview, NY: Cold Springs Harbor Laboratory Press, 2001), 225.

9. Peters, "Human Genome Project."

10. Ibid.

11. Richard Sherlock, *Nature's End: The Theological Meaning of the New Genetics* (Wilmington, DE: ISI Books, 2010), 104.

12. Aquinas, *Summa theologica* I-II, q. 90, ad. 1, trans. Fathers of the English Dominican Province (hereafter *ST*).

13. *ST* I-II, q. 91, art. 4, *respondeo*.

14. *ST* I-II, q. 90, art. 4, ad. 1.

15. *ST* I-II, q. 91, art. 2, *respondeo*.

16. *ST* I-II, q. 94, art. 2.

17. *ST* I-II, q. 94, art. 2.

18. *ST* I, q. 79, art. 13.

19. Benedict Ashley, "Elements of a Catholic Conscience," in *Catholic Conscience Foundation and Formation,* ed. Russell E. Smith (Philadelphia: National Catholic Bioethics Center, 1991), 48–52.

20. For more on these disagreements, see Todd A. Salzman and Michael G. Lawler, "Natural Law and Perspectivism: A Case for Plural Definitions of Objective Morality," *Irish Theological Quarterly* 82, no. 1 (2017): 31–38.

21. See Germain Grisez, Joseph Boyle and John Finnis, "Practical Principles, Moral Truth and Ultimate Ends," *American Journal of Jurisprudence* 99 (1987): 99–151.

22. Ralph McInerny, "The Principles of Natural Law," *American Journal of Jurisprudence* 25 (1980): 1–15.

23. Christopher Tollefsen, "The New Natural Law Theory," *Lyceum* 10, no. 1 (2008): 1–17.

24. George Khushf, "What Hope for Reason?," *Christian Bioethics* 22, no. 2 (2016): 238–64.

25. Jean Porter, *Nature as Reason: A Thomistic Theory of Natural Law* (Grand Rapids, MA: Eerdmans, 2005), 27.

26. Ibid., 27.

27. Matthew Levering, *Biblical Natural Law: A Theocentric and Teleological Approach* (Oxford: Oxford University Press, 2012), 231–32.

28. Ibid., 232.

29. Eugene F. Rogers, "Aquinas on Natural Law and the Virtues in Biblical Context: Homosexuality as a Test Case," *Journal of Religious Ethics* 27, no. 1 (1999): 45.

30. John Calvin, *Institutes* 14.2, trans. Battles, ed. McNeill, vol. 1.

31. Sherlock, *Nature's End*, 108.

32. See Karl Barth, *A Letter to Great Britain from Switzerland* (Eugene, OR: Wipf and Stock, 2014).

33. Karl Barth, *Church Dogmatics*, vol. 3, pt. 1, *The Doctrine of Creation*, ed. G. W. Bromily and T. F. Torrance (Edinburgh: T. & T. Clark, 1960), 39–41.

34. David Bentley Hart, "Is, Ought, and Nature's Laws," *First Things*, February 28, 2013, www.firstthings.com/web-exclusives/2013/02/is-ought-and-natures-laws.

35. Rogers, "Aquinas on Natural Law," 31.

36. For disability-positive interpretations of the Bible, see Melcher, Parsons, and Yong, *Bible and Disability*.

37. Bethany McKinney Fox, *Disability and the Way of Jesus: Holistic Healing in the Gospels and the Church* (Downers Grove, IL: IVP Academic, 2019).

38. See David F. Watson, "Luke—Acts," in Melcher, Parsons, and Yong, *Bible and Disability*, 303–32.

39. George A. Lindbeck, "Natural Law in the Thought of Paul Tillich: Note," *Natural Law Forum* 7 (1962): 85. In general, the naturalistic fallacy is not a problem for the natural law tradition, which seeks to derive moral norms from nature.

40. Paul Tillich, *Theology of Culture*, ed. Robert C. Kimball (New York: Oxford University Press, 1959), 137.

41. Ibid., 143.

42. Ibid., 137–38.

43. Paul Tillich, *Love, Power, and Justice: Ontological Analyses and Ethical Applications* (New York: Oxford University Press, 1954), 25.

44. Ibid., 25.

45. Lindbeck, "Natural Law," 89.

46. Ibid.

47. Tillich, *Love, Power, and Justice*, 57.

48. Tillich, *Theology of Culture*, 189.

49. Tillich, *Love, Power, and Justice*, 63. Tillich refers to this as attributive justice.

50. Lindbeck, "Natural Law," 91.

51. Tillich, *Love, Power, and Justice*, 64–65.

52. Ibid., 76–77.

53. Tillich, *The Socialist Decision*, trans. Franklin Sherman (New York: Harper and Row, 1977), 140.

54. Congregation for the Doctrine of the Faith, *Donum vitae*, February 22, 1987, n1, www.vatican.va/roman_curia/congregations/cfaith/documents/rc_con_cfaith_doc_19870222_respect-for-human-life_en.html.

55. Ibid.

56. Ibid.

57. Richard A. McCormick, *Corrective Vision: Explorations in Moral Theology* (Kansas City, MO: Sheed and Ward, 1994), 177.

58. Pope John Paul II, "The Ethics of Genetic Manipulation," *Origins*, November 17, 1983, 388–89n6.

59. William E. May, *Catholic Bioethics and the Gift of Human Life*, 2nd ed. (Huntington, IN: Our Sunday Visitor, 2008), 241.

60. Congregation for the Doctrine of the Faith, *Dignitas personae*, December 8, 2008, n25. See also James J. Delaney, "The Catholic Position on Germ Line Genetic Engineering," *American Journal of Bioethics* 9, no. 11 (November 2009): 33.

61. May, *Catholic Bioethics*, 241.

62. Delaney, "Catholic Position," 33.

63. Congregation for the Doctrine of the Faith, *Donum vitae, I.2.*

64. Ibid., I.2.

65. US Conference of Catholic Bishops, *Ethical and Religious Directives for Catholic Health Care Services*, 5th ed. (Washington, DC: USCCB, 2009), n50.

66. Pope Pius XII, "Moral Aspects of Genetics."

67. Sherlock, *Nature's End*, 12.

68. Celia Deane-Drummond, "Aquinas, Wisdom Ethics and the New Genetics," in *Re-ordering Nature: Theology, Society and the New Genetics*, ed. Celia Deane-Drummond, Bronislaw Szerszynski, and Robin Grove-White (London: T. & T. Clark, 2003), 308.

69. Catholic Church, *Catechism of the Catholic Church*, 2nd ed. (Vatican: Libreria Editrice Vaticana, 2012), sec. 1, chap. 1, art. 4. An act is intrinsically evil if its object is evil; neither good intentions nor circumstances can justify the act. Of course, there are debates in Catholic moral theology over the structure of human acts.

70. Deane-Drummond, "Aquinas, Wisdom Ethics," 308.

71. *ST* I-II, q. 57, art. 2.

72. Deane-Drummond, "Aquinas, Wisdom Ethics," 298.

73. *ST* I-II, q. 57, art. 2.

74. Deane-Drummond, "Aquinas, Wisdom Ethics," 299.

75. Ibid., 300.

CHAPTER SEVEN.   Practical, Embodied Wisdom

1. Pete Shanks, "The Scandal and the Summit: Reactions to the Announcement of Gene-Edited Babies," Center for Genetics and Society, *Biopolitical Times* (blog), December 7, 2018, www.geneticsandsociety.org/bio political-times/scandal-and-summit-reactions-announcement-gene-edited -babies.

2. National Academies of Sciences, Engineering, and Medicine, *Second International Summit on Human Genome Editing: Continuing the Global*

Discussion: Proceedings of a Workshop in Brief (Washington, DC: National Academies Press, 2019).

3. Sharon Begley, "Global Summit Opens Door to Controversial Gene-Editing of Human Embryos," *Stat*, December 3, 2015, www.statnews .com/2015/12/03/gene-editing-human-embryos/.

4. Erika Check Hayden, "Should You Edit Your Children's Genes?," *Nature*, February 23, 2016, www.nature.com/news/should-you-edit-your -children-s-genes-1.19432. CRISPR has already been used to alter the genes of both embryos and adults.

5. Emily Beitiks, "5 Reasons Why We Need People with Disabilities in the CRISPR Debates," Paul K. Longmore Institute on Disability, *Disability Remix* (blog), September 5, 2016, https://longmoreinstitute.sfsu.edu /5-reasons-why-we-need-people-disabilities-crispr-debates.

6. See, for example, the webpages of the Disability Ministries Committee of the United Methodist Church (www.umdisabilityministries.org /resource.html), the United Church Christ Disability Ministries (http:// uccdm.org/), the Episcopal Disability Network (www.disability99.org/), and Presbyterians for Disability Concerns (www.presbyterianmission.org /ministries/phewa/presbyterians-disability-concerns/).

7. Christine Hauskeller, "Genes, Genomes and Identity: Projections on Matter," *New Genetics and Society* 23, no. 3 (2004): 285–99.

8. Ibid., 293.

9. Maureen Junker-Kenny, "Genes and the Self: Anthropological Questions to the Human Genome Project," in *Brave New World? Theology, Ethics, and the Human Genome* (London: T. & T. Clark International, 2003), 120.

10. National Institutes of Health, "*All of Us* Research Program Backgrounder," accessed July 31, 2021, https://allofus.nih.gov/news-events/press -kit/all-us-research-program-backgrounder.

11. Miranda Fricker, *Epistemic Injustice: Power and the Ethics of Knowing* (Oxford: Oxford University Press, 2007).

12. Gary L. Albrecht and Patrick J. Devlieger, "The Disability Paradox: High Quality of Life against All Odds," *Social Science and Medicine* 48, no. 8 (1999): 977–88, and reply by Tom Koch, "The Illusion of Paradox," *Social Science and Medicine* 50, no. 6 (2000): 757–59.

13. Jonathan Glover, *Choosing Children: Genes, Disability, and Design*, Uehiro Series in Practical Ethics (Oxford: Oxford University Press, 2006), 18.

14. Dan Brock, "Preventing Genetically Transmitted Disabilities While Respecting Persons with Disabilities," in *Quality of Life and Human Difference: Genetic Testing, Health Care and Disability*, ed. D. Wasserman,

J. Bickenbach, and R. Wachbroit (New York: Cambridge University Press, 2005), 67–100.

15. Ibid.

16. John Harris, "Is Gene Therapy a Form of Eugenics?," *Bioethics* 7, no. 7 (1993): 178–87.

17. John Harris, *Clones, Genes, and Immortality: Ethics and the Genetic Revolution* (Oxford: Oxford University Press, 1998), 91.

18. Allen Buchanan et al., *From Chance to Choice: Genetics and Justice* (Cambridge: Cambridge University Press, 2000), 257.

19. James Watson, "President's Essay: Genes and Politics," *Cold Springs Harbor Annual Report*, 1996, 1–20, 19.

20. See examples by Michael Gerson, "The Eugenics Temptation," *Washington Post*, October 24, 2007, https://www.washingtonpost.com /wp-dyn/content/article/2007/10/23/AR200 7102301803.html.

21. Robert G. Edwards, *Sunday Times*, July 4, 1999, quoted in John Bryant and Peter Turnpenny, "Genetics and Genetic Modification of Humans: Principles, Practices and Possibilities," in *Brave New World? Theology, Ethics, and the Human Genome*, ed. Celia Deane-Drummond (London: T. & T. Clark International, 2003), 14.

22. John Harris, *Enhancing Evolution: The Ethical Case for Making Better People* (Princeton, NJ: Princeton University Press, 2007), 9.

23. Traditionally, bioethicists have distinguished medical "therapy," which is aimed at curing or alleviating disease, from "enhancement," which is aimed at improving otherwise normal traits. Of course, as many people point out, the ambiguity of what counts as disease makes the blurring of the boundaries between therapy and enhancement inevitable.

24. Norman Daniels, *Just Health Care* (New York: Cambridge University Press, 1985), 43. Daniels acknowledges we live in a pluralistic society that will never agree on an articulation of the human telos or the good life, but even if we cannot agree on what a human being ought to be in any philosophical or theological sense, we may still want to articulate what a human being is *naturally*. Daniels believes the medical sciences, and particularly the biomedical model of health, can accurately describe the "naturalness" of human life.

25. When advocating for the Human Genome Project, the Office of Technology Assessment (OTA) adopted this same rationale in 1988, citing a report claiming, "Individuals have a paramount right to be born with a normal, adequate hereditary endowment." Thus, according to the OTA, "a eugenics of normalcy" can be distinguished from early eugenics programs. US Congress, Office of Technology Assessment, *Mapping Our Genes* (Washington, DC: Government Printing Office, 1988), 85.

26. Buchanan et al., *From Chance to Choice*, 283.

27. Ibid., 288.

28. R. Amundson and S. Tresky, "On a Bioethical Challenge to Disability Rights," *Journal of Medicine and Philosophy* 32, no. 6 (2007): 549.

29. For a fuller disability rights critique of the book, see R. Amundson and S. Tresky, "Bioethics and Disability Rights: Conflicting Values and Perspectives," *Bioethical Inquiry* 5, nos. 2–3 (2008): 111.

30. Margaret Farley, "The Role of Experience in Moral Discernment," in *Christian Ethics: Problems and Prospects*, ed. Lisa Sowle Cahill and James F. Childress (Cleveland, OH: Pilgrim Press, 1996), 136.

31. John M. Hull, *In the Beginning There Was Darkness: A Blind Person's Conversations with the Bible* (Harrisburg, PA: Trinity Press International, 2001).

32. Richard Cross, "Baptism, Faith and Severe Cognitive Impairment in Some Medieval Theologies," *International Journal of Systematic Theology* 14, no. 4 (2012): 420–38.

33. Aquinas, *Summa theologica* II-II, q. 47, art. 4, trans. Fathers of the English Dominican Province (hereafter *ST*).

34. Margaret Farley, *Just Love: A Framework for Christian Sexual Ethics* (New York: Continuum International Publishing Company, 2008), 193–94.

35. Gregory Kellogg et al., "Attitudes of Mothers of Children with Down Syndrome towards Noninvasive Prenatal Testing," *Journal of Genetic Counseling* 23, no. 5 (2014): 805–13.

36. Brian G. Skotko, Susan P. Levine, and Richard Goldstein, "Self-Perceptions from People with Down Syndrome," *American Journal of Medical Genetics* 155, no. 10 (2011): 2360–69.

37. Gerson, "Eugenics Temptation."

38. Barnes, *Minority Body*. Barnes's example is Michael Phelps's marfanoid habitus (14–15).

39. Tobin Siebers, *Disability Theory* (Ann Arbor: University of Michigan Press, 2008).

40. Simo Vehmas, "Live and Let Die? Disability in Bioethics," *New Review of Bioethics* 1, no. 1 (2003): 146.

41. Jackie Leach Scully, *Disability Bioethics: Moral Bodies, Moral Difference* (Lanham, MD: Rowman and Littlefield, 2008), 25.

42. Alison Kafer, *Feminist Queer Crip* (Bloomington: Indiana University Press, 2013).

43. On criticisms of insufficient attentiveness to material conditions, see Tom Shakespeare, *Disability Rights and Wrongs Revisited*, 2nd ed. (New York: Routledge, 2014), 12.

44. Jill Harshaw, *God beyond Words: Christian Theology and the Spiritual Experiences of People with Profound Intellectual Disabilities* (London: Jessica Kingsley, 2016), 1–4.

45. Calvin, *Institutes,* trans. Battles, ed. McNeill, 1.

46. Deborah Creamer, "Toward a Theology That Includes the Human Experience of Disability," *Journal of Religion, Disability and Health* 7, no. 3 (2003): 65.

47. John Swinton, "Who Is the God We Worship? Theologies of Disability: Challenges and New Possibilities," *International Journal of Practical Theology* 14, no. 2 (2011): 296.

48. Elaine Scarry, *The Body in Pain: The Making and Unmaking of the World* (Oxford: Oxford University Press, 1985), 2.

49. Hans S. Reinders, *The Future of the Disabled in Liberal Society: An Ethical Analysis* (Notre Dame, IN: University of Notre Dame Press, 2000).

50. Adrienne Asch, "Why I Haven't Changed My Mind about Prenatal Diagnosis: Reflections and Refinements," in *Prenatal Testing and Disability Rights,* ed. Erik Parens and Adrienne Asch (Washington, DC: Georgetown University Press, 2000), 240.

51. Erik Parens and Adrienne Asch, "The Disability Rights Critique of Prenatal Genetic Testing," in Parens and Asch, *Prenatal Testing and Disability Rights.*

52. Bruce Jennings, "Technology and the Genetic Imaginary," in *Theology, Disability and the New Genetics: Why Science Needs the Church,* ed. John Swinton and Brian Brock (London: T. & T. Clark, 2007), 129–32.

53. Tom Shakespeare, "Arguing about Genetics and Disability," in Swinton and Brock, *Theology, Disability,* 68.

54. Anita Ho, "The Individualist Model of Autonomy and the Challenge of Disability," *Bioethical Inquiry* 5, nos. 2–3 (2008): 197.

55. Alicia Ouellette, "Selection against Disability: Abortion, ART, and Access," *Journal of Law, Medicine, and Ethics* 43, no. 2 (2015): 220.

56. Teresa Blankmeyer Burke, "Rendered Mute," *Atrium* 12 (2014): 1–2.

57. Brian Brock and Stephanie Brock, "Being Disabled in the New World of Genetic Testing," in Swinton and Brock, *Theology, Disability,* 38–39.

58. Robert Spaemann, *Persons: The Difference between "Someone" and "Something,"* trans. Oliver O'Donovan (Oxford: Oxford University Press, 2006), 240.

59. Ibid., 240, 243. Spaemann does go on to describe persons with severe disabilities as "sick," as "patients," and as "broken"—language I find objectionable and unnecessary to his formulation of personhood.

60. Ibid., 244.

61. Ibid.

62. John Milbank, "Can a Gift Be Given? Prolegomena to a Future Trinitarian Metaphysic," *Modern Theology* 11, no. 1 (1995): 136.

63. Ibid., 136–37.

64. Ibid., 135.

65. Ibid., 137. To refuse the gift of our being and reciprocate that gift creates a paradox that alienates us from God and from our true natures, which could be undone only through Christ's incarnation and crucifixion.

66. J. Todd Billings, "John Milbank's Theology of the 'Gift' and Calvin's Theology of Grace: A Critical Comparison," *Modern Theology* 21 no. 1 (2005): 87–105.

CHAPTER EIGHT. Disability Inclusion and Virtue within the Church

1. Robert Song, "Genetic Manipulation and the Body of Christ," *Studies in Christian Ethics* 20, no. 3 (2007): 415.

2. Ibid., 415–16.

3. Ibid., 418.

4. Reynolds, *Vulnerable Communion*, 123. Reynolds adopts these categories from Gabriel Marcel.

5. Eva Feder Kittay, *Love's Labor: Essays on Women, Equality, and Dependency* (New York: Routledge, 1999).

6. Reinders, *Receiving the Gift.*

7. Reynolds, *Vulnerable Communion*, 126.

8. Jason Reimer Greig, *Reconsidering Intellectual Disability: L'Arche, Medical Ethics, and Christian Friendship* (Washington, DC: Georgetown University Press, 2015), 133.

9. Ibid., 133–34.

10. Ibid.

11. Aquinas, *Summa theologica* II-II, q. 23, art. 7, trans. Fathers of the English Dominican Province (hereafter *ST*).

12. *ST* II-II, q. 25, art. 4.

13. *ST* II-II, q. 30, art. 3. Pope Benedict XVI also offers a compelling read of "charity" in which he pairs voluntarily, radical acts of charity with truth in the encyclical letter *Caritas in veritate*, July 7, 2009, www.vatican .va/holy_father/benedict_xvi/encyclicals/documents/hf_ben-xvi_enc _20090629_caritas-in-veritate_en.html.

14. *ST* II-II, q. 30, art. 2.

15. M. Therese Lysaught, "Vulnerability within the Body of Christ: Anointing of the Sick and Theological Anthropology," in *Health and Human Flourishing*, ed. Carol Taylor and Robert Dell-Oro (Washington, DC: Georgetown University Press, 2006), 159–84.

16. Nancy Mairs, *Ordinary Time: Cycles in Marriage, Faith, and Renewal* (Boston: Beacon Press, 1993), 163.

17. Therese Lysaught, "'Ten Decades to a More Christ-Like You!': Liturgy as God's Workout Plan for the Church," *Liturgy* 24, no. 1 (2008): 8.

18. L. Edward Phillips, "Ethics and Worship," in *The New Westminster Dictionary of Liturgy and Worship*, ed. Paul Bradshaw (Louisville, KY: Westminster John Knox Press, SCM Press, 2002), 167–69.

19. See Julia Watts Belser and Melanie S. Morrison, "What No Longer Serves Us: Resisting Ableism and Anti-Judaism in New Testament Healing Narratives," *Journal of Feminist Studies in Religion* 27, no. 2 (2011): 153–70.

20. Susan Sontag, "Illness as Metaphor," *New York Review of Books*, January 26, 1978, www.nybooks.com/articles/1978/01/26/illness-as-meta phor/.

21. Andrew Sung Park, *The Wounded Heart of God: The Asian Concept of Han and the Christian Doctrine of Sin* (Nashville, TN: Abingdon Press, 1993).

22. Thomas Kocik, "[Re]Turn to the East?," *Adoremus Bulletin* 5, no. 8 (1999).

23. After Vatican II many Catholic churches adopted the part of Pope Paul VI's *Novus Ordo* mass in which priests "turn toward the people," though conciliar and postconciliar documents have not demanded this. The stance *ad orientem*, however, is still used in some Roman Catholic rites.

24. Barbara J. Newman, *Accessible Gospel, Inclusive Worship* (Wyoming, MI: CLC Network, 2015), 18.

25. Newman describes these eight "vertical habits" first articulated by Dr. John Witvliet in 2005. Ibid., 36.

26. Margaret Farley, "Beyond the Formal Principle: A Reply to Ramsey and Saliers," *Journal of Religious Ethics* 7, no. 2 (1979): 195.

27. Greig, *Reconsidering Intellectual Disability*, 4.

28. Ibid., 202.

29. Ibid.

30. Ibid, 159.

31. Ibid, 227.

32. Paul Tillich, "The Permanent Significance of the Catholic Church for Protestants," *Protestant Digest* 3, no. 10 (1941): 23–31.

33. Ibid., 25.

34. Louise A. Gosbell, "Banqueting and Disability in the Ancient World: Reconsidering the Parable of the Great Banquet (Luke 14:15–24)," in *Theology and the Experience of Disability: Interdisciplinary Perspectives from Voices Down Under*, ed. Andrew Picard and Myk Habets (New York: Routledge, 2016): 129–44.

35. Interestingly, Gosbell notes how most biblical interpreters have focused on the inclusion of the "poor" being that of Gentiles and not persons

with disabilities, who are described as "the poor, the crippled, the blind, and the lame" in the text. Ibid., 130–31.

36. Bethany McKinney Fox, "About Us," Beloved Everybody Church, 2019, www.belovedeverybody.org/about-us.

37. Bethany McKinney Fox, *Disability*, 151–52.

38. Ibid., 152.

39. Bethany McKinney Fox to author, July 23, 2019.

40. Stanley Hauerwas, "The Church and the Mentally Handicapped: A Continuing Challenge to the Imagination," in *Critical Reflections on Stanley Hauerwas' Theology: Disability Society, Enabling Theology*, ed. John Swinton (New York: Routledge, 2005), 60.

41. Tracy A. Balboni et al., "A Scale to Assess Religious Beliefs in End-of-Life Medical Care," *Cancer* 125, no. 9 (2019): 1527–35.

42. T. McNichol, "The New Faith in Medicine," *USA Today Weekend*, April 5–7, 1996, 4–5 (survey conducted February 1996 by ICR Research Group).

43. See US Conference of Catholic Bishops, *Ethical and Religious Directives for Catholic Health Care Services*, 5th ed., www.usccb.org/issues -and-action/human-life-and-dignity/health-care/upload/Ethical-Religious -Directives-Catholic-Health-Care-Services-fifth-edition-2009.pdf.

44. Evangelical Lutheran Church in America, "The Church in Society: A Lutheran Perspective," Social teaching statement adopted at the second biennial Churchwide Assembly, August 28–September 4, 1991, 6, http:// download.elca.org/ELCA%20Resource%20Repository/Church_Society SS.pdf?_ga=1.79757461.320553945.1430960137.

45. Ibid.

46. United Methodist Church, *Social Principles*, II J (Washington, DC: General Board of Church and Society, 2012).

47. Ibid., II B, C, G.

48. Richard M. Gula, *Moral Discernment* (New York: Paulist Press, 1997), 120.

49. Laurie A. Jungling, "Conscience-Bound or Conscience-Liberated: What's Best for the ELCA?," *Journal of Lutheran Ethics* 5, no. 7 (2005), www.elca.org/JLE/Articles/653.

50. Wolfhart Pannenberg, *Anthropology in Theological Perspective*, trans. Matthew J. O'Connell (Philadelphia: Westminster, 1985). Pannenberg cautions Christians not to allow their conscience to be bound too much to one's personal understanding of God's Word to the exclusion of other persons' experiences, or to be bound to "the world" or the claims of one's particular society.

51. Ted Peters, *For the Love of Children: Genetic Technology and the Future of the Family* (Louisville, KY: Westminster John Knox Press, 1996), 118.

52. Dollar, *No Easy Choice*, 77.

CONCLUSION

1. Silver, *Remaking Eden*, 4.
2. Ibid., 6.

BIBLIOGRAPHY

Albrecht, Gary L., and Patrick J. Devlieger. "The Disability Paradox: High Quality of Life against All Odds." *Social Science and Medicine* 48, no. 8 (1999): 977–88.

Amundson, Ron, and Shari Tresky. "Bioethics and Disability Rights: Conflicting Values and Perspectives." *Bioethical Inquiry* 5, nos. 2–3 (2008): 111–23.

———. "On a Bioethical Challenge to Disability Rights." *Journal of Medicine and Philosophy* 32, no. 6 (2007): 541–61.

Andrews, Edmund L. "Religious Leaders Prepare to Fight Patents on Genes." *New York Times*, May 13, 1995. www.nytimes.com/1995/05/13 /us/company-news-religious-leaders-prepare-to-fight-patents-on -genes.html.

Aquinas, Thomas. *On Evil*. Translated by Richard Regan. Edited by Brian Davies. Oxford: Oxford University Press, 2003.

———. *The Sermon-Conferences of St. Thomas Aquinas on the Apostles' Creed*. Translated by and edited by Nichola Ayo. Eugene, OR: Wipf and Stock, 2005.

———. *Summa contra Gentiles*. Translated by Anton C. Pegis. Edited by Joseph Kenny. New York: Hanover House, 1955–57. http://dhspriory .org/thomas/ContraGentiles.htm.

———. *Summa theologica*. Translated by Fathers of the English Dominican Province. Oxford: New Advent, 2008. www.newadvent.org/summa/.

Aristotle. *On the Soul*. Translated by W. S. Hett. Loeb Classic Library. Cambridge, MA: Harvard University Press, 1957. www.loebclassics.com/view /aristotle-soul/1957/pb_LCL288.9.xml?rskey=sj2Vp3 &result=3.

———. *Physics*. In *Aristotle: Complete Works*, edited by Jonathan Barnes, 2:1–267. Princeton, NJ: Princeton University Press, 1984.

Asch, Adrienne. "Why I Haven't Changed My Mind about Prenatal Diagnosis Reflections and Refinements." In *Prenatal Testing and Disability Rights*, edited by Eric Parens and Adrienne Asch, 234–59. Washington, DC: Georgetown University Press, 2000.

Ashley, Benedict. "Elements of a Catholic Conscience." In *Catholic Conscience Foundation and Formation*, edited by Russell E. Smith, 39–58. Philadelphia: National Catholic Bioethics Center, 1991.

Augustine. *City of God*. Edited by G. R. Evans. Translated by Henry Bettenson. London: Penguin, 1987.

———. *Confessions*. Translated by R. S. Pine-Coffin. London: Penguin Books, 1961.

———. *Enchiridion on Faith, Hope, and Charity*. Translated and edited by Albert C. Outler. www.tertullian.org/fathers/augustine_enchiridion_02_trans.htm.

———. *The Literal Meaning of Genesis*. Vol. 1. Translated by John Hammond Taylor. Edited by Johannes Quasten, Walter J. Burghardt, and Thomas Comerford Lawler. New York: Newman Press, 1982.

———. *On Christian Doctrine*. Translated by D. W. Robertson Jr. Indianapolis: Bobbs-Merrill, 1958.

———. *On Genesis*. Translated by Edmund Hill. Edited by John E. Rotelle. Hyde Park, NY: New City Press, 2002.

———. *The Trinity*. 2nd ed. Translated by Edmund Hill. Edited by John E. Rotelle. Hyde Park, NY: New City Press, 2016.

Bacon, Francis. "Magnalia Naturae." In *The Advancement of Learning and New Atlantis*, edited by Arthur Johnston, 249–50. Oxford: Clarendon Press, 1974.

———. "New Organon." In *The Works of Francis Bacon*, edited by James Spedding, Robert Ellis, and Douglas Heath, 70–366. London: Longman, 1857–74.

Balboni, Tracy A., Holly G. Prigerson, Michael J. Balboni, Andrea C. Enzinger, Tyler J. VanderWeele, and Paul K. Maciejewski. "A Scale to Assess Religious Beliefs in End-of-Life Medical Care." *Cancer* 125, no. 9 (2014): 1527–35.

Balthasar, Hans Urs von. *Cosmic Liturgy: The Universe According to Maximus the Confessor*. San Francisco: Ignatius Press, 2003.

Bard, Bernard, and Joseph Fletcher. "The Right to Die." *Atlantic Monthly*, April 1968, 59–64.

Barnes, Elizabeth. *The Minority Body: A Theory of Disability*. Oxford: Oxford University Press, 2016.

Barr, James. *Biblical Faith and Natural Theology: The Gifford Lectures for 1991, Delivered in the University of Edinburgh.* Oxford: Oxford University Press, 1993.

Barth, Karl. *Church Dogmatics.* Vol. 3. *The Doctrine of Creation.* Edited by G. W. Bromily and T. F. Torrance. Edinburgh: T. & T. Clark, 1960.

———. *A Letter to Great Britain from Switzerland.* Eugene, OR: Wipf and Stock, 2014.

Barzilay, Judge Judith M. Slip Opinion No. 03-2, Court No. 96-10-02291, Toy Biz, Inc. v. United States. January 3, 2003. United States Court of International Trade. www.cit.uscourts.gov/sites/cit/files/slip-op%20 03-2.pdf.

Begley, Sharon. "Global Summit Opens Door to Controversial Gene-Editing of Human Embryos," *Stat,* December 3, 2015. www.statnews .com/2015/12/03/gene-editing-human-embryos/.

Beitiks, Emily. "5 Reasons Why We Need People with Disabilities in the CRISPR Debates." Paul K. Longmore Institute on Disability, *Disability Remix* (blog), September 5, 2016. https://longmoreinstitute.sfsu.edu/5 -reasons-why-we-need-people-disabilities-crispr-debates.

Belser, Julia Watts. "God on Wheels: Disability and Jewish Feminist Theology." *Tikkun* 24 no. 4 (2014): 27–28.

Belser, Julia Watts, and Melanie S. Morrison. "What No Longer Serves Us: Resisting Ableism and Anti-Judaism in New Testament Healing Narratives." *Journal of Feminist Studies in Religion* 27, no. 2 (2011): 153–70.

Bentham, Jeremy. *The Principles of Morals and Legislation.* Oxford: Clarendon Press, 1789.

Berkman, John. "Are Persons with Profound Intellectual Disabilities Sacred Icons of Heavenly Life? Aquinas on Impairment." *Studies in Christian Ethics* 26, no. 1 (2013): 83–96.

Betcher, Sharon V. *Spirit and the Politics of Disablement.* Minneapolis, MN: Fortress Press, 2007.

Beurton, P. J. "A Unified View of the Gene, or How to Overcome Reductionism." In *The Concept of the Gene in Development and Evolution: Historical and Epistemological Perspectives,* edited by Peter Beurton, Raphael Falk, and Hans-Joerg Rheinberger, 286–314. Cambridge: Cambridge University Press, 2000.

Billings, J. Todd. *Calvin, Participation, and the Gift: The Activity of Believers in Union with Christ.* Oxford: Oxford University Press, 2007.

———. "John Milbank's Theology of the 'Gift' and Calvin's Theology of Grace: A Critical Comparison." *Modern Theology* 21, no. 1 (2005): 87–105.

Bishop, Edwin W. "Eugenics and the Church." *Eugenics: A Journal of Race Betterment* 2 (1929): 8. www.eugenicsarchive.org/eugenics/topic_images .pl?theme=32&search=&matches=&dpage=1.

Bishop, Jeffrey Paul. *The Anticipatory Corpse: Medicine, Power, and the Care of the Dying.* Notre Dame, IN: University of Notre Dame Press, 2011.

Bock, Walter J. "Multiple Explanations in Darwinian Evolutionary Theory." *Acta Biotheoretica* 58 (2010): 65–79.

Boelsche, Wilhelm. *The Evolution of Man.* Translated by Ernest Untermann. Chicago: Charles H. Kerr, 1905.

Bognar, Greg. "Is Disability Mere Difference?" *Journal of Medical Ethics* 42, no. 1 (2016): 46–49.

Boorse, Christopher. "On the Distinction between Disease and Illness." *Philosophy and Public Affairs* 5, no. 1 (1975): 49–68.

Botoseneanu, Adana, Jeffrey A. Alexander, and Jane Banaszak-Holl. "To Test or Not to Test? The Role of Attitudes, Knowledge, and Religious Involvement among U.S. Adults on Intent-to-Obtain Adult Genetic Testing." *Health Education Behavior* 38, no. 6 (2011): 617–28.

Boyle, Robert. *The Works of the Honourable Robert Boyle.* Edited by Thomas Birch. 6 vols. 1772. Reprint, Hildesheim: George Olms, 1966. https://archive.org/details/bub_gb_LqYrAQAAMAAJ/page/n10.

Brock, Brian, and Stephanie Brock. "Being Disabled in the New World of Genetic Testing." In *Theology, Disability, and the New Genetics: Why Science Needs the Church*, edited by John Swinton and Brian Brock, 29–43. London: T. & T. Clark, 2007.

Brock, Dan. "Preventing Genetically Transmitted Disabilities While Respecting Persons with Disabilities." In *Quality of Life and Human Difference: Genetic Testing, Health Care and Disability*, edited by D. Wasserman, J. Bickenbach, and R. Wachbroit, 67–100. New York: Cambridge University Press, 2005.

Brooke, John Hedley. *Science and Religion: Some Historical Perspectives.* New York: Cambridge University Press, 1991.

Bruehl, Charles P. *Birth Control and Eugenics in the Light of Fundamental Ethical Principles.* New York: Joseph F. Wagner, 1928.

Brunner, Emil. *The Christian Doctrine of Creation and Redemption.* Philadelphia: Westminster, 1952.

Bryan, William Jennings. "Text of the Closing Statement of William Jennings Bryan at the Trial of John Scopes, Dayton, Tennessee, 1925." California State University, Dominguez Hills, website. www2.csudh.edu /oliver/smt310-handouts/wjb-last/wjb-last.htm.

Bryan, William Jennings. *Orthodox Christianity versus Modernism.* New York: Fleming Revell, 1923.

Bryant, John, and Peter Turnpenny. "Genetics and Genetic Modification of Humans: Principles, Practices and Possibilities." In *Brave New World? Theology, Ethics, and the Human Genome*, edited by Celia Deane-Drummond, 5–26. London: T. & T. Clark International, 2003.

Buchanan, Allen, Dan W. Brock, Norman Daniels, and Daniel Wikler. *From Chance to Choice: Genetics and Justice*. Cambridge: Cambridge University Press, 2000.

Burke, Teresa Blankmeyer. "Rendered Mute." *Atrium* 12 (2014): 1–2.

Burkhardt, Richard W., Jr. "Lamarck, Evolution and the Inheritance of Acquired Characters." *Genetics* 194, no. 4 (2013): 793–805.

Burtt, Edwin A. *Metaphysical Foundations of Modern Physical Science*. Garden City, NY: Doubleday, 1954.

Calvin, John. *Commentary on Genesis*. Translated by John King. 2 vols. Grand Rapids, MI: Baker, 1996. www.ccel.org/ccel/calvin/calcom01.pdf.

———. *Institutes of the Christian Religion*. Translated by Ford Lewis Battles. Edited by John T. McNeill. Louisville, KY: Westminster John Knox Press, 1960.

Cameron, Nigel M. de S. "Bioethics: The Twilight of Christian Hippocratism." In *God and Culture: Essays in Honor of Carl F. H. Henry*, edited by D. A. Carson and John D. Woodbridge, 321–40. Grand Rapids, MI: Eerdmans, 1993.

Carel, Havi. *Illness: The Cry of the Flesh*. Durham, NC: Acumen, 2007.

Carey, Nessa. *The Epigenetics Revolution: How Modern Biology Is Rewriting Our Understanding of Genetics, Disease, and Inheritance*. New York: Columbia University Press, 2012.

Catholic Church. *Catechism of the Catholic Church*. 2nd ed. Vatican: Libreria Editrice Vaticana, 2012.

Chapp, Larry S. *The God of Covenant and Creation: Scientific Naturalism and Its Challenge to the Christian Faith*. London: T. & T. Clark, 2011.

Chesterton, G. K. *Eugenics and Other Evils*. London: Cassell, 1922.

Chial, Heidi. "DNA Sequencing Technologies Key to the Human Genome Project." *Nature Education* 1, no. 1 (2008): 219. www.nature.com/scitable/topicpage/dna-sequencing-technologies-key-to-the-human-828.

Childress, Kelly Dahlgren. "Genetics, Disability, and Ethics: Could Applied Technologies Lead to a New Eugenics?" *Journal of Women and Religion* 19, no. 20 (2003): 157–78.

Church, Dawson. *The Genie in Your Genes: Epigenetic Medicine and the New Biology of Intention*. Santa Rosa, CA: Energy Psychology Press, 2009.

Clayton, Philip. "Theology and the Physical Sciences." In *The Modern Theologians: An Introduction to Christian Theology since 1918*, edited by David F. Ford and Rachel Muers, 342–56. Malden, MA: Blackwell, 2005.

Clifton, Shane. "Theodicy, Disability, and Fragility: An Attempt to Find Meaning in the Aftermath of Quadriplegia." *Theological Studies* 76, no. 4 (2015): 765–84.

Clinton, William J. "Remarks at Robert Morris College in Corapolis, Pennsylvania, September 25, 1996." In *Public Papers of the Presidents of the United States: William J. Clinton* (1996, Book II). Washington, DC: US Government Printing Office, 1997.

Cloud, John. "Why Genes Aren't Destiny." *Time*, January 18, 2010, 48–53. http://content.time.com/time/magazine/article/0,9171,1952313,00 .html.

Congregation for the Doctrine of the Faith. *Dignitas personae.* December 8, 2008.

———. *Donum vitae.* February 22, 1987. www.vatican.va/roman_curia /congregations/cfaith/documents/rc_con_cfaith_doc_19870222 _respect-for-human-life_en.html.

Council Fathers. *Fourth Lateran Council.* 1215 AD. Papal Encyclicals Online. www.papalencyclicals.net/councils/ecum12-2.htm.

Creamer, Deborah. "Toward a Theology That Includes the Human Experience of Disability." *Journal of Religion, Disability and Health* 7, no. 3 (2008): 57–67.

Cross, Richard. "Aquinas on Physical Impairment: Human Nature and Original Sin." *Harvard Theological Review* 110, no. 3 (2017): 317–38.

———. "Baptism, Faith and Severe Cognitive Impairment in Some Medieval Theologies." *International Journal of Systematic Theology* 14, no. 4 (2012): 420–38.

Cunningham, Connor. *Darwin's Pious Idea: Why Ultra-Darwinists and Creationists Both Get It Wrong.* Grand Rapids, MI: Eerdmans, 2010.

Curran, Charles E. *The Development of Moral Theology: Five Strands.* Washington, DC: Georgetown University Press, 2013.

Daly, Ann K., and Ingolf Cascorbi. "Opportunities and Limitations: The Value of Pharmacogenetics in Clinical Practice." *British Journal of Clinical Pharmacology* 77, no. 4 (2014): 583–86.

Daniels, Norman. *Just Health Care.* New York: Cambridge University Press, 1985.

Darwin, Charles. *The Origin of Species.* 6th ed. 1872. Reprint, Amherst, MA: Prometheus Books, 1991.

———. *The Variation of Animals and Plants under Domestication.* Vol. 2. London: John Murray, 1868.

Davis, John Jefferson. "Christian Reflections on the Genetic Revolution." *Evangelical Review of Theology* 28, no. 1 (2004): 65–79.

Dawkins, Richard. *The Blind Watchmaker: Why the Evidence of Evolution Reveals a Universe.* New York: Norton, 1986.

————. *The Selfish Gene.* Oxford: Oxford University Press, 1989.

————. *The Selfish Gene.* 30th anniversary ed. Oxford: Oxford University Press, 2006.

de Alminana, Margaret English. "Aimee Semple McPherson's Pentecostalism, Darwinism, Eugenics, the Disenfranchised, and the Scopes Monkey Trial." *Pneuma* 41, no. 2 (2019): 255–78.

Deane-Drummond, Celia. "Aquinas, Wisdom Ethics and the New Genetics." In *Re-ordering Nature: Theology, Society and the New Genetics*, edited by Celia Deane-Drummond, Bronislaw Szerszynski, and Robin Grove-White, 293–311. London: T. & T. Clark, 2003.

Delaney, James J. "The Catholic Position on Germ Line Genetic Engineering." *American Journal of Bioethics* 9, no. 11 (2009): 33–34.

Dennett, Daniel. *Brainstorms: Philosophical Essays on Mind and Psychology.* Cambridge: MIT Press, 1978.

Descartes, René. *Oeuvres.* Edited by Charles Adam and Paul Tannery. 2nd ed. 11 vols. Paris: Vrin, 1974–86.

————. *Meditation from First Philosophy* (1641). In *The Philosophical Writings of Descartes*, translated by John Cottingham, Robert Stoothoff, and Dugald Murdoch, 2:1–62. Cambridge: Cambridge University Press, 1984.

Dodds, Michael J. *Unlocking Divine Action: Contemporary Science and Thomas Aquinas* Washington, DC: Catholic University of America Press, 2012.

Dollar, Ellen Painter. *No Easy Choice: A Story of Disability, Parenthood, and Faith in an Age of Advanced Reproduction.* Louisville, KY: Westminster John Knox Press, 2012.

Drees, Willem B., ed. *Is Nature Ever Evil? Religion, Science and Value.* London: Routledge, 2003.

Dvořák, Petr. "The Concurrentism of Thomas Aquinas: Divine Causation and Human Freedom." *Philosophia* 41 (2013): 617–34.

Eberl, Jason T. "Disability, Enhancement, and Flourishing." Paper presented at the annual meeting of the International Academy of Bioethical Inquiry, July 17, 2018.

————. *Thomistic Principles and Bioethics.* New York: Routledge, 2006.

Eiesland, Nancy L. *The Disabled God: Toward a Liberatory Theology of Disability.* Nashville, TN: Abingdon Press, 1994.

Episcopal Church. *Journal of the General Convention of the Protestant Episcopal Church in the United States of America: Otherwise Known as the Episcopal Church. Held in Anaheim, California, from September Seventh to Fourteenth, Inclusive, in the Year of Our Lord 1985.* New York: General Convention, 1986. www.episcopalarchives.org/sites/default/file/publications/1985_GC_Journal.pdf.

————. *Journal of the General Convention of the Protestant Episcopal Church in the United States of America: Otherwise Known as the Episcopal Church. Held in Phoenix, Arizona, from July Eleventh to Twentieth, Inclusive, in the Year of Our Lord 1991.* New York: General Convention, 1992.

————. *Journal of the General Convention of the Protestant Episcopal Church in the United States of America: Otherwise Known as the Episcopal Church. Held in Minneapolis, Minnesota, from July Thirtieth to August Eighth, Inclusive, in the Year of Our Lord 2003.* New York: General Convention, 2004. www.episcopalarchives.org/sites/default /files /publications/2003_GC_Journal.pdf.

Evangelical Lutheran Church in America. "The Church in Society: A Lutheran Perspective." Social teaching statement adopted at the Second Biennial Churchwide Assembly, August 28–September 4, 1991. http:// download.elca.org/ELCA%20Resource%20Repository/Church _SocietySS.pdf?_ga=1.79757461.320553945.1430960137.

Evans, John Hyde. *Playing God? Human Genetic Engineering and the Rationalization of Public Bioethical Debate.* Chicago: University of Chicago Press, 2002.

Evans, John Hyde, and Kathy Hudson. "Religion and Reproductive Genetics: Beyond Views of Embryonic Life?" *Journal for the Scientific Study of Religion* 46, no. 4 (2007): 565–81.

Farley, Margaret. "Beyond the Formal Principle: A Reply to Ramsey and Saliers." *Journal of Religious Ethics* 7, no. 2 (1979): 191–202.

————. "The Role of Experience in Moral Discernment." In *Christian Ethics: Problems and Prospects,* edited by Lisa Sowle Cahill and James F. Childress, 134–51. Cleveland, OH: Pilgrim Press, 1996.

Fletcher, Joseph F. *The Ethics of Genetic Control: Ending Reproductive Roulette.* Garden City, NY: Anchor Press, 1974.

————. *Humanhood: Essays in Biomedical Ethics.* Buffalo, NY: Prometheus Books, 1979.

————. *Medicine and Morals: The Moral Problems of the Patient's Right to Know the Truth, Contraception, Artificial Insemination, Sterilization, and Euthanasia.* Princeton, NJ: Princeton University Press, 1954.

Fosdick, Henry Emerson. *Christianity and Progress.* New York: Fleming H. Revell, 1922.

Foster, Morris W., and Richard R. Sharp. "Race, Ethnicity and Genomics: Social Classification as Proxies of Biological Heterogeneity." *Genome Research* 12, no. 6 (2002): 844–50.

Fox, Bethany McKinney. "About Us." Beloved Everybody Church, 2019. www.belovedeverybody.org/about-us.

————. *Disability and the Way of Jesus: Holistic Healing in the Gospels and the Church.* Downers Grove, IL: IVP Academic, 2019.

Fricker, Miranda. *Epistemic Injustice: Power and the Ethics of Knowing.* Oxford: Oxford University Press, 2007.

Funkenstein, Amos. *Theology and the Scientific Imagination from the Middle Ages to the Seventeenth Century.* Princeton, NJ: Princeton University Press, 1986.

Gallup. "Gay and Lesbian Rights." Gallup News, May 2019. https://news.gallup.com/poll/1651/gay-lesbian-rights.aspx.

Galton, Francis. *English Men of Science: Their Nature and Nurture.* London: Macmillan, 1874.

Gaukroger, Stephen. *The Collapse of Mechanism and the Rise of Sensibility: Science and the Shaping of Modernity: 1680–1760.* Oxford: Oxford University Press, 2010.

————. *The Emergence of a Scientific Culture: Science and the Shaping of Modernity, 1210–1685.* Oxford: Oxford University Press, 2009.

Gayon, Jean. "From Mendel to Epigenetics: History of Genetics." *Comptes Rendus Biologies* 339 (2016): 225–30.

Gerson, Michael. "The Eugenics Temptation." *Washington Post,* October 24, 2007. https://www.washingtonpost.com/wp-dyn/content/article/2007/10/23/AR2007102301803.html.

Gilbert, Walter. "A Vision of the Grail." In *The Code of Codes: Scientific and Social Issues in the Human Genome Project,* edited by Daniel J. Kevles and Leroy E. Hood, 83–97. Cambridge, MA: Harvard University Press, 1992.

Gilkey, Langdon. *Maker of Heaven and Earth: The Christian Doctrine of Creation in the Light of Modern Knowledge.* Lanham, MD: University Press of America, 1985.

————. "Religion and Science in an Advanced Scientific Culture." *Zygon* 22, no. 2 (1987): 165–78.

Glass, H. Bentley. *Science and Ethical Values.* Chapel Hill: University of North Carolina Press, 1965.

Glover, Jonathan. *Choosing Children: Genes, Disability, and Design.* Oxford: Oxford University Press, 2006.

Goldberg, Steven. *Seduced by Science: How American Religion Has Lost Its Way.* New York: New York University Press, 1999.

Gosbell, Louise A. "Banqueting and Disability in the Ancient World: Reconsidering the Parable of the Great Banquet (Luke 14:15–24)." In *Theology and the Experience of Disability: Interdisciplinary Perspectives from Voices Down Under,* edited by Andrew Picard and Myk Habets, 129–44. New York: Routledge, 2016.

Gould, Stephen Jay. *Rock of Ages: Science and Religion in the Fullness of Life.* New York: Ballantine, 1999.

Gregory of Nazianzus. "Letter CI ('To Cledonius against Apollinaris')." In *Christology of the Later Fathers*, edited by Edward R. Hardy, 215–32. Philadelphia: Westminster Press, 1954.

Greig, Jason Reimer. *Reconsidering Intellectual Disability: L'Arche, Medical Ethics, and Christian Friendship.* Washington, DC: Georgetown University Press, 2015.

Grisez, Germain, Joseph Boyle, and John Finnis. "Practical Principles, Moral Truth and Ultimate Ends." *American Journal of Jurisprudence* 99 (1987): 99–151.

Gula, Richard M. *Moral Discernment.* New York: Paulist Press, 1997.

Gustafson, James M. *Ethics from a Theocentric Perspective.* Chicago: University of Chicago Press, 1981.

———. "Theology Confronts Technology and the Life Sciences." In *On Moral Medicine: Theological Perspectives on Medical Ethics*, edited by M. Therese Lysaught, Joseph Kotva, Stephen E. Lammers, and Allen Verhey, 46–52. Grand Rapids, MI: Eerdmans, 2012.

Haeckel, Ernst. *Evolution of Man: A Popular Scientific Study.* New York: G. P. Putnam's Sons, 1905.

———. *Monism as Connecting Religion and Science: A Man of Science.* Translated by J. Gilchrist. Project Gutenberg Ebook, 2003. www.gutenberg.org/files/9199/9199-h/9199-h.htm.

———. "Ueber die Naturanschauung von Darwin, Göthe und Lamarck." In *Tageblatt der 55. Versamm-lung Deutscher Naturforscher und Aerzte in Eisenach, von 18. bis 22. September 1882.* Eisenach: Hofbuchdruckerei von H. Kahle, 1882. Translated by Robert J. Richards in "Ernest Haeckel and the Struggles over Evolution and Religion," *Annals of the History and Philosophy of Biology* 10 (2005): 89–115.

Hall, Amy Laura. "To Form a More Perfect Union: Mainline Protestantism and the Popularization of Eugenics." In *Theology, Disability and the New Genetics: Why Science Needs the Church*, edited by John Swinton and Brian Brock, 75–95. London: T. & T. Clark, 2007.

Hanby, Michael. *No God, No Science? Theology, Cosmology, Biology.* Oxford: Wiley-Blackwell, 2013.

Häring, Bernard. *Manipulation: Ethical Boundaries of Medical, Behavioral, and Genetic Manipulation.* Slough, UK: St. Paul Publications, 1975.

Harmon, Katherine. "How Useful Is Whole Genome Sequencing to Predict Disease?" *Scientific American*, April 2, 2012. www.scientificamerican.com/article/whole-genome-sequencing-predict-disease/.

Harris, John. *Clones, Genes, and Immortality: Ethics and the Genetic Revolution.* Oxford: Oxford University Press, 1998.

———. *Enhancing Evolution: The Ethical Case for Making Better People.* Princeton, NJ: Princeton University Press, 2007.

———. "Is Gene Therapy a Form of Eugenics?" *Bioethics* 7, nos. 2–3 (1993): 178–87.

Harris, Sam. *The End of Faith: Religion, Terror and the Future of Reason.* New York: Norton, 2004.

Harrison, Peter. *The Bible, Protestantism and the Rise of Natural Science.* Cambridge: University of Cambridge Press, 1998.

———. *The Fall of Man and the Foundations of Science.* Cambridge: Cambridge University Press, 2007.

———. *The Territories of Science and Religion.* Chicago: University of Chicago Press, 2015.

Harshaw, Jill. *God beyond Words: Christian Theology and the Spiritual Experiences of People with Profound Intellectual Disabilities.* London: Jessica Kingsley, 2016.

Hart, David Bentley. *The Doors of the Sea: Where Was God in the Tsunami.* Grand Rapids, MI: Eerdmans, 2005.

———. "Is, Ought, and Nature's Laws." *First Things*, February 28, 2013. www.firstthings.com/web-exclusives/2013/02/is-ought-and-natures-laws.

———. "Providence and Causality: On Divine Innocence." In *The Providence of God: Deus Habet Consilium*, edited by Francesa Aran Murphy and Philip G. Ziegler, 34–56. London: T. & T. Clark, 2009.

Haslam, Nick, Brock Bastian, Paul Bain, and Yoshihisa Kashima. "Psychological Essentialism, Implicit Theories, and Intergroup Relations." *Group Processes and Intergroup Relations* 9, no. 1 (2006): 63–76.

Hauerwas, Stanley. "The Church and the Mentally Handicapped: A Continuing Challenge to the Imagination." In *Critical Reflections on Stanley Hauerwas' Theology: Disability Society, Enabling Theology*, edited by John Swinton, 53–62. New York: Routledge, 2005.

———. *Naming the Silences: God, Medicine, and the Problem of Suffering.* Grand Rapids, MI: Eerdmans, 1990.

Hauskeller, Christine. "Genes, Genomes and Identity: Projections on Matter." *New Genetics and Society* 23, no. 3 (2004): 285–99.

Hayden, Erika Check. "Should You Edit Your Children's Genes?" *Nature*, February 23, 2016. www.nature.com/news/should-you-edit-your-children-s-genes-1.19432.

Hegarty, P. "'It's Not a Choice, It's the Way We're Built': Symbolic Beliefs about Sexual Orientation in the US and Britain." *Journal of Community and Applied Social Psychology* 12, no. 3 (2002): 723–35.

Heine, Steven J., Ilan Dar-Nimrod, Benjamin Y. Cheung, and Travis Proulx. "Essentially Biased: Why People Are Fatalistic about Genes." *Advances in Experimental Social Psychology* 55 (2017): 137–92.

Herrnstein, Richard J., and Charles A. Murray. *The Bell Curve: Intelligence and Class Structure in American Life*. New York: Simon and Schuster, 1996.

Ho, Anita. "The Individualist Model of Autonomy and the Challenge of Disability." *Bioethical Inquiry* 5, nos. 2–3 (2008): 193–207.

Hobbes, Thomas. "Human Nature." In *The English Works of Thomas Hobbes of Malmesbury*, edited by Sir William Molesworth, 4:1–76. London: John Bohn, 1839–45.

———. "Leviathan." Vol. 3 of *The English Works of Thomas Hobbes of Malmesbury*, edited by Sir William Molesworth. London: John Bohn, 1839–45.

———. "Seven Philosophical Problems." In *The English Works of Thomas Hobbes of Malmesbury*, edited by Sir William Molesworth, 7:1–68. London: John Bohn, 1839–45.

Hollands, Gareth J., David P. French, Simon J. Griffin, A. Toby Prevost, Stephen Sutton, Sarah King, and Theresa M. Marteau. "The Impact of Communicating Genetic Risks of Disease on Risk-Reducing Health Behavior: Systematic Review with Meta-analysis." *British Medical Journal* 352, no. 1102 (2016): 1–11.

Hull, John M. *In the Beginning There Was Darkness: A Blind Person's Conversations with the Bible*. Harrisburg, PA: Trinity Press International, 2001.

Human Rights Campaign. "HRC Welcomes Scientific Study Exploring Genetic Basis of Sexual Orientation and Gender Identity." Press release, October 20, 2003. Collected on Enviroshop site. https://enviro shop.com/hrc-welcomes-scientific-study-exploring-genetic-basis -of-sexual-orientation-and-gender-identity/.

Hume, David. *An Enquiry into the Principles of Morals*. Edited by L. A. Selby-Bigge. 3rd ed. Revised by P. H. Nidditch. Oxford: Oxford University Press, 1975.

Huxley, Thomas Henry. *Lay Sermons, Addresses, and Reviews*. Cambridge: Cambridge University Press, 2009.

———. *Science and Christian Tradition: Essays*. New York: D. Appleton, 1896. https://archive.org/details/sciencechristian00huxlrich.

Irenaeus of Lyons. *Against Heresies*. Translated by Dominic J. Unger. New York: Newman Press, 1992.

Jackson, Nick. "Against the Grain: There Are Questions That Science Cannot Answer." *The Independent*, September 20, 2007. www.independent.co.uk/news/science/against-the-grain-there-are-questions-that-science-cannot-answer-402864.html.

Jahme, Carole. "Richard Dawkins Wants Evolutionary Science to Be 'the New Classics.'" *The Guardian*, June 12, 2012. www.theguardian.com/science/blog/2012/jun/12/richard-dawkins-evolution-new-classics.

James, William. *Is Life Worth Living?* Philadelphia: S. Burns Weston, 1896.

Jaroff, Leon. "The Gene Hunt." *Time*, March 20, 1989. http://content.time.com/time/magazine/article/0,9171,957263,00.html.

Jayaratne, Toby Epstein, Susan A. Gelman; Merle Feldbaum, Jane P. Sheldon, Elizabeth M. Petty, and Sharon L. R. Kardia. "The Perennial Debate: Nature, Nurture, or Choice? Black and White Americans' Explanations for Individual Differences." *Review of General Psychology* 13, no. 1 (2009): 24–33.

Jayaratne, Toby Epstein, Oscar Ybarra, Jane P. Sheldon, Tony N. Brown, Merle Feldbaum, Carla A. Pfeffer, and Elizabeth M. Petty. "White Americans' Genetic Lay Theories of Race Differences and Sexual Orientation: Their Relationship with Prejudice toward Blacks, and Gay Men and Lesbians." *Group Processes and Intergroup Relations* 9, no. 1 (2006): 77–94.

Jennings, Bruce. "Technology and the Genetic Imaginary." In *Theology, Disability and the New Genetics: Why Science Needs the Church*, edited by John Swinton and Brian Brock, 129–32. London: T. & T. Clark, 2007.

Jones, Evan, and Blaine Smith. "Epigenetics and Pastoral Counseling the Science behind What We Preach." *European Journal of Science and Theology* 8, no. 2 (2012): 47–52.

Jones, L. "Social Darwinism Revisited." *History Today* 48 (1998): 7–8.

Jonsen, Albert R. *The Birth of Bioethics*. Oxford: Oxford University, 1998.

Julian of Norwich. "Revelations of Divine Love." In *Medieval Writings on Female Spirituality*, edited by Elizabeth Spearing, 183–205. London: Penguin Books, 2002.

Jungling, Laurie A. "Conscience-Bound or Conscience-Liberated: What's Best for the ELCA?" *Journal of Lutheran Ethics* 5, no. 7 (2005). www.elca.org/JLE/Articles/653.

Junker-Kenny, Maureen. "Genes and the Self: Anthropological Questions to the Human Genome Project." In *Brave New World? Theology, Ethics, and the Human Genome*. London: T. & T. Clark International, 2003.

Kafer, Alison. *Feminist Queer Crip*. Bloomington: Indiana University Press, 2013.

Kant, Immanuel. *Groundwork for the Metaphysics of Morals*. Translated by Thomas E. Hill and Arnulf Zweig. Oxford Philosophical Texts. Oxford: Oxford University Press, 2002.

Kate, Leo P. Ten. "Victims of Nature Cry Out." In *Is Nature Ever Evil? Religion, Science and Value*, edited by Willem B. Drees, 170–72. London: Routledge, 2003.

Keefe, Donald J. *Thomism and the Ontological Theology of Paul Tillich: A Comparison of Systems*. Leiden: E. J. Brill, 1971.

Keller, Evelyn Fox. "Nature, Nurture, and the Human Genome Project." In *The Code of Codes: Scientific and Social Issues in the Human Genome Project*, edited by Daniel J. Kevles and Leroy Hood, 281–99. Cambridge, MA: Harvard University Press, 1992.

Keller, Mitch. "The Scandal at the Zoo." *New York Times*, August 6, 2006. www.nytimes.com/2006/08/06/nyregion/thecity/06zoo.html.

Kellogg, Gregory, Leah Slattery, Louanne Hudgins, and Kelly Ormond. "Attitudes of Mothers of Children with Down Syndrome towards Noninvasive Prenatal Testing." *Journal of Genetic Counseling* 23, no. 5 (2014): 805–13.

Kemp, Kenneth. "Science, Theology, and Monogenesis." *American Catholic Philosophical Quarterly* 85, no. 2 (2011): 217–36.

Kevles, David J. "Out of Eugenics: The Historical Politics of the Human Genome." In *The Code of Codes: Scientific and Social Issues in the Human Genome Project*, edited by Daniel J. Kevles and Leroy Hood, 3–36. Cambridge, MA: Harvard University Press, 1992.

Kevles, Daniel J., and Leroy Hood, eds. *The Code of Codes: Scientific and Social Issues in the Human Genome Project*. Cambridge, MA: Harvard University Press, 1992.

Kevles, Daniel J., and Leroy Hood. Preface to *The Code of Codes: Scientific and Social Issues in the Human Genome Project*, edited by Daniel J. Kevles and Leroy Hood. Cambridge, MA: Harvard University Press, 1992.

Khushf, George. "What Hope for Reason?" *Christian Bioethics* 22, no. 2 (2016): 238–64.

Kilner, John F. *Dignity and Destiny: Humanity in the Image of God*. Grand Rapids, MI: Eerdmans, 2015.

Kittay, Eva Feder. *Love's Labor: Essays on Women, Equality, and Dependency*. New York: Routledge, 1999.

Koch, Tom. "The Illusion of Paradox." *Social Science and Medicine* 50, no. 6 (2000): 757–59.

Kocik, Thomas. "[Re]Turn to the East?" *Adoremus Bulletin* 5, no. 8 (1999).

Kuhse, Helga, and Peter Singer. *Should the Baby Live? The Problem of Handicapped Infants.* Oxford: Oxford University Press, 1985.

Larsen, Timothy. *Crisis of Doubt: Honest Faith in Nineteenth-Century England.* Oxford: Oxford University Press, 2009.

Latour, Bruno. *We Have Never Been Modern.* Translated by Catherine Porter. Cambridge, MA: Harvard University Press, 1993.

Lebacqz, Karen. "Dignity and Enhancement in the Holy City." In *Transhumanism and Transcendence: Christian Hope in an Age of Technological Enhancement*, edited by Ronald Cole-Turner, 51–62. Washington, DC: Georgetown University Press, 2011.

Levering, Matthew. *Biblical Natural Law: A Theocentric and Teleological Approach.* Oxford: Oxford University Press, 2012.

Lewontin, Richard C. *It Ain't Necessarily So: The Dream of the Human Genome and Other Illusions.* New York: New York Review of Books, 2000.

Lewontin, Richard C., Steven P. R. Rose, and Leon J. Kamin. *Not in Our Genes: Biology, Ideology, and Human Nature.* New York: Pantheon Books, 1984.

Lindbeck, George A. "Natural Law in the Thought of Paul Tillich: Note." *Natural Law Forum* 7 (1962): 84–96.

Lipinski, Kamil A., Louise J. Barber, Matthew N. Davies, Matthew Ashenden, Andrea Sottoriva, and Marco Gerlinger. "Cancer Evolution and the Limits of Predictability in Precision Cancer Medicine." *Trends in Cancer* 2, no. 1 (2016): 49–63. www.sciencedirect.com/science/article/pii/S2405803315000692.

Lui, Yongsheng. "A New Perspective on Darwin's Pangenesis." *Biological Review* 83, no. 2 (2008): 141–49.

Luria, S. E. "Directed Genetic Change: Perspectives from Molecular Geneticists." In *The Control of Human Heredity and Evolution*, edited by Tracy M. Sonneborn, 1–19. New York: Macmillan, 1965.

Luther, Martin. "On the Bondage of the Will." In *Martin Luther's Basic Theological Writings*, 3rd ed., edited by Timothy F. Lull and William R. Russell, 138–70. Minneapolis, MN: Fortress Press, 2012.

———. *Sermons I.* Vol. 51 of *Luther's Works*, edited by John W. Doberstein and Helmult T. Lehmann. Minneapolis MN: Fortress Press, 1959.

Lysaught, M. Therese. "'Ten Decades to a More Christ-Like You!': Liturgy as God's Workout Plan for the Church." *Liturgy* 24, no. 1 (2009): 3–15.

———. "Vulnerability within the Body of Christ: Anointing of the Sick and Theological Anthropology." In *Health and Human Flourishing,* edited by Carol Taylor and Robert Dell-Oro, 159–84. Washington, DC: Georgetown University Press, 2006.

MacIntyre, Alasdair. "Is Understanding Religion Compatible with Believing?" In *Rationality*, edited by Bryan R. Wilson, 62–77. Oxford: Basil Blackwell, 1977.

Madden, Ward. *The Timely and the Timeless: The Interrelationships of Science, Education and Society.* New York: Basic Books, 1980.

Mahoney, Jack. "Christian Doctrines, Ethical Issues, and Human Genetics." *Theological Studies* 64, no. 4 (2003): 719–49.

Mairs, Nancy. *Ordinary Time: Cycles in Marriage, Faith, and Renewal.* Boston: Beacon Press, 1993.

Marsden, George M. *Fundamentalism and American Culture.* 2nd ed. Oxford: Oxford University Press, 2006.

Masci, David. "Public Opinion on Religion and Science in the United States." Pew Research Religion and Public Life Project, November 5, 2009. www.pewforum.org/2009/11/05/public-opinion-on-religion-and-science-in-the-united-states/.

Mathisen, Robert R. "The Encounter between Religion and Science." In *Critical Issues in American Religious History: A Reader*, edited by Robert R. Mathisen, 375–76. Waco, TX: Baylor University Press, 2006.

May, William E. *Catholic Bioethics and the Gift of Human Life.* 2nd ed. Huntington, IN: Our Sunday Visitor, 2008.

Mayr, Ernst. "Darwin's Influence on Modern Thought." *Scientific American*, November 24, 2009. www.scientificamerican.com/article/darwins-influence-on-modern-thought/.

McCabe, Linda L., and Edward R. B. McCabe. *DNA: Promise and Peril.* Berkeley: University of California Press, 2008.

McCarty, Maclyn. "Discovering Genes Are Made of DNA." *Nature* 42 (2006). www.nature.com/articles/nature01398.

McClay, Wilfred. "Chesterton's Warning." *American Interest* 6, no. 1 (2010). www.the-american-interest.com/2010/09/01/chestertons-warning/.

McCormick, Richard A. *Corrective Vision: Explorations in Moral Theology.* Kansas City, MO: Sheed and Ward, 1994.

McFarland, Ian A. "Fallen or Unfallen? Christ's Human Nature and the Ontology of Human Sinfulness." *International Journal of Systematic Theology* 10, no. 4 (2008): 399–415.

———. *From Nothing: A Theology of Creation.* Louisville, KY: Westminster John Knox Press, 2014.

———. "The Problem with Evil." *Theology Today* 74, no. 4 (2018): 321–39.

McGrath, Alister E. *A Scientific Theology.* Vol. 1, *Nature.* Grand Rapids, MI: W. B. Eerdmans, 2003.

McInerny, Ralph. "The Principles of Natural Law." *American Journal of Jurisprudence* 25 (1980): 1–15.

McKenny, Gerald P. *To Relieve the Human Condition: Bioethics, Technology, and the Body*. Albany: State University of New York Press, 1997.

McNichol, T. "The New Faith in Medicine." *USA Today Weekend*, April 5–7, 1996, 4–5.

Melanchthon, Philip. *Orations of Philosophy and Education*. Translated by S. Kusukawa. Cambridge: Cambridge University Press, 1999.

Melcher, Sarah J., Mikeal C. Parsons, and Amos Yong, eds. *The Bible and Disability: A Commentary*. Waco, TX: Baylor University Press, 2017.

Midgley, Mary. "Criticizing the Cosmos." In *Is Nature Ever Evil? Religion, Science and Value*, edited by Willem B. Drees, 11–26. London: Routledge, 2003.

Milbank, John. "Can a Gift Be Given? Prolegomena to a Future Trinitarian Metaphysic." *Modern Theology* 11, no. 1 (1995): 119–61.

———. "The Second Difference: For a Trinitarianism without Reserve." *Modern Theology* 2 (April 1986): 213–34.

Miller, Hugh. *The Testimony of the Rocks*. Edinburgh: T. Constable, 1857.

Moltmann, Jürgen. *The Crucified God: The Cross of Christ as the Foundation and Criticism of Christian Theology*. London: SCM Press, 1974.

Monterosso, John, Edward B. Royzman, and Barry Schwartz. "Explaining Away Responsibility: Effects of Scientific Explanation on Perceived Culpability." *Ethics and Behavior* 15, no. 2 (2005): 139–58.

Muller, Herman J. *Out of the Night: A Biologist's View of the Future*. New York: Vanguard Press, 1935.

Muray, Leslie A. *Liberal Protestantism and Science*. Edited by Richard Olson. Westport, CT: Greenwood Press, 2008.

National Academies of Sciences, Engineering, and Medicine. *Second International Summit on Human Genome Editing: Continuing the Global Discussion: Proceedings of a Workshop in Brief*. Washington, DC: National Academies Press, 2019.

National Human Genome Research Institute. "The Ethical, Legal and Social Implications Research Program." Accessed July 31, 2021. www.genome .gov/10002329/elsi-research-program-fact-sheet/.

National Human Genome Research Institute. "What Is the Human Genome Project?" National Institutes of Health. Updated October 28, 2018. www.genome.gov/human-genome-project/What.

National Institutes of Health. "*All of Us* Research Program Backgrounder." Accessed July 31, 2021. https://allofus.nih.gov/news-events/press-kit /all-us-research-program-backgrounder.

————. "An Overview of the Human Genome Project." Accessed July 31, 2021. www.genome.gov/12011239/a-brief-history-of-the-human -genome-project/.

Nederman, Cary J. "The Puzzle of the Political Animal: Nature and Artifice in Aristotle's Political Theory." *Review of Politics* 56, no. 2 (1994): 283–304.

Nelkin, Dorothy, and M. Susan Lindee. *The DNA Mystique: The Gene as a Cultural Icon.* Conversations in Medicine and Society. Ann Arbor: University of Michigan Press, 2004.

Newman, Barbara J. *Accessible Gospel, Inclusive Worship.* Wyoming, MI: CLC Network, 2015.

Newport, Frank. "In U.S., 46% Hold Creationist View of Human Origins." Gallup Politics, June 1, 2012. www.gallup.com/poll/155003/Hold -Creationist-View-Human-Origins.aspx.

Nicholas of Cusa. *On Not-Other (De Li Non Aliud).* Translated by Jasper Hopkins. Minneapolis, MN: Arthur J. Banning Press, 1987.

Niebuhr, H. Richard. *The Meaning of Revelation.* Louisville, KY: Westminster John Knox Press, 2006.

Niebuhr, Reinhold. "Ten Years That Shook My World." *Christian Century,* April 26, 1939, 542–46.

Nola, Michael. "Aristotelian Background to Aquinas' Denial That 'Woman Is a Defective Male.'" *The Thomist* 64, no. 1 (2000): 21–69.

Oakley, Francis. "The Absolute and Ordained Power of God and King in the Sixteenth and Seventeenth Centuries: Philosophy, Science, Politics, and Law." *Journal of the History of Ideas* 59, no. 4 (1998): 669–90.

Office of the Press Secretary. "Fact Sheet: President Obama's Precision Medicine Initiative." News release, January 30, 2015. www.whitehouse .gov/the-press-office/2015/01/30/fact-sheet-president-obama-s -precision-medicine-initiative.

Oliver, Simon. *Philosophy, God, and Motion.* London: Routledge, 2005.

Onori, Luciano, and Guido Visconti. "The GAIA Theory: From Lovelock to Margulis. From a Homeostatic to a Cognitive Autopoietic World-view." *Rendiconti Lincei* 23, no. 4 (2012): 375–86.

Ottati, Douglas F. *Theology for Liberal Protestants: God the Creator.* Grand Rapids, MI: William B. Eerdmans, 2013.

Ouellette, Alicia. "Selection against Disability: Abortion, ART, and Access." *Journal of Law, Medicine, and Ethics* 43, no. 2 (2015): 211–23.

Paley, William. *Natural Theology.* Boston: Lincoln and Edmans, 1829.

Pannenberg, Wolfhart. *Anthropology in Theological Perspective.* Translated by Matthew J. O'Connell. Philadelphia: Westminster, 1985.

————. *Metaphysics and the Idea of God.* Grand Rapids, MO: William B. Eerdmans, 1990.

————. *Systematic Theology.* London: T. & T. Clark International, 2004.

Parens, Erik, and Adrienne Asch. "The Disability Rights Critique of Prenatal Genetic Testing." In *Prenatal Testing and Disability Rights,* edited by Erik Parens and Adrienne Asch, 3–43. Washington, DC: Georgetown University Press, 2000.

Park, Andrew Sung. *The Wounded Heart of God: The Asian Concept of Han and the Christian Doctrine of Sin.* Nashville, TN: Abingdon Press, 1993.

Paynter, Nina P., Daniel Chasman, Guillaume Pare, Julie E. Buring, Nancy R. Cook, Joseph P. Miletich, and Paul M. Ridker. "Association between a Literature-Based Genetic Risk Score and Cardiovascular Events in Women." *JAMA* 303, no. 7 (2010): 631–37.

Peters, Ted. *For the Love of Children: Genetic Technology and the Future of the Family.* Louisville, KY: Westminster John Knox Press, 1996.

————. "Human Genome Project." In *Encyclopedia of Science and Religion.* New York: Macmillan, 2003.

————. "Patenting Life: Yes." *First Things: A Journal of Religion, Culture, and Public Life* 63 (May 1996): 18–20.

Petersen, Arthur C. "Contingency and Risk: Comment on Smit." In *Is Nature Ever Evil? Religion, Science and Value,* edited by Willem B. Drees, 98–100. London: Routledge, 2003.

Phillips, L. Edward. "Ethics and Worship," In *The New Westminster Dictionary of Liturgy and Worship,* edited by Paul Bradshaw, 167–69. Louisville, KY: Westminster John Knox Press, SCM Press, 2002.

Pope Benedict XVI. *Caritas in veritate.* July 7, 2009. www.vatican.va/holy _father/benedict_xvi/encyclicals/documents/hf_ben-xvi_enc _20090629_caritas-in-veritate_en.html.

Pope John Paul II. "The Ethics of Genetic Manipulation." *Origins,* November 17, 1983, 388–89.

Pope Paul VI. *Humanae vitae,* July 25, 1968. Translated by US Conference of Catholic Bishops. Washington, DC: USCCB, 1968.

Pope Pius XI. *Casti connubii.* December 31, 1930.

————. *Quadragesimo anno.* May 15, 1931.

Pope Pius XII. "Moral Aspects of Genetics." Address to those attending the Primum Symposium Geneticae Medicae, September 7, 1953. In *The Human Body: Papal Teachings,* edited by Monks of Solesmes, 246–60. Boston: Daughters of Saint Paul, 1960.

Popper, Karl Raimund. *Objective Knowledge: An Evolutionary Approach.* Oxford: Clarendon Press, 1972.

Porter, Jean. *Nature as Reason: A Thomistic Theory of Natural Law.* Grand Rapids, MI: Eerdmans, 2005.

PCUSA (Presbyterian Church USA). "The Covenant of Life and the Caring Community and Creation: Theological Reflections on Contraception and Abortion." 195th General Assembly, 1983. www.pcusa.org/site _media/media/uploads/_resolutions/covenant-of-life-and-covenant -and-creation.pdf.

———. "On Providing Just Access to Reproductive Health Care." 220th General Assembly, 2012. www.presbyterianmission.org/resource/pres byterian-church-us-general-assembly-resolution/.

———. *Our Confessional Heritage: Confessions of the Reformed Tradition with a Contemporary Declaration of Faith.* Atlanta, GA: Materials Distribution Service of the PCUSA, 1978.

Reich, David. "How Genetics Is Changing our Understanding of 'Race.'" *New York Times,* March 23, 2018. www.nytimes.com/2018/03/23 /opinion/sunday/genetics-race.html.

Reimer, A. James. *Paul Tillich: Theologian of Nature, Culture and Politics.* New Brunswick, NJ: Transaction, 2004.

Reinders, Hans S. *Disability, Providence, and Ethics: Bridging Gaps, Transforming Lives.* Waco, TX: Baylor University Press, 2014.

———. *The Future of the Disabled in Liberal Society: An Ethical Analysis.* Notre Dame, IN: University of Notre Dame Press, 2000.

———. *Receiving the Gift of Friendship: Profound Disability, Theological Anthropology, and Ethics.* Grand Rapids, MI: Eerdmans, 2008.

———. "Understanding Humanity and Disability: Probing an Ecological Perspective." *Studies in Christian Ethics* 26, no. 1 (2013): 37–49.

Reynolds, Thomas E. *Vulnerable Communion: A Theology of Disability and Hospitality.* Grand Rapids, MI: Brazos Press, 2008.

Robinette, Brian D. "The Difference Nothing Makes: Creatio ex Nihilo, Resurrection, and Divine Gratuity." *Theological Studies* 72, no. 3 (2011): 525–57.

Robinson, Ann. "Genomics: The Future of Healthcare and Medicine." *Prescriber,* April 2016. http://onlinelibrary.wiley.com/doi/10.1002/psb.1454 /pdf.

Rogers, Eugene F. "Aquinas on Natural Law and the Virtues in Biblical Context: Homosexuality as a Test Case." *Journal of Religious Ethics* 27, no. 1 (1999): 29–56.

Rosen, Christine. *Preaching Eugenics: Religious Leaders and the American Eugenics Movement.* Oxford: Oxford University Press, 2004.

Roth, Stephen M. *Genetics Primer for Exercise and Health.* Champaign, IL: Human Kinetics, 2007.

Salzman, Todd A., and Michael G. Lawler. "Natural Law and Perspectivism: A Case for Plural Definitions of Objective Morality." *Irish Theological Quarterly* 82, no. 1 (2017): 31–38.

Sandel, Michael J. *The Case against Perfection: Ethics in the Age of Genetic Engineering*. Cambridge, MA: Belknap Press of Harvard University Press, 2007.

Sanger Center. "The First Draft of the Book of Humankind Has Been Read, The Wellcome Trust and the Sanger Centre in Cambridge, Together with International Partners, Are Announcing Today." Press release, June 26, 2000. www.sanger.ac.uk/news_item/first-draft-book-human kind-has-been-read/.

Scarry, Elaine. *The Body in Pain: The Making and Unmaking of the World*. Oxford: Oxford University Press, 1985.

Schleiermacher, Friedrich. *The Christian Faith*. Edited by H. R. Mackintosh and James Stuart Stewart. Edinburgh: T. & T. Clark, 1928.

Scully, Jackie Leach. *Disability Bioethics: Moral Bodies, Moral Difference*. Lanham, MD: Rowman and Littlefield, 2008.

Shakespeare, Tom. "Arguing about Genetics and Disability." In *Theology, Disability and the New Genetics: Why Science Needs the Church*, edited by John Swinton and Brian Brock, 67–71. London: T. & T. Clark, 2007.

———. *Disability Rights and Wrongs Revisited*. 2nd ed. New York: Routledge, 2014.

Shanks, Pete. "The Scandal and the Summit: Reactions to the Announcement of Gene-Edited Babies." Center for Genetics and Society, *Biopolitical Times* (blog), December 7, 2018. www.geneticsandsociety.org /biopolitical-times/scandal-and-summit-reactions-announcement -gene-edited-babies.

Shapin, Steven, and Simon Schaffer. *Leviathan and the Air-Pump: Hobbes, Boyle, and the Experimental Life*. Princeton, NJ: Princeton University Press, 2018.

Shapiro, Adam R. "William Paley's Lost 'Intelligent Design.'" *History and Philosophy of the Life Sciences* 31, no. 1 (2009): 55–77.

Sherlock, Richard. *Nature's End: The Theological Meaning of the New Genetics*. Wilmington DE: ISI Books, 2010.

Shostak, S., J. Freese, B. G. Link, and J. C. Phelan. "The Politics of the Gene: Social Status and Beliefs About Genetics for Individual Outcomes." *Social Psychology Quarterly* 72, no. 1 (2009): 77–93.

Shuman, Joel James, and Keith G. Meador. *Heal Thyself: Spirituality, Medicine, and the Distortion of Christianity*. Oxford: Oxford University Press, 2003.

Siebers, Tobin. *Disability Theory.* Ann Arbor: University of Michigan Press, 2008.

Silva, Ignacio. "Thomas Aquinas Holds Fast: Objections to Aquinas within Today's Debate on Divine Action." *Heythrop Journal* 54, no. 4 (2011): 658–67.

Silver, Lee. *Remaking Eden: Cloning and Beyond in a Brave New World.* New York: Avon Books, 1997.

Singer, Peter. *Practical Ethics.* Cambridge: Cambridge University Press, 1979.

———. *Practical Ethics.* 2nd ed. Cambridge: Cambridge University Press, 1993.

Skotko, Brian G., Susan P. Levine, and Richard Goldstein. "Self-Perceptions from People with Down Syndrome." *American Journal of Medical Genetics* 155, no. 10 (2011): 2360–69.

Smith, Timothy L. *Thomas Aquinas' Trinitarian Theology: A Study in Theological Method.* Washington, DC: Catholic University of America Press, 2003.

Song, Robert. "Genetic Manipulation and the Body of Christ." *Studies in Christian Ethics* 20, no. 3 (2007): 399–420.

Sontag, Susan. "Illness as Metaphor." *New York Review of Books,* January 26, 1978. www.nybooks.com/articles/1978/01/26/illness-as-metaphor/.

Spaemann, Robert. *Persons: The Difference between "Someone" and "Something."* Translated by Oliver O'Donovan. Oxford: Oxford University Press, 2006.

Sparkes, Russell. "The Enemy of Eugenics." *Chesterton Review* 25, nos. 1/2 (1999). www.secondspring.co.uk/articles/sparkes.htm.

Spinoza, Benedict. *Theological-Political Treatise.* 2nd ed. Translated by Samuel Shirley. Indianapolis, IN: Hackett, 2001.

Spiro, Jonathan Peter. *Defending the Master Race: Conservation, Eugenics, and the Legacy of Madison Grant.* Burlington: University of Vermont Press, 2009.

Stahl, Devan. "A Christian Ontology of Genetic Disease and Disorder." *Journal of Disability and Religion* 19, no. 2 (2015): 119–45.

———. "Moral Evaluations of Genetic Technologies: The Need for Catholic Social Doctrine." *National Catholic Bioethics Quarterly* 15, no. 3 (2015): 155–59.

Stahl, Devan, and John Kilner. "The Image of God, Bioethics, and Persons with Profound Intellectual Disabilities." *Journal of the Christian Institute on Disability* 6, nos. 1–2 (2017): 19–40.

Surin, Kenneth. *Theology and the Problem of Evil.* Oxford: Blackwell, 1986.

Swinburne, Richard. *Providence and the Problem of Evil.* Oxford: Oxford University Press, 1998.

Swinton, John. *Becoming Friends of Time: Disability, Timefulness, and Gentle Discipleship*. Waco, TX: Baylor University Press, 2016.

———. "Introduction: Hauerwas on Disability." In *Critical Reflections on Stanley Hauerwas' Theology of Disability: Disabling Society, Enabling Theology*, edited by John Swinton, 1–10. New York: Haworth Pastoral Press, 2004.

———. *Raging with Compassion: Pastoral Responses to the Problem of Evil*. Grand Rapids, MI: Eerdmans, 2007.

———. "Who Is the God We Worship? Theologies of Disability: Challenges and New Possibilities." *International Journal of Practical Theology* 14 (2011): 273–301.

Swinton, John, and Brian Brock, eds. *Theology, Disability and the New Genetics: Why Science Needs the Church*. London: T. & T. Clark, 2007.

Szerszynski, Bronislaw. *Nature, Technology and the Sacred*. Malden, MA: Blackwell, 2005.

Talbott, Steve. "Getting over the Code Delusion." *New Atlantis* 28 (2010): 14–23.

Taylor, Mark Kline. "Introduction: The Theological Development and Contribution of Paul Tillich." In *Paul Tillich: Theologian of the Boundaries*, edited by Mark Kline Taylor, 11–34. Minneapolis, MN: Fortress Press, 1991.

Tillich, Paul. "Heal the Sick; Cast Out the Demons." In *The Eternal Now*, edited by Religion Online. New York: Charles Scribner's Sons, 1963.

———. *Love, Power, and Justice: Ontological Analyses and Ethical Applications*. New York: Oxford University Press, 1954.

———. "The Permanent Significance of the Catholic Church for Protestants." *Protestant Digest* 3, no. 10 (1941): 23–31.

———. *The Socialist Decision*. Translated by Franklin Sherman. New York: Harper and Row, 1977.

———. *Systematic Theology*. 3 vols. Chicago: University of Chicago Press, 1951–63.

———. *The System of the Sciences According to Objects and Methods*. Translated by Paul Wiebe. Lewisburg, PA: Bucknell University Press, 1981.

———. *Theology of Culture*. Edited by Robert C. Kimball. New York: Oxford University Press, 1959.

Tollefsen, Christopher. "The New Natural Law Theory." *Lyceum* 10, no. 1 (2008): 1–17.

23andMe. "Learn More About 23andMe's New Genetic Health Risk Reports." *23andMeBlog*, May 19, 2017. https://blog.23andme.com/health-traits/learn-23andmes-new-genetic-health-risk-reports/.

United Church of Christ. "A Call for the Study of Our Church's Involvement in the Eugenics Movement (A Prudential Resolution)." Approved 2009 at the 27th General Synod of the UCC. https://uccfiles.com/pdf /gs27minutes.pdf.

———. "The Church and Genetic Engineering: A Pronouncement and Proposal for Action." 17th General Synod, Resolution 15, 1989. Available on request from Common Services Ministry, Mr. Edward C. Cade, Archivist and Records Manager, United Church of Christ, 700 Prospect Ave., Cleveland, OH 44115.

———. "Resolution on Concern about Moral and Ethical Implications of Genetic Engineering." 14th General Synod, Resolution 19, 1983. Available on request from Common Services Ministry, Mr. Edward C. Cade, Archivist and Records Manager, United Church of Christ, 700 Prospect Ave., Cleveland, OH 44115.

United Methodist Church. *The Book of Resolutions of the United Methodist Church 1992*. Nashville, TN: United Methodist Publishing House, 1992.

———. *Social Principles*. Washington, DC: General Board of Church and Society, 2012.

US Conference of Catholic Bishops. *Ethical and Religious Directives for Catholic Health Care Services*. 5th ed. Washington, DC: USCCB, 2009.

US Congress, Office of Technology Assessment. *Mapping Our Genes*. Washington, DC: Government Printing Office, 1988.

US National Library of Medicine. "What Are Some of the Challenges Facing Precision Medicine and the Precision Medicine Initiative?" *Genetics Home Reference*, August 28, 2018. https://ghr.nlm.nih.gov/primer/pre cisionmedicine/challenges.

———. "What Is Precision Medicine?" *Genetics Home Reference,* August 28, 2018. https://ghr.nlm.nih.gov/primer/precisionmedicine/definition.

Vatican Council II. *Gaudium et spes.* December 7, 1965.

Vehmas, Simo. "Live and Let Die? Disability in Bioethics." *New Review of Bioethics* 1, no. 1 (2003): 145–57.

Velde, Rudi te. *Aquinas on God: The Divine Science of the Summa Theologiae.* Burlington, VT: Ashgate, 2006.

Wade, Nicholas. "A Decade Later, Genetic Map Yields Few New Cures." *New York Times*, June 12, 2010. www.nytimes.com/2010/06/13/health /research/13genome.html?pagewanted=all.

Watson, David F. "Luke—Acts." In *The Bible and Disability: A Commentary*, edited by Sarah J. Melcher, Mikeal C. Parsons, and Amos Yong, 303–32. Waco, TX: Baylor University Press, 2017.

Watson, James D. *The Double Helix: A Personal Account of the Discovery of the Structure of DNA.* New York: Touchstone, 2001.

———. *A Passion for DNA: Genes, Genomes, and Society*. Plainview, NY: Cold Springs Harbor Laboratory Press, 2001.

———. "President's Essay: Genes and Politics." *Cold Springs Harbor Annual Report*, 1996, 1–20.

Watson, James D., and Andrew Berry. *DNA: The Secret of Life*. New York: Alfred A. Knopf, 2004.

Weinberg, Steven. *The First Three Minutes: A Modern View of the Origin of the Universe*. Updated ed. New York: Basic Books, 1993.

"What They Said: The Genome in Quotes." *BBC News*, June 26, 2000. http://news.bbc.co.uk/2/hi/science/nature/807126.stm.

Williams, Thomas. "Biblical Interpretation." In *The Cambridge Companion to Augustine*, edited by Eleonore Stump and Norman Kretzmann, 59–70. Cambridge: Cambridge University Press, 2001.

Wilson, E. O. "Human Decency Is Animal." *New York Times Magazine*, October 12, 1975, 38–50.

INDEX

Holy Spirit, 133, 174, 191, 206,
227–28, 234
hospitality, 150, 214
human enhancement, 146–48, 185,
237–38, 270n23
Human Genome Project (HGP), 57,
67–69, 73, 75, 77–79, 123,
155–56, 179–81, 183, 194
human nature
and dependency, 143, 145,
199–202
fallen, 135, 137–40
and finitude, 57, 79, 110, 136,
139–43, 152, 188
implications of, 35–36, 52, 158–59,
160–61, 165
and limitations, 7–8, 136
and reason, 127–28, 159
relational model of, 196–98
and science, 65, 74–76
teleological/essential model of,
115, 118–19, 125, 163, 166–67,
198–99
and vulnerability, 110, 139–40, 200,
224
See also cocreatorship; law(s):
natural
Humanae Vitae, 20, 160, 170
Hume, David, 8, 158, 164

imago Dei (image of God), 128–31,
146, 163, 200, 224
in vitro fertilization (IVF), 18,
170–71, 183–84
incarnation. *See* Christ
International Human Genome
Sequencing Consortium, 67
Irenaeus, 101, 147

Jesus. *See* Christ
John Paul II, Pope, 170–71
Julian of Norwich, 112

Kant, Immanuel, 8, 50–51
Kilner, John, 128–29
Kingdom of God, 11, 80, 125,
142–45, 148, 151, 163, 169,
225–26, 228, 239

Lamarck, Jean-Baptiste, 59–60
Last Judgment, 143
law(s)
divine, 159, 162, 166–67
eternal, 35, 159, 161–62, 165–67
human, 159
natural, 15–16, 20, 35–38, 61, 99,
147, 157–70, 173, 229, 267n39
of nature, 37–38, 44–45, 49, 110
Lewontin, Richard, 80–81
LGBT issues, 155–56, 265n6
liturgy, 219–28, 233
Luther, Martin, 134, 162

Mairs, Nancy, 218–19
materialism, 75–76, 152
McFarland, Ian, 101, 119, 139
McKenny, Gerald, 77
mechanist theory, 42–46, 50, 67,
70–71, 74, 124
medicine, models of, 40, 48, 77–78,
158
Mendel, Gregor, 66–67
metaphysics, xi–xii, 123–25
analogical, 93
and Christianity, 28, 32, 80,
123–25, 175, 209, 230
of creation, 83–84, 99–101, 105–6
of disability, 108, 120, 143, 203
and ethics, 36–38, 40, 74–75, 89,
166, 168, 174–75, 192, 211–12,
224, 230, 238–39
of medicine, 78, 180, 187, 224, 234
of nature, 95–96
participatory, 92–93
and philosophy, 35

DEVAN STAHL is an assistant professor of religion at Baylor University and editor of *Imaging and Imagining Illness: Becoming Whole in a Broken Body.*

CPSIA information can be obtained
at www.ICGtesting.com
Printed in the USA
LVHW081120300822
727162LV00005B/141